# A Vade-Mecum

## Third Edition

Edited by

**Brian Speidel** MD FRCP FRCPCH
Consultant Neonatologist, Southmead Hospital, Bristol

**Peter Fleming** PhD FRCP FRCP(C) FRCPCH
Professor of Infant Health and Developmental Physiology,
St Michael's Hospital, Bristol

**John Henderson** MD FRCP FRCPCH
Senior Lecturer in Paediatric Intensive Care, Royal Hospital
for Sick Children, Bristol

**Alison Leaf** MD MRCP FRCPCH
Consultant Neonatologist, Southmead Hospital, Bristol

**Neil Marlow** DM FRCP FRCPCH
Professor of Neonatal Medicine, University of Nottingham,
Nottingham

**Glynn Russell** FRCP FCP(SA) FRCPCH
Consultant Neonatologist, St Michael's Hospital, Bristol

**Peter Dunn** MD FRCP FRCOG FRCPCH
Emeritus Professor of Perinatal Medicine and Child Health,
University of Bristol, Bristol

ARNOLD

A member of the Hodder Headline Group
LONDON · SYDNEY · AUCKLAND
Copublished in the United States of America by
Oxford University Press Inc., New York

First published in Great Britain in 1998 by
Arnold, a member of the Hodder Headline group,
338 Euston Road, London NW1 3BH
**http://www.arnoldpublishers.com**

Co-published in the United States of America by Oxford University Press, Inc.,
198 Madison Avenue, New York, NY10016
Oxford is a registered trademark of Oxford University Press

*British Library Cataloguing in Publication Data*
A catalogue record for this book is available from the British Library

*Library of Congress Cataloging-in-Publication Data*
A catalog record for this book is available from the Library of Congress

ISBN 0 340 691409    1190\438

Publisher: Annalisa Page
Production Editor: James Rabson
Production Controller: Rose James
Cover designer: Terry Griffiths

Typeset in  9.5/11 Minion by Photoprint Typesetters, Torquay, Devon
Printed and bound in Great Britain by J W Arrowsmith, Bristol.

# CONTENTS

# PREFACE TO THE THIRD EDITION

In preparing this third edition of the *Vade-Mecum* we have tried to maintain the practical nature of the book, which is intended to be a ward guide to the care of the newborn infant for medical and nursing staff. All the chapters have been revised, and some have been extensively re-written to take into account the many changes that have occurred in neonatal care since 1991; this particularly applies to the chapters on Resuscitation, Respiratory Disorders, Nutrition and Metabolism. We are especially pleased to have an obstetrician join us in writing the chapter on High-Risk Pregnancy. The order in which the chapters occur has been rearranged so that related topics are grouped together for ease of reference. We have combined Follow-Up and Audit into a single new chapter and our neonatal nurse practitioners have provided a combined chapter on Nursing Care and The High-Risk Infant.

Once again we would like to express our gratitude to Mrs Angela Burge, whose skills with the word processor have made the preparation of this edition so much easier.

# CONTRIBUTORS TO THE THIRD EDITION

Jeremy Berry, FRCPath, FRCPCH, Professor of Paediatric Pathology, St Michael's Hospital, Bristol.

Eleri Cusick, FRCS, Consultant Paediatric Surgeon, Royal Hospital for Sick Children, Bristol.

Gillian Gill, BA, CQSW, Medical Social Worker, St Michael's Hospital, Bristol.

Cameron Kennedy, FRCP, Consultant Dermatologist, Royal Hospital for Sick Children, Bristol.

Peter Lunt, MSC, FRCP, Consultant Clinical Geneticist, Royal Hospital for Sick Children, Bristol.

Richard Markham, MRCP, FRCS, Consultant Ophthalmologist, Bristol Eye Hospital, Bristol.

Robert Martin, FRCP, FRCPCH, Consultant Paediatric Cardiologist, Royal Hospital for Sick Children, Bristol.

Mary McGraw, FRCP, FRCPCH, Consultant Paediatric Nephrologist, Southmead Hospital, Bristol.

Helen Noblett, FRACS, FRCS, Consultant Paediatric Surgeon, Royal Hospital for Sick Children, Bristol.

Charles Pennock, MD, FRCPath, FRCPCH, Consultant Senior Lecturer in Child Health (Clinical Pathology), St Michael's Hospital, Bristol.

Mary Pillai, MRCP, MRCOG, MD, Consultant Obstetrician, The General Hospital, Cheltenham.

Marie Rymill, BSc, RGN, RM, ENBA19, Advanced Neonatal Nurse Practitioner, St Michael's Hospital, Bristol.

Richard Spicer, FRCS, Consultant Paediatric Surgeon, Royal Hospital for Sick Children, Bristol.

Martin Ward Platt, MD, FRCP, FRCPCH, Consultant Paediatrician, Royal Victoria Infirmary, Newcastle upon Tyne.

Sharon Winterbottom, BSc, RGN, RSCN, ENBA19, Advanced Neonatal Nurse Practitioner, St Michael's Hospital, Bristol.

# CONTRIBUTORS TO THE SECOND EDITION

Jeremy Berry, MRCPath, Consultant Perinatal and Paediatric Pathologist, Bristol Maternity Hospital, Bristol.

Mark Drayton, MA, MD, MRCP, Consultant Neonatologist, University Hospital of Wales, Cardiff.

Timothy French, MB BS, MSc, MRCP, Consultant Paediatrician, Musgrove Park Hospital, Taunton.

Cameron Kennedy, MD, FRCP, Consultant Dermatologist, Royal Hospital for Sick Children, Bristol.

Peter Lunt, MA, MSc, MRCP, Consultant Clinical Geneticist, Royal Hospital for Sick Children, Bristol.

Richard Markham, MD, FRCS, Consultant Ophthalmologist, Bristol Eye Hospital and Royal Hospital for Sick Children, Bristol.

Robert Martin, MB, MRCP, Consultant Paediatric Cardiologist, Royal Hospital for Sick Children, Bristol.

Mary McGraw, MB, ChB, MRCP, DCH, Consultant Paediatrician, Southmead Hospital, Bristol.

Helen Noblett, MB BS, FRACS, FRCS, Consultant Paediatric Surgeon, Royal Hospital for Sick Children, Bristol.

Charles Pennock, BSc, MD, FRCPath, Consultant Senior Lecturer in Child Health, University of Bristol, Bristol.

Bhupinda Sandhu, MD, MRCP, Consultant Paediatrician, Royal Hospital for Sick Children, Bristol.

John Walter, MSc, MD, MRCP, Lecturer in Child Health, University of Bristol, Bristol.

Barry Wilkins, MA, MB, BChir, MRCP, DCH, Formerly Research Fellow in Paediatric Intensive Care, Royal Hospital for Sick Children, Bristol.

Michael Woolridge, BSc, DPhil, Lactation Physiologist, University of Bristol, Bristol.

# LIST OF ABBREVIATIONS USED

| | |
|---|---|
| AFP | Alpha-fetoprotein |
| AIDS | Acquired immune deficiency syndrome |
| APH | Antepartum haemorrhage |
| ASD | Atrial septal defect |
| AV | Arterio-venous |
| BP | Blood pressure |
| BPD | Bronchopulmonary dysplasia |
| CAH | Congenital adrenal hyperplasia |
| CDH | Congenital dislocation of the hip |
| CMV | Cytomegalovirus |
| CPAP | Continuous positive airway pressure |
| CSF | Cerebrospinal fluid |
| CT | Computer tomography |
| CTG | Cardiotocograph |
| CVP | Central venous pressure |
| CVS | Chorionic villous sample |
| CXR | Chest X-ray |
| DIC | Disseminated intravascular coagulation |
| EDD | Estimated date of delivery |
| ETT | Endotracheal tube |
| FBC | Full blood count |
| FDP | Fibrin degradation products |
| FHR | Fetal heart rate |
| $FiO_2$ | Fractional inspired oxygen concentration |
| GFR | Glomerular filtration rate |
| HAS | Human albumin solution |
| HCG | Human chorionic gonadotrophin |
| HFOV | High frequency oscillatory ventilation |
| HIV | Human immunodeficiency virus |
| HLA | Human leukocyte antigen |
| ICP | Intracranial pressure |
| IDM | Infant of a diabetic mother |
| IPPV | Intermittent positive-pressure ventilation |
| ITP | Idiopathic thrombocytopenic purpura |
| IUGR | Intrauterine growth retardation |
| IVH | Intraventricular haemorrhage |
| IVIG | Intravenous immunoglobulin |
| IVU | Intravenous urogram |

| | |
|---|---|
| kPa | Kilopascals |
| LBW | Low birthweight ($< 2500$ g) |
| LMP | Last menstrual period |
| LP | Lumbar puncture |
| MAP | Mean airway pressure |
| MCUG | Micturating cystourethrogram |
| MRI | Magnetic resonance imaging |
| NEC | Necrotizing enterocolitis |
| NEFA | Non-esterified fatty acids |
| NICU | Neonatal intensive care unit |
| $PaCO_2$ | Arterial partial pressure of $CO_2$ |
| $PaO_2$ | Arterial partial pressure of $O_2$ |
| PCV | Packed cell volume (= haematocrit) |
| PDA | Patent ductus arteriosus |
| PEEP | Positive end-expiratory pressure |
| PIE | Pulmonary interstitial emphysema |
| PIP | Peak inspiratory pressure |
| PKU | Phenylketonuria |
| PN | Parenteral nutrition |
| PPH | Persistent pulmonary hypertension |
| PTT | Prothrombin time |
| PTV | Patient-triggered ventilation |
| PVH | Periventricular haemorrhage |
| PVL | Periventricular leucomalacia |
| PVR | Pulmonary vascular resistance |
| RDS | Respiratory distress syndrome |
| ROP | Retinopathy of prematurity |
| RTA | Renal tubular acidosis |
| $SaO_2$ | Saturation oxygen level |
| SCBU | Special care baby unit |
| SGA | Small for gestational age |
| SG | Specific gravity |
| SIMV | Synchronized intermittent mandatory ventilation |
| SLE | Systemic lupus erythematosus |
| SPA | Suprapubic aspirate (of urine) |
| SVT | Supraventricular tachycardia |
| $T_4$ | Thyroxine |
| $T_i$ | Inspiratory time |
| $T_e$ | Expiratory time |
| $TcPO_2$ | Transcutaneous oxygen tension |
| TOF | Tracheo-oesophageal fistula |
| TSH | Thyroid-stimulating hormone |

| | |
|---|---|
| TTN | Transient tachypnoea of newborn |
| UTI | Urinary tract infection |
| VLBW | Very low birthweight ($< 1500g$) |
| VSD | Ventricular septal defect |
| WBC | White blood cell (count) |

# The high-risk pregnancy

The focus of antenatal care is the identification of adverse factors that may impair the outcome of pregnancy for the mother or baby, and their management to achieve optimal outcome. The more common maternal and fetal problems are discussed below in limited detail, with particular emphasis on the neonatal consequences.

## PREGNANCY LOSS

The risk of spontaneous miscarriage correlates with maternal age and is relatively independent of the age of the father. About 15% of confirmed pregnancies miscarry, rising to 40% in women aged 40 years, and exponentially thereafter, at a time when fertility declines rapidly. The risk of trisomy is also dependent on maternal age, but if an older woman conceives by IVF utilizing donor eggs, the risk of trisomy and miscarriage is related to the age of the donor. In contrast, conditions related to the sperm rather than to the eggs, such as sex chromosome anomalies and triploidy, are independent of maternal age.

Women who have previously experienced a bad outcome of pregnancy deserve special consideration. The new pregnancy is a time of great anxiety, and it may be optimal to outline an individualized plan of management with combined input from both obstetrician and paediatrician.

## PRENATAL SCREENING

Prenatal screening commenced in the 1970s with the introduction of maternal serum AFP in mid-trimester to screen for neural tube defects, followed in the early 1990s by various combinations of AFP with human chorionic gonadotrophin (HCG), unconjugated oestriol and occasionally other markers to screen for trisomy 21. Detailed high-resolution mid-trimester scanning has largely replaced bio-chemical screening and amniocentesis for neural tube defects, but these are still widely used for trisomy 21. More recently, some centres have moved towards first-trimester screening by nuchal translucency (an increased thickness of skin oedema at the level of the fetal neck), which indicates increased risk of chromosomal anomaly and other syndromes, particularly structural cardiac defects.

The role of testing is to assist the woman with choice in her pregnancy, and it is undertaken with the informed consent of the woman, as an 'opt in' test. There can be no obligation to undergo diagnostic testing for those who screen positive, and no obligation to terminate for the small minority who ultimately prove to have a chromosomally or structurally abnormal fetus. This has significant resource implications for the provision of consistent and accurate non-directive counselling, and someone with the skill and time to ensure that the information has been understood.

Although in time biochemistry will probably be replaced by ultrasound screening, it may be retained as an adjunct and it may have a role in risk assessment. An elevated maternal serum AFP level (and possibly HCG) with a structurally normal fetus significantly increases the risk of an adverse pregnancy outcome. Elevated levels of AFP have particularly been associated with increased risk of pre-eclampsia and intrauterine growth retardation.

**Diagnostic testing** For chromosome or DNA analysis an invasive test is required, with an intrinsic small risk of pregnancy loss, membrane rupture or prematurity. Fetal or placental cells must be obtained, and this can be achieved by sampling amniotic fluid, placental biopsy (chorionic villous sample) or direct fetal blood sampling.

Amniocentesis is traditionally performed in the second trimester, most often around 16 weeks. Under ultrasound direction the needle should be visualized continuously, avoiding the placenta. Amniocentesis can be performed in the first trimester, but amnion and chorion are not fused and the transplacental approach may be preferred. In the first trimester amniocentesis confers a higher miscarriage rate than CVS and, because there are fewer cells, the risk of failed culture is higher than in the second trimester. CVS prior to 10 weeks has been associated with a small risk of fetal limb reduction anomalies, and most centres offer CVS only from 11 weeks onwards. Fetal blood sampling is difficult prior to 20 weeks, and is most often performed when a rapid karyotype is desired at a relatively advanced stage of pregnancy. Access to the fetal circulation is also utilized for fetal therapy, mostly for anaemia due to alloimmune haemolytic disease, and very rarely for thrombocytopenia due to alloimmune platelet disease.

Karyotypes obtained following CVS may be less accurate than fetal blood or amniotic fluid sampling. Placental mosaicism is found in 1–2% of CVS biopsies, and these cannot be reliably interpreted. By comparison, failure to obtain a result following amniocentesis or fetal blood sampling is exceedingly rare.

The risk of miscarriage following CVS in the first trimester is apparently high compared to testing in the second trimester. Combined with a 1–2 % procedure-related loss, the 3% background pregnancy loss rate at 10–14 weeks gives an overall loss rate of 4–5%. By contrast, the 1–1.5% loss rate following any test in the second trimester seems much lower, but is largely due to a low background loss rate of 0.5%.

## MATERNAL CONDITIONS AFFECTING THE INFANT

### Hypertensive disease

Hypertension (defined as a blood pressure greater than 140/90 mm Hg on two occasions) occurs in about 6% of pregnancies. The development of proteinuria is more serious, and the condition is then termed pre-eclampsia. This is a major cause of maternal and fetal mortality and morbidity, the main fetal risks being impaired growth, placental abruption and prematurity. As the disease process becomes more severe, it is termed eclampsia in the presence of seizures, and, with the development of haemolysis, hepatic dysfunction (elevated liver enzymes) and low platelets, it is termed **HELLP** syndrome. These represent the most severe end of a spectrum of disease for which the only cure is delivery of the fetus and placenta. Control of the blood pressure is aimed at protecting the maternal cerebral circulation from intracranial haemorrhage. Risk of this occurs when usually normotensive individuals develop blood pressures above 170/110 mm Hg or a mean arterial pressure above 125–130 mm Hg. Antihypertensive medication prevents increases in blood pressure, but there is no substantial evidence that therapy modifies any other outcome. Control of hypertension may result in less hospitalization and increase the gestational age at delivery. Care must be taken not to drop the pressure to a level which could impair uteroplacental perfusion; fetal death has occurred with over-zealous treatment of maternal hypertension.

The hypotensive drugs most commonly used and their effects on the fetus and newborn are listed below:

**Methyl dopa** Has been used more than any other antihypertensive in pregnancy, and has not been associated with any increase in congenital malformations. It should be the drug of first choice where long-term therapy is required. A clinically insignificant, mild reduction in neonatal systolic blood pressure has been reported in the first 2 days. There is no contraindication to breast feeding.

**Hydralazine** Most widely used drug for prompt treatment of severe maternal hypertension, without fetal compromise. It is not associated with congenital anomalies. Neonatal thrombocytopenia may occur, but is itself a well-recognized complication of pre-eclampsia. There is no contraindication to breast feeding.

**Nifedepine** Is used for its hypotensive and tocolytic effects. Rapidly absorbed sublingually, it is often used for very labile blood pressure. Interacts with magnesium and combined use is not recommended. Less than 5% of the dose is excreted in breast milk, and thus it is compatible with breast feeding.

**Beta blockers (e.g. labetolol, atenolol, oxprenolol)** These readily cross the placenta, and atenolol may cause a reduction in birthweight. Babies exposed near to delivery should be observed for 24–48 hours for signs of beta-blockade. Small amounts of drug are excreted in breast milk, but are compatible with breast feeding.

**Diuretics** Are usually contraindicated because the maternal circulation is already contracted in pre-eclampsia, but used if pulmonary oedema or left ventricular failure develop.

**Magnesium sulphate** Is the anticonvulsant of choice in eclamptic women. Magnesium sulphate [IV] has not been associated with significant adverse fetal or neonatal effects. Elevated cord calcium concentrations may occur. Neonatal neurological depression and hypotonia are potential side-effects, but are not problematic clinically. With long-term maternal treatment over many weeks, for magnesium's tocolytic effect in preterm labour, rachitic skeletal changes have been reported. Nifedepine and aminoglycoside antibiotics may potentiate the effects of magnesium, and caution is recommended in neonatal use of aminoglycosides for 48 hours after exposure to maternally administered drug.

## Renal disease

The maternal glomerular filtration rate (GFR) increases by about 50% by the end of the first trimester, with increased clearance of creatinine and urea, and lower plasma levels. Protein excretion increases slightly (upper limit 260 mg/L), and due to increased blood flow the kidneys swell and the pelvicalyceal system dilates. The incidence of pyelonephritis in pregnant women with bacteruria is increased. Thus all women are screened once for bacteruria, and those with renal disease should be screened regularly throughout gestation.

Women with primary glomerulonephritis but with normal renal function have a normal pregnancy prognosis. They show a similar decline in renal function over time to those who never become pregnant. In contrast, women with impaired renal function may worsen during pregnancy; the greater the renal impairment, the more likely it is to worsen and for hypertension and proteinuria to supervene. These conditions themselves accelerate the decline in renal function, and it may be impossible to distinguish super-added pre-eclampsia.

In general, end-stage renal failure results in marked suppression of fertility, and perinatal mortality is high in the minority who conceive. By contrast, transplant patients with normal renal function are usually fertile and do well in pregnancy if they stay on their regular immunosuppression.

## Venous thrombosis and anticoagulants

Pulmonary embolism remains a major cause of maternal death. The true incidence of non-fatal venous thrombosis is unknown, but after Caesarean section the incidence is 1–2%. Risk factors include maternal age over 35 years, operative delivery and any underlying thrombophilia disorder, e.g. activated protein C resistance.

Treatment of an identified thrombosis and prophylaxis of high-risk women requires the use of anticoagulants with recognized consequences as follows.

### Warfarin

- Fetal warfarin syndrome: characterized by nasal hypoplasia due to failure of development of the nasal septum, intrauterine growth retardation, visual and hearing problems, stippled epiphyses and developmental delay.
- CNS abnormalities.
- Spontaneous abortion and stillbirth.
- Significant risk of bleeding *in utero*, particularly at the time of delivery.

### Heparin

- Does not cross the placenta, but may cause maternal problems (allergic reactions, thrombocytopenia and osteoporosis (occurs in 2% of women on long-term prophylaxis).

Both drugs may be used during breast feeding.

## Diabetes mellitus

Recognized complications include increased fetal malformations and increased risk of fetal death in late pregnancy, both related to quality of control. Maternal hyperglycaemia is teratogenic, and improved diabetic control is important before conception. Congenital heart disease may occur in 3% of cases where first trimester control is poor; prenatal screening should include fetal echocardiography at 20–22 weeks in addition to the usual detailed scan. Poor first trimester control is associated with growth delay leading to problems in interpretation of AFP and HCG levels, making screening for Down's syndrome unreliable.

Transport of glucose across the placenta is facilitated, so high levels in the mother are mirrored in the fetus, resulting in fetal hyperinsulinaemia. The major fetal effect of insulin is increased metabolic rate with deposition of excessive liver glycogen and subcutaneous tissue. In the macrosomic fetus the abdominal circumference tends to be relatively large proportionate to other dimensions.

Features suggestive of gestational diabetes are:

- obesity;
- family history (first-degree relative or several second-degree relatives);
- maternal polycystic ovary syndrome;
- large-for-dates fetus (above 90th centile);
- hydramnios;
- recurrent or heavy glycosuria.

Women with such features should be screened with a glucose tolerance test at 28 weeks, but sooner if there is earlier evidence of diabetes. There is no increased risk of congenital malformation, as maternal blood sugar levels have usually been normal in the first trimester. However, they are at risk of hyperinsulinaemia, macrosomia and the attendant neonatal complications.

### Antenatal and perinatal care in the diabetic pregnancy

- Fetal growth and amniotic volume should be followed with monthly ultrasound from 24 weeks.
- The presence of hydramnios or accelerated fetal abdominal circumference is indicative of poor diabetic control.
- Hydramnios, although usually not severe, may increase the risk of premature labour.
- Proteinuric hypertension is twice as common in women with diabetes.
- Intrapartum complications are related to macrosomia, but are difficult to predict from ultrasound or fetal weight assessment. They include:
    - intrapartum hypoxia;

- shoulder dystocia;
- fractures of the clavicle and humerus;
- brachial plexus injury and phrenic nerve palsy.

**Breast feeding** Should be encouraged as with non-diabetic women, and has the benefit that it reduces the insulin requirements. Oral hypoglycaemic drugs are excreted in breast milk and may put the baby at risk of hypoglycaemia. Thus if dietary regulation alone is not adequate, insulin must be continued during lactation.

Other neonatal problems include hypoglycaemia (see Chapter 5), jaundice and pulmonary immaturity.

## Thyroid disease

Thyroid physiology changes considerably during pregnancy, secondary to increased thyroid-binding globulin levels and the thyroid-stimulating effects of increased HCG production. Symptoms of thyrotoxicosis are common in women with trophoblastic disease and hyperemesis because of high HCG levels. Interpretation of thyroid function tests must take account of pregnancy-specific reference ranges, but in general the concentration of *free* hormones is little changed.

Autonomous fetal thyroid activity commences early in the first trimester. The placenta is almost impermeable to maternal thyroid hormones. The antithyroid drugs carbimazole and propylthiouracil both cross the placenta, but with low doses the risk of fetal or neonatal hypothyroidism is very small.

Most women with hyperthyroidism have thyroid-stimulating IgG which crosses the placenta and may cause transient fetal or neonatal thyrotoxicosis. The risk to the fetus is small provided that the maternal disease is well controlled throughout pregnancy. If there is significant hyperthyroidism over many weeks, there may be fetal growth retardation and increased perinatal mortality. When the mother is poorly controlled or requiring high doses of antithyroid drugs, it is appropriate to monitor the fetus with serial scans for growth, goitre and heart rate. Neonatal thyrotoxicosis or thyroid crisis occurs rarely (in about 1–2% of babies born to affected women). Management is discussed in Chapter 16.

The use of radioactive iodine for investigation or treatment of thyroid dysfunction is absolutely contraindicated in pregnancy. Iodine freely crosses the placenta and is avidly taken up by the fetal thyroid, resulting in irreversible destruction.

*Breast feeding*  Both carbimazole and propylthiauracil will be present in breast milk at low concentrations. Breast feeding should not be discouraged, but surveillance of the baby's TSH should be considered.

## Platelet disorders (see Chapter 19)

Platelet survival is shortened in pregnancy because of increased destruction within the uteroplacental circulation. This process increases towards term; the finding of mild thrombocytopenia ($100\,000$–$150\,000$/mm$^3$) is common and benign.

### Immune thrombocytopenia

- The most common cause of an isolated low platelet count in early pregnancy.
- Treatment with steroids, and if refractory with intravenous immunoglobulin (IVIG), is used to keep the platelet count above $20\,000$/mm$^3$ or above $50\,000$/mm$^3$ approaching delivery or surgery.
- IgG antiplatelet antibody crosses the placenta and may cause transient fetal/neonatal thrombocytopenia, but there is no correlation between maternal platelet count or antibody level and fetal platelet count.
- The risk of spontaneous haemorrhage in the baby is extremely low, and Caesarean section has not been shown to confer any benefit. Thus there is no indication for invasive fetal testing, and delivery should be by obstetric indication alone.
- The neonatal platelet count tends to fall to a nadir at around 72 hours, and so should be monitored for 3–4 days. The count falls to less than $50\,000$/mm$^3$ in 10–15% of infants. IVIG and platelet transfusion may be considered where the count falls below $20\,000$/mm$^3$ or there is spontaneous haemorrhage respectively. For infants in this more severe category a neonatal brain scan is appropriate.

### Alloimmune thrombocytopenia

- The platelet equivalent of rhesus disease, but fortunately rare. Usually due to PLA1 incompatibility, but several known platelet antigens may be responsible. Unlike rhesus disease, first pregnancies are often affected.
- The antibodies are directed against fetal and not maternal platelets. Maternal counts are normal.

- The diagnosis is most often made during investigation of a thrombocytopenic baby.
- There is significant risk of spontaneous fetal or neonatal intracranial haemorrhage, and it should be considered in any fetus with an unexplained acquired intracranial lesion (ventriculomegaly or porencephaly).
- It is appropriate to examine the serum of mothers of babies with unexplained thrombocytopenia for the presence of platelet-specific antibody (examining the baby's serum is useless because the antibody will be tightly platelet bound).
- Following identification, any first-degree female relative who may undertake pregnancy should also be screened, as it is the HLA type which determines the risk of sensitization in PLA1-negative women. Management of pregnancy in women at risk is exceedingly complex, and should take place in an appropriate fetal medicine centre with expertise in fetal intravascular therapy. The risk of recurrent fetal intracranial haemorrhage following one such affected pregnancy is thought to be high. It is not yet established whether weekly IVIG or weekly fetal platelet transfusion are the optimum management, but certainly steroids to promote lung maturity combined with delivery at around 32 weeks will be appropriate in any pregnancies subsequent to one complicated by fetal intracranial haemorrhage. Surveillance of the fetal brain and consideration of late termination are also appropriate where management fails to prevent this catastrophic complication.

Other perinatal causes of thrombocytopenia are:

- hypertensive disease/pre-eclampsia (risk of haemorrhage is low);
- drugs (aspirin, heparin, non-steroidal anti-inflammatory drugs);
- viral infections (it is now also relevant to establish any associated risk factors for HIV infection and to consider counselling the woman about testing).

## Epilepsy

Pregnancy has no consistent effect on epilepsy. Poorly controlled fits pose more risk to the fetus than drugs used to control epilepsy, and this should be stressed to pregnant women to encourage compliance. Women with poorly controlled epilepsy should be encouraged to bath themselves and their baby only when surveillance is available, and should be warned of the risks of drowning.

### Antiepileptic drugs

- Serum levels of drugs will tend to decline with the increase in plasma volume; however, their dose should only be increased and serum levels monitored if fits occur.
- All anticonvulsants cross the placenta, and all have been associated with a slightly increased risk of fetal abnormality. The most common associated malformations are cardiac, facial clefting and neural tube defects.
- Prophylactic folic acid in a dose of 5mg/day commencing at cessation of contraception is appropriate for women taking folate antagonists, and they should be offered appropriate high-quality mid-trimester scanning to screen for the associated abnormalities.
- Vitamin K given in late pregnancy as well as to the newborn is appropriate with drugs which interfere with its absorption.
- Neonatal withdrawal from antiepileptic drugs is not a problem. Only small amounts of anticonvulsants enter breast milk, and breast feeding is not generally contraindicated (and only relatively in women taking phenobarbitone or primidone).

## Systemic lupus erythematosus (SLE)

SLE is not universally associated with a high fetal loss rate. In women with renal involvement, the need for preterm delivery and the risk of late pregnancy loss is high because of hypertension and renal failure.

The increased risk of fetal loss occurs in the presence of high levels of anti-phospholipid antibodies (APL – anticardiolipin or lupus anticoagulant). Risk is difficult to quantify, although low levels of antibody do not appear to be significant. APL is not confined to SLE, but is found in otherwise healthy women and a wide variety of rheumatic, inflammatory, drug-induced and infectious disorders. A poor obstetric history is an important predictive factor, and there may be a history of venous thrombosis or past thrombotic events. The cause of fetal death is not well understood. Women with recurrent first-trimester miscarriage, unexplained mid-trimester fetal death or growth failure, particularly if there is a past history of venous thrombosis, should be screened for APL. Treatment with low-dose aspirin is advocated, and for those with a history of thrombosis additional daily low-molecular-weight heparin through-out pregnancy. Whether this improves the outcome for the fetus is not clear. Steroids are no longer recommended.

**Heart block**

- Anti-Ro and anti-La antibodies confer a risk of fetal heart block, which occasionally occurs in the presence of other connective tissue disease, such as rheumatoid arthritis. In the presence of anti-Ro, fetal heart block occurs in about one third of pregnancies.
- There is no effective treatment to reduce this risk, despite anecdotal reports of a response to maternal steroids at 20–24 weeks.
- The fetus should be followed carefully from 20 weeks for evidence of bradycardia. Heart block should be diagnosed with detailed echocardiography excluding structural abnormality and M-mode showing dissociation of the atrial and ventricular rates.
- In general the development of heart block will be permanent. Most fetuses with heart block continue to grow and develop unimpaired. At heart rates above 55–60 bpm the fetal cardiac output is maintained, but hydrops is a high risk at slower rates. If the rate is low or the fetus develops any signs of hydrops, treatment with maternal sympathomimetics may increase the fetal heart rate.
- During labour it is not possible to interpret CTG monitoring, and the fetus that is unable to increase its heart rate above 60–80 bpm may be more susceptible to hypoxia. For these empirical reasons, delivery is often by elective Caesarean section.

*Neonatal lupus syndrome* is rare, but presents with haematological and cardiac problems in a baby with skin lesions. The precise antibody that crosses the placenta and causes this syndrome has not been identified, so it cannot be predicted.

## Myasthenia gravis

There are specific anaesthetic considerations in affected women, but the disease itself does not contraindicate normal labour and delivery. About 20% of babies will experience a transient myasthenic illness which may have a delayed onset and last for up to 5 weeks. Neonatal myasthenia causes hypotonia, breathing and feeding difficulties. Symptoms are relieved by a test dose of edrophonium (Tensilon) 0.5 mg/kg i.m. Maintenance is with neostigmine 1 mg/kg 6-hourly orally with feeds.

## Haemoglobinopathies

These comprise the thalassaemias and sickle cell disease, which are autosomal recessive inherited conditions affecting the structure or synthesis of haemoglobin. All 'at risk' women (Asian, Mediterranean, African and West Indian) should be screened antenatally. The heterozygous (trait) condition manifests anaemia, but is relatively asymptomatic and does not require any special management in pregnancy apart from screening the partner. Where both parents are heterozygous they should be counselled about the 1 in 4 risk of homozygous disease in their children, and offered invasive diagnostic prenatal testing.

The thalassaemias are hereditary microcytic anaemias caused by defects in haemoglobin synthesis. Beta thalassaemia is common, and women of Mediterranean and Asian origin should be screened at booking. Alpha thalassaemia is rare, and mainly affects people of South East Asian (Chinese) origin.

Cord blood screening of babies at risk of haemoglobinopathy is undertaken in some areas.

**Alpha-thalassaemia major** A lethal fetal disorder; live birth is extremely rare. Lethal hydrops fetalis occurs in the second trimester, which often results in maternal pre-eclampsia. Prenatal diagnosis was originally by fetal blood sampling, but now recombinant DNA techniques allow diagnosis from villus tissue in the first trimester.

**Beta thalassaemia minor** More common. The heterozygous state is characterized only by microcytic anaemia. The homozygous state requires regular blood transfusion and chelation therapy to prevent iron overload. These impact significantly on quality of life.

**Sickle cell disease** African and West Indian women should be screened for heterozygous 'trait' status. Survival to adult life is usual in homozygous individuals, and fertility is usually unaffected. For an affected woman with a carrier partner, the risk that her baby will inherit the disease is 50%, so again identification of the carrier status of the partner and, where appropriate, making available prenatal diagnosis must form part of the management.

In pregnancy the frequency of infections and sickling crises is increased, with a significant risk of maternal death, intrauterine growth retardation and perinatal fetal loss. A personalized plan of management for crises needs to be identified in the antenatal clinical notes, and care should be co-ordinated by a team with experience of managing this disease in pregnancy.

## DISORDERS OF AMNIOTIC FLUID VOLUME

Both severe oligohydramnios and severe polyhydramnios in the *second* trimester are associated with substantial perinatal morbidity and mortality. This reflects the underlying aetiology and complications. Conversely, a mild reduction in amniotic volume during the *third* trimester is relatively common, and may be idiopathic without adverse sequelae.

### Polyhydramnios

Causes are shown in Table 1.1. Fetal anaemia is commonly cited as a cause, but the volume of amniotic fluid is a very poor guide to the degree of anaemia. Around 40% of infants born to women with

**Table 1.1** Conditions associated with polyhydramnios

**Neurological impairment of fetal swallowing**

- Anencephaly
- Myotonic dystrophy
- Fetal akinesia sequence (arthrogryposis)
- Maternal myasthenia gravis
- Spinal muscular atrophy (Werdnig-Hoffmann syndrome)

**Mechanical impairment of fetal swallowing**

- Facial tumor (epignathus)
- Macroglossia (Beckwith-Wiedemann syndrome)
- Fetal goitre (maternal antithyroid drugs)

**Gastrointestinal obstruction**

- Oesophageal atresia (commonly with tracheal-oesophageal fistula)
- Duodenal atresia (aetiology may be Down's syndrome)
- Small intestinal atresia (aetiology may be a vascular accident)

**High fetal urine output**

- Recipient of twin-twin transfusion
- Fetal/placental tumors
  Sacrococcygeal teratoma
  Large placental chorioangioma
- Fetal macrosomia (maternal diabetes or Beckwith-Wiedemann syndrome)

**Congenital infection**

- Cytomegalovirus, syphilis, viral hepatitis, parvovirus

**Table 1.2** Conditions associated with oligohydramnios

---

**Anomalies**

 (1) Renal
    - Agenesis
    - Dysplasia
 (2) Bladder outlet obstruction
    - Posterior urethral valves (males)
    - Urethral agenesis

**Other conditions**

 - Ruptured membranes
 - Severe intrauterine growth retardation
 - Post-dates pregnancy

**Deformations**

 - Dolichocephaly
 - Low-set ears
 - Arthrogryposis
 - Talipes
 - Pulmonary hypoplasia

---

polyhydramnios have major anomalies. Antenatal tapping of excess fluid may produce temporary relief, but carries a risk of abruption or preterm labour. Indomethacin is occasionally used, as it crosses the placenta and causes a reduction in fetal urine output. After birth the child should be examined carefully and the patency of the oesophagus confirmed by passing a gastric tube and confirming that the aspirate is acidic.

### Oligohydramnios

Variously defined as a deepest pool of less than 1, 2 or 3 cm or an amniotic index of less than 5 cm. Common associations of oligohydramnios are shown in Table 1.2. Severe oligohydramnios in the second trimester has a poor prognosis, with fetal loss rates of up to 88%. In this group the increased risk of aneuploidy should be appreciated and karyotyping considered.

 Severe oligohydramnios poses a diagnostic challenge, because it impairs ultrasound resolution. Amnioinfusion facilitates visualization of fetal anatomy and may help in diagnosis of membrane rupture.

***Deformations and oligohydramnios*** Dependent on gestational age at presentation; abnormal reduction of amniotic volume can interfere with fetal development, leading to structural deformation (Table 1.2), including cranial, facial and skeletal deformations and pulmonary hypoplasia.

**Pulmonary hypoplasia** Results from impaired lung growth, leading to small lungs with diminished vasculature. This is not simply a feature of compression, but rather low amniotic pressure leading to reduced positive tracheal pressure distending the terminal air sacs. Accurate prediction of pulmonary hypoplasia is very difficult.

- The development of pulmonary hypoplasia depends on the gestation of onset, severity and duration of oligohydramnios. When a severe degree of oligohydramnios occurs between 16 and 26 weeks, during the cannalicular phase of lung development, postnatal survival may be compromised. Oligohydramnios commencing after 26 weeks does not result in this complication.
- The degree of oligohydramnios that will result in lung hypoplasia is difficult to ascertain. Where there is no fluid, e.g. in renal agenesis, lethal lung hypoplasia is certain. Where the volume fluctuates, e.g. with membrane rupture early in the middle trimester, lung hypoplasia is difficult to predict, and some fetuses do well. The best predictor is the size of pockets measured serially, but even this is imprecise.
- In the presence of ruptured membranes the prognosis for the fetus correlates best with gestation at delivery.
- Improvement in lung growth by restoring amniotic volume has been attempted by either bladder drainage (successful) or by serial amnioinfusion (uncertain success).

### Fetal renal tract anomalies and oligohydramnios (Table 1.2)

- **Renal agenesis** is especially difficult to identify because the lack of amniotic fluid results in loss of the acoustic window which normally permits ultrasound delineation of fetal structure. Amnioinfusion or instillation of fluid into the fetal peritoneal cavity may be required if renal agenesis is suspected. Care must be taken not to mistake the adrenal glands for kidneys. Frusemide and a fluid load given by cordocentesis to promote fetal diuresis and filling of the bladder can confirm the absence of renal function.
- **Bladder outlet obstruction** may be relieved by vesico-amniotic shunting. However, this has a very limited role, as irreversible renal damage is likely by the time of diagnosis. Despite drainage and the promotion of lung development, the pre-existing degree

of renal impairment will persist; it is usually severe by 18 weeks if obstruction is complete.

- **Severe uteroplacental insufficiency** is considered when gestation is beyond 24 weeks. The associated renal hypoperfusion results in severe oliguria, which may not carry such a grave prognosis as oliguria due to intrinsic renal causes. Doppler ultrasound may demonstrate abnormal high-resistance uteroplacental waveforms, in contrast to a low-resistance picture with renal causes of oliguria or ruptured membranes.

- **Preterm prelabour rupture of the membranes** affects 6% of pregnancies and is responsible for 30% of premature births. Ultrasound assessment of the amniotic volume is useful for predicting risk to the fetus; the incidence of chorioamnionitis and fetal heart rate abnormalities is increased in cases where the residual amniotic volume is consistently low. In the absence of evidence of infection before 34 weeks' gestation, the pregnancy should be managed conservatively following administration of steroids, which probably further enhance fetal lung maturation without increasing the risk of infection in this situation. However, if labour supervenes, tocolysis is not indicated. After 34 weeks, consideration should be given to delivery if labour has not commenced within 24 hours.

- **Amnioinfusion in labour** Third-trimester oligohydramnios may be associated with cord compression with resultant fetal heart rate abnormalities and meconium staining of the amniotic fluid, most commonly during labour. Intrapartum saline amnioinfusion may reduce the incidence of emergency Caesarean section for fetal distress, when fetal heart rate abnormalities are consistent with cord compression. This approach has not gained wide use in the UK.

## MANAGEMENT OF PRETERM LABOUR

Delivery before 37 completed weeks of gestation accounts for 5–10% of births but 85% of neonatal deaths. Almost any complication of pregnancy increases the risk of preterm delivery, particularly multiple pregnancies (especially those of high order, i.e. triplets and above).

- Where preterm delivery is anticipated, maternal steroid therapy should be given to promote fetal lung maturation once the gestation is beyond 23 weeks. This is most effective when given 24 hours to 7 days before delivery, although shorter treatment-delivery intervals are effective in reducing the risk of perinatal death, RDS and IVH.

- The use of drugs to inhibit contractions is controversial. It is unclear whether tocolytics improve perinatal outcome. Currently they are most frequently used for a limited interval to allow time for steroid administration to benefit the fetal lungs (usually 48 hours).

Communication with the neonatal unit and consultant paediatrician is vital whenever preterm labour or delivery seems likely. Provision of intensive or special care of the anticipated level must be established. If this is not available locally then consideration must be given to transfer, and whether this is safer before or after delivery. Where possible, a senior paediatrician should meet the parents and discuss what is likely to happen in the event of their baby being delivered prematurely.

## ASSESSMENT OF FETAL WELL-BEING

**Antenatal fetal monitoring** Clinical evaluation of fetal growth by measurement of symphysis fundal height is routine at all antenatal visits after 24 weeks. Where there is a discrepancy between the size and gestational age, more objective evaluation is performed by ultrasound measurement of the fetus and amniotic fluid, although this still carries a considerable margin of error.

All women are asked to take notice of their baby's movements in the second half of pregnancy and to report any reduction in activity.

More formal antenatal assessment of well-being is usually only applied to high-risk pregnancy, and is achieved by a combination of fetal heart rate monitoring and ultrasound, including assessment of amniotic fluid volume and fetal movements. A low amniotic fluid volume, even when associated with a reactive fetal heart rate pattern, is associated with a less favourable outcome for the fetus. Observation of fetal tone, fetal movements and fetal breathing together with amniotic fluid volume and fetal heart rate reactivity comprise the *biophysical profile*. Two points are awarded for each of the five variables which satisfy predetermined criteria, giving a score out of 10. This is often shortened to an amniotic volume assessment together with fetal heat rate monitoring, the other variables only being considered when these are unsatisfactory.

Evaluation of umbilical artery diastolic flow velocity using Doppler ultrasound is established as a predictor of risk in those fetuses confirmed as being small for gestational age and in pregnancy complicated by pre-eclampsia and oligohydramnios. The role of Doppler assessment in other circumstances is less well established; in particular, Doppler indices have no predictive value after antepartum haemorrhage, or in the diabetic or post-term pregnancy.

**Intrapartum fetal monitoring** This is largely dependent on continuous electronic fetal heart rate monitoring. Continuous monitoring in all low-risk cases has not been shown to improve perinatal outcome compared to intermittent auscultation. However, for labour in high-risk cases, continuous monitoring is routine, despite equally inconclusive data. When significant fetal heart rate abnormalities occur, further evaluation of fetal condition is indicated, usually by measuring the pH of fetal scalp blood.

Unfortunately, the widespread introduction of intrapartum heart rate monitoring over the last 25 years has been associated with an increase in intervention, particularly in delivery by Caesarean section, with no apparent reduction in the incidence of perinatal hypoxia or children with cerebral palsy. This reinforces the impression that most insults resulting in cerebral palsy have occurred before birth.

## BIBLIOGRAPHY

Briggs, G.G., Freeman, R.K. and Yaffe, S.J. (1994) *Drugs in pregnancy and lactation*, 4th edn. Williams and Wilkins.

James, D.K., Steer, P.J., Wiener C.P. and Gonik, B. (1994) *High risk pregnancy*. London: W.B. Saunders.

**2**

# In the delivery room

'Every maternity unit, whether or not Neonatal Intensive Care is undertaken, must have clearly established arrangements for the prompt, safe and effective resuscitation of babies and for the care of babies who require continuing support, either in the maternity unit or by safe transfer elsewhere.' (Extract from *British Paediatric Association Working Party on Neonatal Resuscitation*, 1993 and *Standards for Hospitals Providing Neonatal Intensive Care, British Association of Perinatal Medicine*, January 1996).

## ORGANIZATION

Delivery-room resuscitation is the most important responsibility of the paediatric staff. Much neonatal morbidity and mortality may be prevented by prompt and efficient action.

**Table 2.1** Deliveries at which paediatric staff should routinely be present

Caesarean section (all emergencies and elective under general anaesthetic)
Breech delivery
Forceps (except simple 'lift outs')
Twins
Preterm delivery
Delivery after significant antepartum haemorrhage (APH)
Prolonged (> 24 hours) rupture of membranes, or suspected amnionitis (e.g. foul liquor or maternal fever)
Polyhydramnios
Fetal distress (see Chapter 1)
Mother with severe pregnancy-induced hypertension
Fetal disease or abnormality known or suspected
Rhesus disease if suspected hydrops
Delivery under heavy sedation or general anaesthesia
Mother with history of diabetes mellitus, myasthenia gravis, thrombocytopenia, thyrotoxicosis, or other disease known to affect the fetus (see Chapter 1)

**Two or more paediatric medical staff should attend:**

Multiple births (especially preterm or high risk)
Delivery before 32 weeks' gestation (or if the baby is thought to be < 1.5 kg)
Preterm (< 37 weeks) Caesarean section

## Responsibilities of the neonatal medical team

**1** Ensure that *all* medical and nursing staff are familiar with and experienced in *neonatal resuscitation*. This includes preparation of appropriate protocols.
**2** Ensure that a *roster of trained staff* immediately available for resuscitation is posted in the delivery suite, the telephonists' office, and the paediatric department.
**3** Ensure that delivery room staff *summon assistance in good time* whenever a resuscitation problem may be anticipated (see Table 2.1).
**4** Ensure that *resuscitation equipment is available and working* (see Appendix 2.1).

## Transitional pathophysiology

The reader should be familiar with the normal respiratory and cardiovascular transition at birth. Acute severe peripartum hypoxia in animals results in primary apnoea. This is associated with

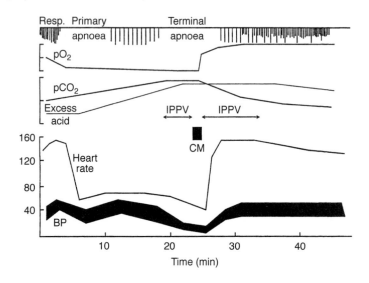

**Fig. 2.1** Physiological changes during asphyxia and resuscitation. (Reproduced with permission from *Principles of Resuscitation at Birth*, 5th edn, Northern Neonatal Network ISBN 0 9527448 0 5.) After Dawes, G.S. (1968) *Foetal and Neonatal Physiology.*

bradycardia and a rise in blood pressure. Redistribution of blood flow occurs, with essential organs (brain and heart) being perfused at the expense of others (skin and kidneys, etc.). If the hypoxic insult persists, deep slow gasping occurs every 10–20 sec before a further period of apnoea occurs – terminal apnoea. Hypotension, more profound bradycardia and decreased cardiac output result in organ damage and death unless active resuscitation is commenced. A similar sequence of changes seems to occur in the human fetus (Fig. 2.1). As it is not always possible to differentiate primary from terminal apnoea, one should assume that the baby is in terminal apnoea, and not delay initiating respiratory and cardiovascular resuscitation.

## Anticipation

It is possible to anticipate many babies that may require resuscitation after birth. Table 2.1 lists many of the higher risk deliveries at which personnel skilled in resuscitation should be present. It is also important to appreciate that the need for resuscitation cannot always be anticipated, and thus all staff should be competent at basic neonatal resuscitation. However, 20% of infants in poor condition at birth and who require resuscitation are not predicted.

## PREPARATION BEFORE DELIVERY

### The parents

Paediatric staff should ensure that they are called to the delivery suite sufficiently early to introduce themselves to parents, explain what is happening or likely to happen, and answer parents' questions.

*Always* introduce yourself to the parents as soon as possible after your arrival in the delivery room.

### The obstetric history

Obtain as full a history as possible from the mother, midwife or obstetrician and examine the mother's notes (see Chapter 1). Note:

- any drugs given to mother?
- gestation? (was the estimation corrected by early scan?)
- evidence of fetal distress?
- prolonged rupture of membranes?
- any relevant past obstetric or medical history?

### Check and prepare the resuscitation equipment
(See Appendix 2.1)

- Ensure that the delivery room is warm ($> 24°C$) and free of draughts.
- Check that equipment is available and in working order.
- Turn on the overhead heater.
- Ensure that warmed towels and/or gamgee in a plastic bag are available.
- Ensure that the transport incubator is switched from 'stand-by' to 'ON'
- Make other preparations, e.g. draw up naloxone into a syringe if the mother has recently received a narcotic such as pethidine.

## INITIAL ASSESSMENT AND MANAGEMENT AT BIRTH

### (1) Time at birth

Start the stop-watch.

### (2) Thermal care (see Chapter 5)

Even healthy infants have difficulty in maintaining body temperature soon after delivery. Small, sick and sedated infants are particularly likely to become chilled. Their problems are greatly exacerbated by cold stress. Even mild chilling may double oxygen requirements and significantly impair prospects for intact survival.

Heat loss is minimized by immediately drying and wrapping the infant in a warm towel. In breech presentations this may be done even before the baby is fully delivered.

Other measures to keep the infant warm include the overhead heater, the incubator and gamgee and plastic sleeping bag and silver swaddler. The latter should not be used under an overhead heater as they reflect radiant heat and reduce the effectiveness of the heater.

**NB** A clothed infant may lose up to 85% of its total heat loss through the head; therefore use a bonnet to reduce heat loss during all prolonged resuscitations.

### (3) Assessment of condition at birth

Initial assessment occurs after the baby has been dried and wrapped, and traditionally consists of the Apgar score (Table 2.3). However, the three essential components common to the Apgar score and to the evaluation of any critically ill patient are:

- **breathing** – assess the rate and *quality* of respiration and note the presence of gasping;
- **heart rate** – palpate base of cord or listen over praecordium;.
- **colour** – note *central* colour (cyanosis, pallor or pink).
  Peripheral vasoconstriction results in a pale appearance.

Based on these three fundamental observations, babies may be grouped into four categories reflecting their condition at birth and the need for resuscitation.

## (4) Initial resuscitation

This depends on the condition at birth, and the basic categories and summary of management are shown in Table 2.2. Babies who require resuscitation may have suffered intrapartum asphyxia, but many will have other reasons for transitional compromise, such as prematurity and sedation.

The condition of the infant at birth is traditionally assessed using the Apgar score (Table 2.3).

The Apgar score is recorded at 1 and 5 min after birth and at subsequent 5 min intervals as a measure of the response to resuscitation as long as the infant requires resuscitation.

If ventilated but breathing spontaneously, record 1 for respiratory effort.

**Table 2.2**  Summary of management at birth

|  | Normal or good condition | Mild/ moderate compromise | Severe compromise | Fresh stillbirth |
|---|---|---|---|---|
| Breathing | Spontaneous | Inadequate | Apnoea | Apnoea |
| Heart rate | > 100/min | > 100/min | < 100/min | No pulse |
| Colour (central) | Pink | Cyanosed | Pale or cyanosed | Pale |
| Management summary | • Dry<br>• Give to mother | • Dry<br>• Stimulation<br>• Oxygen | • Dry<br>• Bag-and-mask | • Dry<br>• Bag-and-mask<br>• Early endotracheal intubation and IPPV<br>• ECM |

**Table 2.3**  The Apgar score

| Sign | Score 0 | Score 1 | Score 2 |
|---|---|---|---|
| Heart rate | Absent | Below 100/min | Above 100/min |
| Respiratory effort | Absent | Weak | Good, crying |
| Muscle tone | Flaccid | Some flexion of extremeties | Well flexed |
| Reflex irritability | No response | Grimace | Cough or sneeze |
| Colour | Pale or blue | Body pink, blue extremities | Completely pink |

### (5) Cord blood acid-base

For babies born after fetal distress (see Chapter 1) or for those needing resuscitation, the cord blood acid-base may be an indicator of the severity of intrapartum asphyxia. However, some infants may have suffered significant intrapartum asphyxia despite having a normal pH.

### (6) Management of the normal infant at birth

Provided that a quick inspection reveals no major resuscitation difficulty or other problem, the baby should be handed at once to the mother. This may be done even before dividing the umbilical cord. The baby may be wrapped in a warmed towel or nursed skin-to-skin on the mother's body and then covered with a towel. If the mother intends to breast feed, the baby should be put to the breast. Such a practice not only improves the success of lactation, but also helps to speed delivery of the placenta through the reflex release of oxytocin (see Chapter 13).

### (7) Dividing the umbilical cord

Clamping the umbilical cord not only determines the distribution of blood between the infant and placenta but may also, while pulsation persists, cause major haemodynamic changes in the circulation.

Modern obstetric practice usually involves division of the cord while the placenta is still *in utero*. In these circumstances, the optimum distribution of blood volume and the least haemodynamic disturbance are likely to be achieved by clamping the cord 30 sec after delivery of the baby. By this time the infant will usually have taken his first breath and will have received a partial placental transfusion.

After division the cord should be firmly occluded about 2 cm from the umbilicus using either a rubber band or a plastic disposable umbilical cord clamp.

## RESUSCITATION (see Fig. 2.2)

### Thermal care

Drying the baby and reducing heat loss is an essential first step. See above.

# NEONATAL RESUSCITATION
## Summary of advanced resuscitation

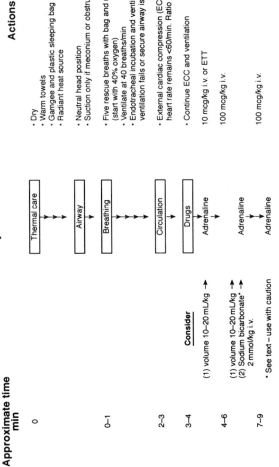

| Approximate time min | | Actions |
|---|---|---|
| 0 | **Thermal care** | • Dry<br>• Warm towels<br>• Gamgee and plastic sleeping bag<br>• Radiant heat source |
| | **Airway** | • Neutral head position<br>• Suction only if meconium or obstruction |
| 0–1 | **Breathing** | • Five rescue breaths with bag and mask (start with 40% oxygen)<br>• Ventilate at 40 breaths/min<br>• Endotracheal incubation and ventilation if bag-and-mask ventilation fails or secure airway is required |
| 2–3 | **Circulation** | • External cardiac compression (ECC) at 120/min, if heart rate remains <60/min. Ratio of 3–5:1 with respiration |
| 3–4 | **Drugs**<br>Adrenaline | • Continue ECC and ventilation<br>10 mcg/kg i.v. or ETT |
| 4–6 | Adrenaline | 100 mcg/kg i.v. |
| 7–9 | Adrenaline | 100 mcg/kg i.v. |

**Consider**

(1) volume 10–20 mL/kg

(1) volume 10–20 mL/kg
(2) Sodium bicarbonate* 2 mmol/kg i.v.

* See text – use with caution

**Fig. 2.2** Flow chart for advanced resuscitation of the newborn.

## Care of the airway

- **Move to resuscitation platform** If the infant is of very low birthweight, or is clearly in poor condition, or has not breathed within 1 min of birth, then move the child to the resuscitation area.
- **Positioning the baby** Place the infant in a gentle head-up position with support under the shoulders so that the head is in the *neutral position* (the neck is neither flexed nor extended).

  *Do not* place the baby in a head-down position. This common practice may itself be responsible for resuscitation difficulty by impairing diaphragmatic action because of the weight of the abdominal contents, by reducing pulmonary lymphatic drainage because of the raised central venous pressure, and by delaying the recovery of normal cerebral activity by causing raised cerebral venous blood pressure. Venous return to the heart, and hence cardiac output, may also be reduced in the head-down position, further contributing to cerebral venous congestion.
- **The upper airway** Obstruction of the upper airway is uncommon (although it may occur after birth because of thick meconium, a congenital abnormality or infected secretions), but this is not a *primary* cause of apnoea. Clinical signs of airway obstruction are inspiratory retraction of the chest wall with poor or absent air entry.

  The majority of babies do *not* require aspiration of the upper airway with a mucus suction catheter. It is usually sufficient to wipe the lips and nose with a piece of gauze. The use of a mucus catheter should normally be confined to aspiration of the nose or mouth. The tip of the catheter should *not* be inserted into the pharynx unless there is clear evidence of obstruction, in which case it should be done under direct vision with the aid of a laryngoscope. *More resuscitation problems are caused than are resolved by blind probing of the sensitive area around the entry to the larynx with a mucus catheter; the practice can lead to activation of reflex bradycardia, apnoea and hypotension.*

  There is also no indication for passing a catheter into the stomach except to rule out suspected oesophageal atresia.

  When the upper airway is obstructed, the blockage is usually located in the nose and is due either to debris or to choanal atresia/stenosis. The patency of the nasal passages may be quickly tested by listening to each nostril in turn with the bell of a stethoscope, the opposite nostril being temporarily occluded.

- **Distal airway obstruction may occur if meconium is aspirated** – see later.
- **Reassess the infant's status** If the infant is still apnoeic, proceed to Breathing.

## Breathing

### Positive-pressure ventilation

Air/oxygen is delivered by a self-inflating bag (500 mL Laerdal or Ambu) or an anaesthetic bag and T-piece. Some favour a finger-controlled T-piece. (Mouth to mouth and nose resuscitation should not be forgotten when equipment is not immediately available.) Recent data suggests that in term infants resuscitation using 100% oxygen has little advantage over air, and that in preterm infants a significant reduction in cerebral blood flow occurs during hyperoxia. Start resuscitation with about 40% oxygen and increase if required.

*Using bag and mask* All medical and midwifery staff in the delivery suite should know how to use the available bag and mask. Five rescue breaths are delivered with deliberate compression of a 500 mL self-inflating bag and soft mask, usually with a maximum inflation pressure of 30 cm $H_2O$. This manoeuvre may provoke onset of respiration by reflex stimulation of pressure receptors in the lower airway (Head's paradoxical inflation reflex). In more compromised babies in 'secondary apnoea' when all reflex activity is severely depressed, inflation of the chest may initially require high (30–40 cm $H_2O$) pressures with prolonged inflation time (2–5 sec). After the rescue breaths, 30–40 inflations/min should be continued until regular spontaneous respiration and a stable heart rate occur. If cardiac compression is also required, a ratio of breaths:compressions of 1:3–5 is suggested.

*Endotracheal intubation* (see Chapter 27) May be required to secure the airway or to help to deliver improved lung inflation. Ventilation via an endotracheal tube is the preferred method for infants who do not respond within 1 min to bag-and-mask ventilation (rise in heart rate, improved colour, onset of respiration), and for those with more severe birth asphyxia. In addition, immediate intubation is preferred when a diaphragmatic hernia is suspected or diagnosed.

*Intubation should be carried out as a calm elective procedure. After stopping ventilation, only 30 secs should elapse before recommencing ventilation. If the first attempt is unsuccessful recommence bag-and-mask resuscitation for 30–60 secs before a further attempt at intubation.*

**DO NOT ALLOW THE BABY TO BECOME COLD OR MORE HYPOXIC AS A RESULT OF REPEATED UNSUCCESSFUL AT-TEMPTS AT INTUBATION.**

If the baby does not respond to intermittent positive-pressure ventilation (IPPV) within 30 secs, check that the tube is correctly placed and is not blocked or dislodged.

**ALWAYS** use a resuscitation bag or air/oxygen supply, with a blow-off set at 30–35 cm $H_2O$. **DO NOT** exceed flow rates recommended by the manufacturer (usually only 2–3 L/min).

Once spontaneous regular respiration is established and the baby is pink and active, the endotracheal tube may be removed. The transfer of preterm babies to the neonatal intensive care unit may be more safely effected by continuing ventilation until it is clear that respiratory support is no longer required. **DO NOT** leave an open ETT in place, as this will impair respiration and may lead to apnoea by reducing functional residual capacity, increasing airway resistance and preventing grunting.

## Circulation

### Cardiac massage (see Chapter 27)

If the heart beat is undetectable or the heart rate remains below 60/min despite positive-pressure ventilation, then cardiac massage should be commenced. This is done most efficiently by placing the fingers around the chest, with one or both thumbs on the lower sternum, which is then depressed by about 2 cm (or about half the diameter of the chest) 100–120 times a minute. A ratio of 1 lung inflation to 3–5 cardiac compressions is recommended. Compression of the sternum must not be violent, especially in preterm infants, to avoid damage to the chest wall, heart or liver.

Ventilation and cardiac compressions should continue until the pulse can be palpated at a rate of 140–160/min. Ventilation should only cease when spontaneous regular respiration is established.

The commonest reason for failure of the heart rate to respond to resuscitation is inadequate ventilation.

## Drugs

### Adrenaline

Give adrenaline 10 mcg/kg (0.1 mL/kg of 1 in 10 000 dilution) intravenously if asystole or bradycardia (< 80/min and not rising) persist after 2 min of effective chest inflations and cardiac compressions. CPR should continue for a further 1 min before a repeat higher dose is given (100 mcg/kg or 1 mL/kg of the 1 in 10 000 dilution). If no response is obtained after a further 1 min, a third dose of adrenaline (100 mcg/kg intravenously) may be given, possibly preceded by sodium bicarbonate 4.2% 2 mL/kg intravenously. In the absence of secure i.v. access adrenaline in larger doses may be given via the endotracheal tube (10–100 mcg/kg). The efficacy of this route is questionable.

*Naloxone* If the mother has received pethidine, morphine, heroin or other related opiates within the previous 8 hours, give naloxone promptly by i.m. injection into the thigh (0.5 mL of 'Adult' Narcan 400 mcg/mL) in term babies and 0.25 mL in babies of < 1.5 kg. Do not waste valuable time trying to inject naloxone intravenously. This specific antagonist given i.m. usually produces a response within 2 min. This dose will be effective for 24 hours.

*Volume expansion* If the infant remains poorly perfused despite adequate ventilation, give 10 mL/kg of fresh frozen plasma or 4.5% human albumin solution over 20 min. Repeat once if necessary.

## Important considerations

### Use of sodium bicarbonate

Intravenous alkali (NaHCO$_3$ or THAM) has been recommended for the asphyxiated infant, as it may dilate the coronary arteries and enhance the efficacy of adrenaline. Intravenous sodium bicarbonate, especially given as a bolus to a poorly ventilated asphyxiated acidotic infant, may exacerbate hypercarbia and intracellular acidosis whilst lowering blood pressure via its vasodilator and negative inotropic actions.

*Resuscitation difficulty* If the resuscitative measures discussed above fail or are inadequate, then consideration should be given to the following diagnoses:

- meconium aspiration syndrome;
- diaphragmatic hernia;
- pneumothorax/pneumomediastinum;

- pleural/pericardial effusion;
- congenital pneumonia/sepsis;
- pulmonary oedema/haemorrhage;
- pulmonary hypoplasia;
- congenital heart disease;
- persistent fetal circulation;
- hypovolaemia due to blood loss;
- cerebrospinal trauma/hypoxia/malformation;
- cerebral depression from drugs;
- severe metabolic disturbance;
- extreme prematurity;
- malformation of the respiratory tract, such as congenital lobar emphysema.

Some of these special problems are considered later in this section or elsewhere as indicated.

**Failed resuscitation** If, despite ventilation, cardiac compression and 3 doses of adrenaline, there is no heart beat at 10 min, resuscitation should be stopped. Despite an improvement in heart rate, if the baby remains apnoeic, profoundly depressed and unresponsive, consideration must be given to the appropriateness of continuing intensive care. The critical question is whether the infant has suffered irreversible damage or has a severely handicapping congenital anomaly. *The most senior paediatrician available should be summoned or informed and the situation discussed fully with the parents. If there is any doubt about the prognosis, intensive care efforts should be continued.* If resuscitation is to be discontinued, the parents may wish the baby to be baptized first. They may then wish to be left with their child during the final minutes.

**Summoning assistance** Neonatal resuscitation may present challenges requiring great experience. *Junior members of the staff should never hesitate to summon the assistance of senior colleagues (sooner rather than later).* When the problem occurs or may be anticipated in a GP maternity unit or at home, then the neonatal transfer team should be called without delay.

## Important points to avoid in neonatal resuscitation

- Cold stress.
- Head-down position.
- Repeated blind aspiration of pharynx.
- Over-flexion or over-extension of the neck.

- Repeated unsuccessful attempts at intubation.
- $NaHCO_3$ infusions (see above).
- Open endotracheal tubes.
- Delay in calling for assistance.

## SPECIAL RESUSCITATION PROBLEMS

### (1) Meconium aspiration

Inhalation of meconium may lead to severe respiratory distress. Partial airway obstruction by sticky meconium ('ball-valve effect') leads to patchy atelectasis and over-inflation of the lungs which, combined with the chemical pneumonitis caused by meconium and the commonly associated persistent fetal circulation, makes this a *very* difficult condition to treat and leads to substantial mortality and long-term morbidity, with a high risk of pneumothorax (see Chapter 10).

Paediatric staff should attend *all* deliveries with fresh meconium-staining of the liquor. A competent assistant is needed.

**NB** Apparent meconium staining may be due to vomited bile or to infection with *Listeria*.

#### Delivery room procedure

- Briefly outline to the parents what is to be done (preferably before the baby is born).
- After delivery of the face, before delivery of the chest, gently clear meconium from the nose and mouth using an oral mucus extractor.
- Quickly dry and wrap the infant.
- Gently suck meconium out of the mouth, pharynx and nose. Use a laryngoscope to see the vocal cords and suck out the posterior pharynx and larynx under direct vision. This may be performed on the delivery bed before cutting the cord, to reduce the risk of early gasping.
- If meconium is present in the posterior pharynx or larynx, transfer the child to the resuscitation trolley and intubate. Apply gentle suction to the ETT whilst removing the tube. If a plug of meconium is removed with the ETT, repeat the process. We can no longer recommend mouth suction because of the risk of HIV.
- Resuscitate the infant with bag-and-mask ventilation or endotracheal IPPV.

**NB**

**1** Do not use IPPV before clearing the airway: meconium may be forced into the bronchial tree.

**2** If the infant cries vigorously before the trachea has been intubated and suctioned, abandon the attempt. A forced intubation may injure the infant's mouth and airways.

**3** Tracheal lavage with saline is *not* recommended and has been shown to worsen the outcome. With practice, the process of clearing the airways should not greatly delay resuscitation.

All babies from whom meconium is aspirated from below the cords should be kept under close observation for 4–6 hours. If no respiratory signs (e.g. tachypnoea, grunting, temperature instability, hypoglycaemia, cyanosis) develop within 6 hours, the infant may go to a normal postnatal ward with its mother, but should be kept under observation for 24 hours, as pneumothorax and infection can occur later. If any respiratory signs develop, transfer to SCBU or NICU, X-ray the chest and manage as described in Chapter 10.

## (2) Hypovolaemia due to fetal blood loss

Such infants present as pale, hypotensive and apnoeic, and have weak pulses that may be slow or rapid. If the infant does not respond to IPPV, give a rapid transfusion (10–20 mL/kg over 5–10 min) of unmatched fresh O Rh-negative blood (or blood cross-matched against the mother's blood) and reassess. A second similar transfusion may be necessary (see Chapter 19).

## (3) Hydrops fetalis

Generalized oedema, ascites, pleural effusions, anaemia and hepatosplenomegaly may occur with severe fetal anaemia (e.g. rhesus disease – Chapter 18; thalassaemia – Chapter 19), congenital infections (syphilis, toxoplasma, CMV – Chapter 17), maternal diabetes (Chapter 5), cardiac failure (Chapter 11), hypoproteinaemia (e.g. congenital hepatitis or nephrotic syndrome) or twin-to-twin transfusion.

Initial problems are similar, whatever the cause:

### Respiration

Sustained IPPV through an ETT is always needed (often with frequent suction to clear pulmonary fluid). Drain ascites and pleural effusions immediately if they are embarrassing respiration. High peak inspiratory pressure may be required to inflate the lungs, and positive end expiratory pressure (PEEP) may help to reduce pulmonary oedema.

### Anaemia and hypoproteinaemia
Correct the anaemia *slowly* with repeated small exchange transfusions of packed red cells (20–40 ml/kg) to avoid major fluid shifts and pulmonary oedema from a rapid rise in oncotic pressure.

### Haemorrhage
Risk is decreased by giving 1 mg i.v. vitamin $K_1$ immediately after birth (Chapter 4), and by exchange transfusion with fresh blood (Chapter 19 and Chapter 27).

### Cardiac failure and poor urine output
Give frusemide 1–2 mg/kg and continue 12-hourly. Create a fluid deficit (10–20 mL/kg) during exchange transfusion (see Chapter 27). Crystalloid fluid infusion should initially be limited to about 60 mL/kg/day.

### Hypoglycaemia
Monitor blood sugar 2 to 4-hourly. Give i.v. glucose at 4–6 mg/kg/min (see Chapter 16.)

### Investigation

- Examine placenta carefully.
- Take blood from placenta for blood group Coombs' test, Hb and PCV, bilirubin (direct and total), serum proteins, transaminase levels and congenital infection screening (see Chapter 17). If placental blood is not available, take blood from the baby *before* transfusion.

## (4) Diaphragmatic hernia (see Chapter 9)

Clues include a history of maternal hydramnios (50%), signs of mediastinal shift, a difference in air entry between the two sides of the chest, and a relatively 'empty' or scaphoid abdomen. When this diagnosis is suspected it is especially important to position the infant tilted head-up, and to avoid bag-and-mask resuscitation. If antenatal diagnosis has been made, early intubation, early use of muscle relaxants and early nasogastric suction on the delivery suite if not adjacent to NICU is indicated.

## (5) Preterm infants

These babies may have poor respiratory drive, compliant chest wall, increased airway resistance and reduced respiratory muscle power. Early support may be necessary, and safe transfer to and stabilization on the SCBU/NICU is essential before withdrawing ventilation and removal of an endotracheal tube. If in doubt, intubate.

*Preterm infants delivered by Caesarean section* are at considerable risk of cardiopulmonary maladaptation. In addition to reduced respiratory muscle power, clearance of lung fluid is often inadequate when a preterm infant is delivered by Caesarean section (particularly when the latter is elective). Dunn has described a technique for the management of preterm Caesarean section to optimize fetal-placental blood distribution (Dunn, 1989).

## AFTERCARE IN THE DELIVERY ROOM

Following successful resuscitation and the establishment of respiration, the infant should be examined for other problems, then wrapped in a warm towel and handed without delay to the mother and father with an explanation for the need for resuscitation. If the infant is very small or sick, or has suffered from severe asphyxia, he or she should be shown to and held briefly by the parents before being placed in the transport incubator and transferred to the special care baby unit (see Chapter 5).

## The placenta

This should be weighed and examined carefully for abnormalities such as vasa praevia, clots, infarction, amnion nodosum, single umbilical artery, etc. In multiple births it is particularly important to examine the membranes for zygosity and the placental vessels for evidence of twin-to-twin transfusion. A placenta weighing > 25% of the infant's birthweight is suggestive of congenital nephrotic syndrome (see Chapter 15).

If the mother is rhesus negative or has blood group isoimmunization, placental blood should be sent to the laboratory at once for grouping, Coombs' test, and haemoglobin and serum bilirubin measurement.

Placental blood for serology should be collected if intrauterine infection is suspected.

## The records

The details of resuscitation and examination should be recorded at once in the infant's notes, together, when necessary, with instructions for further investigation and care in the nursery or SCBU. In particular, watch for signs of hypoglycaemia, hypothermia and cerebral dysfunction in the postasphyxiated infant (see Chapter 12). Order *immediate* antibiotic therapy if infection is suspected. *All infants* should receive vitamin $K_1$ soon after birth (see Chapter 4).

## Transfer to the SCBU/NICU (see Chapter 5)

All infants who still require respiratory support and are being transferred to the nursery should be accompanied by a doctor or nurse. Never transfer an intubated infant without IPPV or CPAP (4–5 cm $H_2O$). Every precaution should be taken to prevent hypothermia or hypoxaemia during transport (see Chapter 7).

## The parents

If it is necessary to transfer the baby to the SCBU/NICU, the parents should be given a full explanation and arrangements made for them to visit. When it is not possible for the mother to visit, a Polaroid photograph of her baby should be made available (see Chapter 23).

---

**Appendix 2.1** Delivery-room resuscitation equipment

---

**Equipment**

- Warmed towels and gamgee in plastic bag or silver swaddler
- Gloves
- Resuscitation trolley with overhead heater, lighting and stop-clock
- Oxygen and air supply (with reducing valve, flow-meter, pressure blow-off device (set at 30 cm $H_2O$), pressure-measuring device (e.g. manometer)), connecting tubes to supply air/oxygen to bag and mask and (with side hole) to endotracheal tube
- Face masks (e.g. Laerdal, sizes 00, 01)
- 500 ml resuscitation bag with fitting for face mask and ETT adaptor and blow-off valve (e.g. Ambu, Laerdal)
- Laryngoscopes, with preterm- and term-sized straight blades (e.g. Wisconsin or Magill) and spare bulbs and batteries

- Endotracheal tubes (2.5, 3.0 and 3.5 mm) and connectors and fixation devices and endotracheal tube introducer (nylon or metal)
- Oropharyngeal airways (sizes 00 and 0)
- Nasogastric tubes (5 and 8)
- Suction device and suction catheters (FG 4, 6, 8)
- Oral mucus extractors
- Stethoscope
- Sterile towel, scissors, cord clamps
- Antiseptic cleaning solution (e.g. povidone-iodine, chlorhexidine)
- Intravenous cannulae, 3-way taps, connecting tubing
- Sterile syringes (2, 5 and 10 mL) and needles
- Adhesive tapes
- Capillary blood sugar test strips (e.g. 'Dextrostix', 'BM Test')
- Alcohol swabs
- Sterile containers; specimen bottles for blood tests (e.g. FBC, PCV, electrolytes, sugar, bilirubin, blood group and Coomb's test)
- Equipment for umbilical catheterization
- Pneumothorax drains + Heimlich valves
- Intravenous giving sets (paediatric)
- Intravenous infusion pumps

*Drugs and fluids*

| | |
|---|---|
| • Adrenaline | 1:10 000 (10 mL ampoule) |
| • Dextrose | 10% solution |
| • Sodium chloride | 0.9% solution for injection |
| • Water for injection | |
| • Naloxone | 400 mcg/mL |
| • Volume expanders | Plasma, albumin solutions |
| • Blood | Fresh Group O Rh-negative (CMV-negative) |

## BIBLIOGRAPHY

Advanced Life Support Group (1997) *Advanced Paediatric Life Support (UK) The practical approach.* London: BMJ Publishing Group.

Dunn, P.M. (1989) Perinatal factors influencing adaptation to extrauterine life. In Belfort, P., Pinotti, J.A. and Eskes, T.K. A.B.

(eds), *Advances in gynaecology and obstetrics. Vol.5. Pregnancy and labour.* Carnforth: Parthenon Press, 119–23.

Freeman, J.M. and Nelson, K.B. (1988) Intrapartum asphyxia and cerebral palsy. *Pediatrics* **82**,240–49.

Lundstrom, K.E., Pryds, O. and Greisen, G. (1995) Oxygen at birth and prolonged cerebral vasoconstriction in preterm infants. *Arch. Dis. Child.* **73**,F81–F86.

Milner, A.D. and Vyas, H. (1982) Lung expansion at birth. *J. Pediatr.* **101**,879–86.

Ramji, S., Ahuja, S., Thiupuram, S. *et al.* (1993) Resuscitation of asphyxic newborn infants with room air or 100% oxygen. *Pediatr. Res.* **34**,809–12.

*Resuscitation of babies at birth. Report of a Multidisciplinary Working Party* (1997) London: BMJ Publishing Group.

# 3

# Birth trauma

Obstetric events predisposing to birth trauma
Injuries to the scalp and skull
Injuries to the face
Brachial plexus injuries
Fracture of the clavicle
Fracture of the cervical spine
Fractures of the long bones of the limbs
Visceral intra-abdominal trauma
Trauma to external genitalia
Generalized bruising

All newborn infants should be examined carefully at birth for evidence of birth injury. *Any findings, even minor ones, should be shown to and discussed with the parents with appropriate explanation and reassurance.*

## OBSTETRIC EVENTS PREDISPOSING TO BIRTH TRAUMA

The following obstetric events are particularly likely to be associated with birth trauma to the baby.

- Fetomaternal disproportion: dystocia with head, shoulders or abdomen.
- Malpresentation: breech, brow, face.
- Instrumental delivery or manual extraction, especially Kielland's forceps.
- Vacuum extraction.
- Preterm delivery.
- Precipitate delivery.

- In association with fetal distress causing cerebral venous congestion and rapid obstetric delivery.
- Twins:
  vaginal delivery of second, larger twin; use of oxytocic agent before delivery of undiagnosed second twin.
- Caesarean delivery:
  scalpel incision.

It is particularly important that infants showing evidence of birth trauma should receive vitamin K, 0.1 mg i.m., following delivery.

## INJURIES TO THE SCALP AND SKULL

### Caput succedaneum

The boggy appearance of the 'presenting' scalp quickly subsides. No treatment is required.

### 'Chignon'

This is the oedematous part of the scalp that has been sucked into a vacuum extractor. There may be haemorrhage and necrosis of the skin. Local toilet may be required. Scars may result occasionally.

### Subaponeurotic haemorrhage

Very considerable haemorrhage may occur beneath the epicranial aponeurosis, with little to show except for a boggy feel to the scalp. The infant may suffer from haemorrhagic shock, anaemia and, later, from jaundice. Infants delivered by ventouse extraction are particularly at risk. Treatment is as for acute haemorrhage (see Chapter 19).

### Lesions due to scalp electrode clips or scalp blood sampling

These small lesions usually require local toilet at the most. Occasionally they may lead to infection and abscess formation. They should not be confused with cutis aplasia (congenital scalp defects).

### Cephalhaematoma

These subperiosteal haemorrhages usually occur over one or other of the parietal bones, and less frequently over the occipital bone. They occur in about 1% of infants, especially at and after term. Frequently there is an associated hairline fracture of the outer table of the bone, while the extent of the haemorrhage is limited by the suture lines. The swelling usually becomes obvious and fluctuant on the second day. A hard, calcified rim around the edge gives the false impression of a hole in the skull. Especially when bilateral, cephalhaematoma may cause anaemia and jaundice. Associated intracranial trauma is rare, and no treatment is required for the actual haematoma. Aspiration should not be undertaken.

### Depressed fractures of the skull

These are very rare. Surgical advice should be sought.

### Intracranial haemorrhage and traumatic brain damage (see Chapter 12).

## INJURIES TO THE FACE

### Traumatic cyanosis

Cyanosis, bruising and petechial haemorrhages of the face may follow pressure on the neck from the cervix or a nucal umbilical cord during delivery. Pinkness of the rest of the body rules out cyanotic heart disease. No treatment is needed, although jaundice may develop.

### Superficial injuries

Fat necrosis over the zygoma and facial paralysis may be caused by forceps. Subconjunctival haemorrhages and bruising of the face may be associated with face and brow presentations. All resolve rapidly within days or weeks. No specific treatment is needed.

### Scalpel incisions

Occurring accidentally during Caesarean delivery, scalpel incisions may affect any part of the body and require suturing. When they are on the face, it is wise to obtain the help of a plastic surgeon. A photographic record should be made.

### Facial nerve palsy

Some cases are caused by pressure on the nerve during forceps delivery. The paralysis is usually unilateral. When the infant cries, the eye on the affected side remains open and the mouth is drawn to the opposite side. No treatment is required except perhaps the use of artificial tears for the open eye. Differential diagnosis includes intrauterine pressure neuropraxia and congenital defects of the 7th nerve (often bilateral). Recovery is usually complete within days or weeks.

## BRACHIAL PLEXUS INJURIES

The brachial plexus may be injured during lateral flexion of the neck while trying to deliver the shoulders with vertex presentation or traction on the body or arms during breech delivery. The injuries may be associated with fracture of the clavicle, or with phrenic nerve damage causing unilateral diaphragmatic paralysis, or with damage to the cervical sympathetic nerves leading to Horner's syndrome (myosis, ptosis and enophthalmos), or very rarely with fracture dislocation of the shoulder.

Injuries to the brachial plexus may be very varied, but are usually divided into those affecting the upper plexus (Erb's palsy) and those affecting the lower plexus (Klumpke's paralysis).

**Erb's palsy** Involves mainly the C5 and C6 nerve roots, and accounts for most cases of brachial-plexus injury. The arm is maintained limply alongside the body with the forearm pronated ('waiter's tip' position). There is loss of movement.

**Klumpke's paralysis** Involves mainly C8 and T1 nerve roots. The small muscles of the hand and the wrist flexors are affected, causing a 'claw hand'. Besides the signs of the lower motor neuron paralysis, there may be loss of sensation and sweating.

X-ray of the spine, shoulder and arm should be undertaken to exclude fracture. Electromyelography and MRI may be indicated in severe cases. Treatment consists mainly of gentle full-range passive movement of the affected joints several times a day. This may be taught to the parents. Splinting is of little value and may delay recovery. Recovery occurs spontaneously in two-thirds of cases, usually commencing within 6 weeks. Improvement may continue for 12 or more months.

Neuropraxia of facial, radial, sciatic and obturator nerves, sterno-mastoid torticollis and other deformities due to intrauterine pressure are discussed in Chapter 7.

## FRACTURE OF THE CLAVICLE

This is usually associated with shoulder dystocia or with delivery of the arms in breech presentation. It may be detected by palpation of the break and crepitus and by pseudoparalysis of the arm on that side. It should be distinguished from the rare pseudoarthrosis of the clavicle in which there is no pain, tenderness or callus formation. Confirm the diagnosis by X-ray. Minimal treatment is required except for gentle handling and analgesia. A gauze pad in the axilla and a crêpe figure-of-eight bandage may relieve discomfort during the 2 to 3 weeks required for the fracture to unite.

## FRACTURE OF THE CERVICAL SPINE

This rare injury is usually associated with breech extraction. Typically there is a fracture dislocation in the C6–8 region with damage to the cord, which may be diagnosed on MRI scan. Diaphragmatic breathing is maintained through the phrenic nerves. There is a flaccid quadriplegia and urinary retention. The prognosis is gloomy.

## FRACTURES OF THE LONG BONES OF THE LIMBS

These are usually of the mid-shaft and sustained during manipulation of the arms or legs in breech delivery; twisting manipulations may cause avulsion of the lower epiphyses of either femur or tibia. Diagnosis is made because of angulation or shortening, through palpation or because of pseudoparalysis. Diagnosis should be confirmed by X-ray. Treatment consists of light splinting in good alignment. When the infant has been lying *in utero* as a breech presentation with extended legs, then alignment of the femur may be best achieved by bandaging the legs over the abdomen, but be careful not to obstruct respiration. Union is usually achieved within 3 weeks or so. The bones of the newborn exhibit a great capacity for remodelling.

## VISCERAL INTRA-ABDOMINAL TRAUMA

Birth trauma to the liver, the spleen, or to some other abdominal organ is rare. Typically, it is associated with breech extraction or with abdominal dystocia due to hepatosplenomegaly, but it may occur spontaneously in infants of mothers on anticonvulsants. The signs of haemorrhagic shock may be delayed for 2 to 3 days until a subcapsular haematoma ruptures. A primary or secondary coagulopathy may be present. Always give vitamin $K^1$, 0.1 mg i.m. Manage as for acute haemorrhage (see p. 326). Surgery may be indicated.

## TRAUMA TO EXTERNAL GENITALIA

### Testicular birth trauma

Significant scrotal bruising and testicular enlargement may be found in approximately 10% of male infants delivered by breech. Typically the infant is a large singleton born at or after term. The external genitalia are very tender and severe cases with haemorrhagic infarction may lead to testicular hypoplasia and sterility. It is inadvisable to discuss this remote possibility with the parents. Discrete examination of the testicles at follow-up is recommended. At birth no treatment is required except perhaps analgesia in severe cases and minimal handling.

*Differential diagnosis* Congenital torsion of the testicle. Usually delivery is by the vertex; minimal scrotal bruising; unilateral stony hard testicular enlargement; typically painless unless of recent origin, in which case urgent surgery is indicated.

### Vulval haematoma

Female breech-born infants may suffer bruising and haematoma of the vulva. Spontaneous recovery may be expected within days.

## GENERALIZED BRUISING

This is particularly likely to occur following breech delivery of the very low birthweight infant. There is also often extensive associated haemorrhage into the muscles. Hypovolaemic shock, oliguria, anaemia and jaundice are complications to be anticipated.

## BIBLIOGRAPHY

Dunn, P.M. (1981) Breech delivery: a paediatric view. In Beared, R.W. and Paintin, D. B. (eds), *Outcomes of obstetric intervention in Britain.* Proceedings of the Royal College of Obstetrics and Gynaecology Scientific Meeting, London.

Roberton, N.R.C. (1992) *Textbook of neonatology,* 2nd edn. Edinburgh: Churchill Livingstone.

Sharrad, W.J.W. (1972) *Paediatric orthopaedics and fractures*, 2nd edn. Oxford: Blackwell Scientific Publications.

# 4

# Routine care of the newborn infant

In the delivery room
On the postnatal ward

## IN THE DELIVERY ROOM (see Chapter 2)

- Ensure that delivery rooms are warm (23–28°C) and free of draughts.
- Carefully dry baby after delivery and wipe secretions, etc., from the face; then wrap in warmed towel or blanket and hand him or her to the mother, with appropriate reassurance.
- Most babies should be put to the breast within a few minutes of delivery.
- Mother's body heat will keep baby warm if he or she is directly against the mother's skin.
- Avoid cold stress – use radiant warmer if the baby is exposed.

### Vitamin K

All infants should be given vitamin K on the day of birth. This will normally be Konakion, 0.25 mL (0.5 mg vitamin K) orally. Formula milk contains vitamin K supplements, but babies who are breast fed should be given a second oral dose of 0.5 mg at the age of 7 days, and a third oral dose at 4–6 weeks if still fully breast fed. The following groups of infants who are at higher risk of vitamin K deficiency bleeding should be given Konokion, 0.05 mL (100 mcg vitamin K) i.m. or i.v.:

- all babies under 33 weeks' gestation;
- all babies requiring surgery within the neonatal period;
- all babies with severe neonatal illness or bleeding disorder;
- babies of mothers on anticonvulsant therapy (phenytoin, phenobarbitone).

Alternative protocols for administering vitamin K have also been proposed by the British Paediatric Association (1992). A new oral preparation, Konakion M.M., has recently been licensed at a recommended dose of 2 mg orally at birth followed by a second dose at 4–7 days. Exclusively breast-fed babies should receive a third dose at 1 month.

## ON THE POSTNATAL WARD

### Routine examination

A rapid examination of all infants in the delivery room is important, but the infant must not be cold stressed or unnecessarily separated from his or her parents.

All babies must be fully examined by a doctor within 24 hours of birth (Tables 4.1 and 4.2), preferably in the presence of the mother, so that her questions can be answered and any problems discussed.

### Feeding

- Advice on breast feeding should start in the antenatal clinic.
- Mothers may need help and advice on the techniques of feeding and breast care (see Chapter 13).
- The more frequently a baby is put to the breast, the sooner feeding will be established and the lower the risk of sore nipples will be (most babies will feed 8–12 times a day in the first 48 hours).
- Test weighing is inaccurate and likely to increase maternal anxiety.
- If the baby is passing urine once every 3–4 hours, fluid intake is adequate. If necessary, assess hydration by checking urine specific gravity (if < 1.010, hydration is likely to be adequate).
- Bottle feeding (see Chapter 13).

**Table 4.1** Routine first-day assessment of the newborn infant: history

**Mother**

Family history
Previous medical conditions (e.g. diabetes, thyrotoxicosis, drug abuse)
Known social problems
Past obstetric history (e.g. preterm delivery, perinatal deaths)
This preganancy
    Dates (certain?)
    Complications (e.g infections, blood pressure, proteinuria)
Scan results
Blood group (and known antibody status)
Labour and delivery
    Onset (spontaneous/induced)
    Presentation
    Fetal distress (type?)
    Type of delivery
    Membrane rupture-to-delivery interval
    Maternal pyrexia?
    Liquor offensive?

**Baby**

Birthweight/gestation
Apgar score at 1 and 5 min
Resuscitation
Temperature
Feeding – breast or bottle – any problems?
Passed stools/urine yet?
Dextrostix (if birth asphyxia, low birthweight, cold or tachypnoeic, or if $> 4$ kg)
Any problems noted already?

## Prevention of infection (see Chapter 17)

Careful cleaning of equipment and scrupulous hand washing by *all* staff is essential. There is no evidence that the use of gowns or masks reduces infection risk, and no evidence that visiting by healthy adults or other children increases it.

### Umbilical cord care

The umbilicus is rapidly colonized after birth, particularly by *Staphylococcus aureus.* In the past this was a major cause of local and systemic infection, often with nursery outbreaks of cross-infection. Antimicrobical cord care was highly effective in preventing this, and

**Table 4.2** Routine first-day assessment of the newborn infant: examination

| | |
|---|---|
| Age at time of examination | Cardiovascular system (heart sounds, |
| Weight, length and head circumference | murmurs, femoral pulses, liver size) |
| (and plot on centile chart) | Abdomen (liver, spleen, kidney, umbilicus |
| Gestation (by dates and by examination) | – number of vessels) |
| (see Chapter 22) | Genitalia |
| Posture | Anus (site, tone) |
| Colour (cyanosis, pallor, plethora, | Spine (dimple, hairy patches, lipoma, |
| jaundice) | scoliosis) |
| Skin (dry, peeling, vernix, any naevi?) | Arms and hands (including palmar |
| Nutrition (subcutaneous tissue, well or | creases) |
| poorly nourished) | Hips (full movements, not dislocatable or |
| Oedema (and site) | dislocated) |
| Skull (moulding cephalhaematoma, | Legs and feet |
| sutures, fontanelle) | Behaviour and activity (including |
| Facies (anomalies, asymmetry) | response to handling) |
| Ears (size, shape, low-set) | Muscle tone |
| Eyes (and epicanthic folds) | Movements (asymmetry) |
| Nose/nasal airway | Cry |
| Mouth and palate (NB feel for posterior | Reflexes (suck, grasp, Gallant, step, |
| palatal spine) | place, Moro) (NB plantar reflex is |
| Neck (and clavicles, sternomastoid | downgoing in normal infant) |
| contracture) | *Assessment* |
| Chest (shape, respiratory pattern and | ? Normal healthy infant |
| effort, auscultation) | ? Appropriate size for gestation |
| | Discuss any problems with the mother |
| | and reassure her if all is well |

cord infection is now so uncommon that the need for routine prophylactic cord care is being questioned.

Dry cord care still has a high *Staphylococcus aureus* colonization rate, and routine cleaning with chlorhexidine, or hexachorophene is equally effective in reducing colonization. We recommend the use of hexachlorophane powder.

### Weighing

Alternate-day weighing is sufficient for most normal infants. Normal infants may lose up to 10% of birthweight in the first week, and may not regain their birthweight until 10–14 days.

### Temperature

Avoid cold stress (see Chapter 5). Axillary temperature should be routinely checked on admission to the postnatal ward and again at

6–12 and 18–24 hours. Always use a low-reading thermometer, and warm the baby if the axillary temperature is < 36°C, or if the extremities feel cold.

**NB**

- Temperature instability may be a very important sign of sepsis.
- Check capillary blood sugar (e.g. Dextrostix, BM-Test) in all cold infants.

## Passage of urine and meconium

Approximately 25% of infants pass urine in the delivery room, and this may not be noted. Infants who have not passed urine by the time they are 24 hours old should be examined for palpable bladder or kidneys.

**99% of infants pass urine by 48 hours** The remaining 1% may be due to obstruction to urine flow (enlarged bladder present with meatal obstruction, urethral valves, neurogenic bladder, ureterocele) or to decreased urine production (bladder not enlarged, e.g. hypovolaemia, dehydration, renal agenesis, acute tubular necrosis, acute cortical necrosis, or inappropriate antidiuretic hormone (ADH) secretion) (see Chapter 15).

**80% of infants pass meconium in the first 24 hours, and 99% by 48 hours**

- Low-birthweight infants, especially if they are unwell or not enterally fed, may have delayed passage of meconium.
- Infants who have not passed meconium by 48 hours should be examined for evidence of bowel obstruction (vomiting, abdominal distension) or anorectal abnormalities (e.g. imperforate anus, ectopic anus), and should be investigated for possible cystic fibrosis or Hirschsprung's disease (see Chapter 9).
- Gentle digital examination of the rectum may provoke passage of meconium, or a plug of white mucus ('meconium plug') followed by meconium.

## Baths

Early bathing of babies (i.e. < 48 hours of age) is a major cold stress and may increase infection risk. Babies should not be routinely bathed in hospital. The main value of bathing a normal infant in hospital is to teach the mother how to do it.

## Discharge examination

Most babies are now discharged home to the care of a community midwife within 48 hours of birth, and do not need a second or discharge examination at that time. However, such examination is required if the baby remains in hospital for more than 4 days.

Discharge examination is as for the first-day examination (see Table 4.2), but in addition the following specific points must be checked:

- *Feeding and weight* Ensure feeding is established and there has not been excessive weight loss.
- *Jaundice* Significant jaundice must be investigated (Chapter 18). Babies should not go home until the bilirubin level is stable or falling.
- *Arrangements for follow-up* Ensure that the parents know both who to contact if any problems develop and whether any follow-up is needed. In addition, the parents must be reassured and their questions answered.
- *Advice* should be given to the parents on keeping the baby warm, on the use of vitamins, and on the need for immunization.
- *Complete the discharge record* (send copies to obstetric and neonatal records and to the primary health-care team).

## Biochemical screening

There is a national neonatal screening programme for phenyl-ketonuria (PKU) and for congenital hypothyroidism. For PKU, blood spots should be collected on filter-paper forms not earlier than the sixth day, and at least 48 hours after starting milk feeds. Thyroid activity is assessed by measuring TSH on the same blood samples.

Some centres have extended screening to other amino-acid disorders, such as homocystinuria and tyrosinaemia. There is increasing use of immunoreactive trypsin measurement as a screen for cystic fibrosis. Routine testing of infants for haemoglobinopathies can be performed on cord blood, and is recommended for districts with an at-risk population.

# BIBLIOGRAPHY

Changing Childbirth Implementation Team (1997) *Changing childbirth and the baby.* Milton Keynes: NHS Executive Anglia and Oxford Health Care Directorate.

Johnston, P. (1994) *Vulliamy's The newborn child,* 7th edn. London: Churchill Livingstone.

Verber, I.G. and Pagan, F.S. (1993) What cord care – if any? *Arch. Dis. Child.* **68**, 594–6

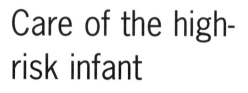

# 5

# Care of the high-risk infant

## DEFINITIONS AND STAFFING

### Definitions of special and intensive care of the newborn

Levels of care have been defined by the British Association for Perinatal Medicine and the Neonatal Nurses Association as follows.

**Maximal intensive care (Level 1)** includes babies:

- receiving assisted ventilation (including endotracheal ventilation and CPAP) and in the first 24 hours following withdrawal. This definition must be extended to include all babies receiving advanced ventilation, e.g. high-frequency oscillation;
- < 27 weeks' gestation and for the first 48 hours post-delivery;
- < 1000 g for 48 hours post-delivery;
- requiring major surgery, for the preoperative period and postoperatively for 48 hours;

- on the day of death;
- during transport, requiring medical and nursing escorts (both within and between hospitals);
- receiving peritoneal dialysis;
- requiring exchange transfusion – complicated by another disease process;
- with severe respiratory disease within 48 hours requiring an $FiO_2 > 0.6$;
- who have recurrent apnoea needing frequent stimulation ($> 5$ in 8 hours or resuscitation with IPPV $> 2$ in 24 hours);
- who have a significant requirement for circulatory support, e.g.:
  inotropes;
  pulmonary vasodilators;
  $> 3$ transfusions of colloid in 24 hours;
  prostaglandin infusion.

**High-dependency intensive care (Level 2)** includes babies:

- requiring parenteral nutrition;
- who have convulsions;
- during transport by an appropriately qualified neonatal nurse;
- who have an indwelling arterial line or chest drain;
- with respiratory disease within 48 hours of life, requiring $FiO_2$ 0.4–0.6;
- with recurrent apnoea requiring stimulation ($< 5$ times in 8-hour period or resuscitation with IPPV);
- who need exchange transfusion alone;
- more than 48 hours post-operation, requiring complex nursing procedures;
- with tracheostomy – for the first 2 weeks.

All other babies requiring admission to the NICU are categorized as **Special Care**, including those:

- requiring continuous monitoring of respiration, heart rate, or by transcutaneous transducers;
- receiving additional oxygen;
- with tracheostomy after the first 2 weeks;
- being given intravenous glucose and electrolyte solutions;
- who are being tube fed;
- who have had minor surgery in the previous 24 hours;
- who require terminal care, but not on the day of death;
- being barrier nursed;
- undergoing phototherapy;

**Table 5.1** Indications for admission to SCBU or Transitional Care Ward

---

(1) *All infants with the following problems*
- Gestation < 36 weeks
- Birthweight < 2200 g
- Major malformations
- Respiratory distress syndrome

  Tachypnoea ( > 70/min) ⎫ Any two at > 1 hour of age
  Grunting             ⎬ or any age if added oxygen is necessary
  Cyanosis           ⎪ to maintain $SaO_2 \geqslant 90\%$
  Recession ⎭

- Severe birth asphyxia
- Apgar store   < 3 at 1 min
                   < 5 at 5 min
- Symptomatic hypoglycaemia (see Chapter 16)
- Symptomatic polycythaemia
- Symptomatic anaemia

(2) *Most of the following infants will require careful observation and/or monitoring*
- Infants with meconium found below the cords
- Infants of narcotic-addicted mothers
- Infants born through offensive smelling liquor
- Rh isoimmunization

(3) *Some of the following infants will require 2- to 4-hourly review for 24 hours*
- Infants needing naloxone to reverse early respiratory depression
- Infants born after premature rupture of membranes (>24 hours) or maternal pyrexia during labour who are asymptomatic

---

- receiving special monitoring (e.g. frequent glucose or bilirubin estimations);
- needing constant supervision (e.g. babies whose mothers are drug addicts);
- being treated with antibiotics.

For indications for admission to Special Care Baby Units (SCBU) and Neonatal Intensive Care Units (NICU) see Tables 5.1 and 5.2.

## Recommended nursing staff

Most units in the UK have a mixture of Intensive Care and Special Care designated cots. Most infants requiring Special Care can be adequately cared for by their mothers on Transitional Care Wards provided that adequately trained staffing levels are maintained.

**Table 5.2** Indications for admission to NICU (or transfer to a hospital with NICU facilities) (see definitions of Level 1 and Level 2 Intensive Care)

Gestation < 32 weeks
Birthweight < 1500 g
Moderate or severe respiratory distress
  Apnoea
  $PaO_2$ < 50 mm Hg in 40% oxygen
  pH < 7.20
  $PaCO_2$ > 60 mm Hg
Complications of respiratory distress
  Shock
  Air leak
      Pneumothorax
      Pneumomediastinum
      Marked interstitial emphysema
Symptomatic meconium aspiration
  Meconium found below cords and infant needs > 40% oxygen to abolish
  cyanosis
Congenital heart disease
  Cyanosis       } in the neonatal period
  Cardiac failure
Major malformations, e.g.
  Diaphragmatic hernia
  Oesophageal atresia/tracheo-oesophageal fistula
  Exomphalos/gastroschisis
  Lobar emphysema
Hydrops fetalis or severe Rh isoimmunization
Convulsions
Bleeding problems
Major trauma

Although there have been recommendations for nurse staffing levels of 5.5 whole-time equivalent nurses per Intensive Care (IC) Level 1 cot, 3.5 whole-time equivalents per IC Level 2 cot, and 1 whole-time equivalent per Special Care cot, these figures do not accurately reflect staffing requirements, and evidence-based recommendations have superseded these (*Standards for hospitals providing neonatal intensive care*, British Association of Perinatal Medicine 1996).

## THERMAL CARE

Thermal care is a critical part of neonatal care, and the responsibility to maintain thermoregulation lies with both medical and nursing staff. The neutral thermal environment is defined as the ambient temperature range which leads to minimum $O_2$ consumption, that is, one in which the body temperature remains normal with the minimum metabolic effort (Fig. 5.1).

The stress associated with allowing an infant to cool is detrimental and can result in an increase in mortality and morbidity. Adverse effects of cold stress include:

- increased $O_2$ consumption and energy expenditure leading to
    hypoxia and acidosis,
    hypoglycaemia,
    increased early weight loss and later slow or delayed weight
    gain;
- pulmonary hypertension;
- increased capillary permeability;
- hypovolaemia and increased blood viscosity;
- general impairment of enzyme efficiency;
- decreased surfactant production.

Cold stress results in a reduction in $O_2$ delivery to vital organs, brain and the heart. Care should therefore be given in infants with

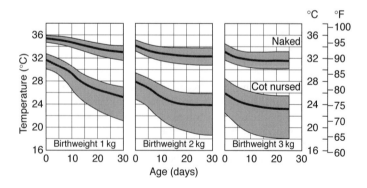

**Fig. 5.1** Neutral thermal ranges for infants of different birthweights and ages. (Reproduced from Hey (1971) *Recent Advances in Paediatrics*, with permission from Churchill Livingstone.)

cardiac or respiratory disease who may already have a compromised ability for $O_2$ delivery. If the oxygen requirement is above that which can be achieved (e.g. in cyanotic heart disease or severe lung disease) the inevitable consequence is progressive acidosis and death, unless the oxygen requirement can be reduced.

Preterm and sick infants have a reduced ability to control their body temperature for several reasons, and are at particular risk.

- The preterm infant (particularly if SGA – see below) has a high surface area to mass ratio, and little subcutaneous fat (which provides important insulation), and thus experiences greater heat loss through the skin than term babies.
- Evaporative losses through the skin of very preterm babies lead to rapid cooling (in effect, the skin is 'not waterproof').
- Small stores of fat (particularly brown fat) and glycogen may be rapidly depleted, with loss of the ability to increase heat generation when needed.
- Temperature regulation by the hypothalamus may be immature, leading to poor feedback mechanisms.

The newborn infant may lose heat in four ways:

**(1) Evaporation** Water is converted to vapour during perspiration and respiration using energy from heat in the superficial tissues; the low birth-weight infant has high transepidermal losses due to increased skin permeability.
*Prevention:*

- dry and wrap in warm towels immediately post-delivery;
- use hats and warm clothing if applicable;
- humidify incubators of babies < 1500 g and < 30 weeks' gestation;
- use incubators rather than cots with radiant heaters.

**(2) Convection** Heat is lost to the surrounding air.
*Prevention:*

- maintain room temperature;
- nurse out of draughts, away from cold air vents;
- nurse clothed rather than naked.

**(3) Conduction** Heat is lost through direct contact with cooler surfaces, e.g. X-ray plates, weighing scales.
*Prevention:*

- warm bedding;
- warm surfaces – cover X-ray plates;
- dress the infant.

*(4) Radiation* The infant radiates heat away from itself to nearby cooler surfaces.

*Prevention:*

- nurse away from windows and external doors;
- avoid direct sunlight;
- use silver swaddlers for transport of small infants;
- (NB do *not* use swaddler between baby and overhead radiant warmer, e.g. during resuscitation).

## ADMISSION TO THE NICU

*Try to give as much warning of potential admissions as possible, to facilitate preparation.*

### (1) Prepare equipment

Check:

- incubator is switched on and at the appropriate temperature within the neutral thermal environment for the anticipated admission;
- air and oxygen supply as appropriate;
- suction tubing and appropriate sized catheters are in working order and to hand;
- humidifier and headbox circuit;
- ventilator/CPAP driver in working order;
- monitors
    cardiorespiratory
    oxygen saturation/transcutaneous monitor
    temperature probes (core + peripheral)
    BP + appropriately sized cuff;
- resuscitation bag and mask;
- intravenous/arterial cannulation and infusion equipment;
- weighing scales – balanced and ready for use – include warm towels.

### (2) Admission procedure

All infants should be transferred in an appropriate transport incubator (see Chapter 6).

- Assess general condition and rectify any urgent problems (temperature, airway, breathing, circulation).

- Note time of admission and perinatal details.
- Weigh.
- Connect to ventilator/CPAP driver/headbox as appropriate.
- Connect to monitors.
- Record:
    axillary or core temperature – adjust incubator temperature accordingly;
    heart rate;
    respiratory rate and pattern.
- Check cord and clamp.
- Check capillary blood glucose.
- Pass gastric tube and aspirate stomach contents.
- Put bonnet and booties on baby as appropriate.
- Cover with bubble wrap if hypothermic or below 1500 g.
- Humidify incubator if < 30 weeks' gestation or < 1500 g.
- Ensure baby is appropriately labelled.
- Take Polaroid photograph for parents.
- Insert cannula as required.
- Give vitamin K.
- Head circumference is measured by Advanced Neonatal Nurse Practitioner (ANNP)/Senior House Officer (SHO) when initial examination is performed.
- Welcome parents, explain treatment, monitors and equipment; outline baby's care; give them NICU booklet and photograph.
- Ensure parents are spoken to by ANNP/medical staff.
- Complete notes, charts, record books, nursing care plans and any relevant audit forms.

## MONITORING

The type and complexity of monitoring used depends on the size, gestation and condition of the infant. Monitoring should not be unnecessarily obtrusive or prolonged beyond when it is needed, the aim being to identify predicted problems. The following are intended to serve as guidelines, and each infant's needs should be assessed individually.

### Temperature
Maintain peripheral (usually toe) temperature between 36°C and 36.5°C, and core (usually axillary) temperature between 36.5°C and 37.5°C, using a probe that is well insulated from the environment.

Peripheral skin temperature may fall before changes in the core temperature, and this may be associated with marked increases in oxygen consumption; significant cold stress may be present with a normal core temperature. Cold peripheries can be an early warning sign of hypovolaemia (due to shock, hypotension or infection) and, if indicated, colloid should be given. In preterm infants peripheral temperature is of more value as an early sign of hypovolaemia than of mild cold stress.

### Cardiorespiratory monitors

These should be used for all infants with significant respiratory distress, < 30 weeks' gestation and all acutely ill infants. For very small and ventilated infants with indwelling arterial lines, heart rate may be taken from the blood pressure trace, thereby avoiding the use of skin electrodes which may damage the skin (note that no respiratory monitoring is used).

Heart rate limits should normally be set at 90–100 (low alarm) and 160–180 (higher alarm), but this may vary according to individual circumstances.

*Apnoea alarms* (abdominal pressure sensors, e.g. Graseby, Densa) may be of value in older infants or in older preterm infants once the acute illness has settled. *Routine impedance respiratory monitoring* from the chest leads is preferable in acutely ill children.

The respiratory alarm delay should be set at 20 sec and the child should be observed to ensure that the monitor is triggered with every breath.

At low cardiac and respiratory rates the increased cardiac impulse may trigger the respiratory monitor, so both respiratory and cardiac alarms should be active.

### Blood pressure

Blood pressure should be monitored continuously in all sick infants by means of an indwelling arterial cannula/catheter. A damped trace will give inaccurate systolic and diastolic values, but the mean is usually accurate if there is a clear oscillation with each ECG impulse.

Non-invasive blood pressure monitoring should be monitored 2- to 6-hourly in all other sick infants, using an oscillometric device (manual or automatic with neonatal algorithms). Appropriate-sized cuffs should be used (i.e., cuff width approximately two-thirds length of upper arm); too large a cuff will give inappropriately low readings and too small a cuff will give too high readings. Blood pressure recordings are made when the infant is quiet, as crying increases the blood pressure (for normal values see Chapter 29).

### Blood glucose

Blood glucose should be measured 4- to 12-hourly in all high-risk infants and maintained between 2.5 and 7 mmol/L (see Chapter 16).

### Continuous measurement of blood gases

***Transcutaneous oxygen monitoring*** Provides invaluable information, especially over the first few days in sick ventilated infants, and remains the route of choice. $TcPO_2$ electrodes measure the oxygen tension of gas that has diffused from the arterialized capillary bed to the skin surface. $TcPO_2$ readings and arterial $PaO_2$ are known to correlate well at values below 90mm Hg (12 kPa), but above this level $TcPO_2$ is less reliable. $TcPO_2$ values are unreliable during periods of hypotension or hypoperfusion. The electrode must be resited every 4 hours, and leaves transient areas of erythema caused by the heating coil.

***Transcutaneous carbon dioxide monitoring*** May be possible in a combined $TcPO_2/TcPCO_2$ probe; recent models are much more reliable and may be calibrated against blood gas results. Diffused transcutaneous $CO_2$ is identified at lower temperatures compared to single oxygen probes, and provides a useful trend monitor for use during ventilation.

***Indwelling oxygen electrodes*** Remain the most accurate method of monitoring umbilical arterial oxygen tension, and are used during the early phase of intensive care, particularly for the very small infant.

***Oxygen saturation monitoring (pulse oxymetry)*** Is the most popular method of monitoring of oxygenation, being non-invasive and easy to apply (care should be taken not to apply the probe too tightly). Saturation monitoring may fail to identify significant hyperoxia, which is critical over the first few days in very preterm infants (see Fig. 10.1), hence transcutaneous monitoring is preferred. If $SaO_2$ is maintained at $< 92\%$, then significant hyperoxaemia is relatively unlikely, but arterial $PaO_2$ must be regularly measured as $SaO_2$ does not have a constant relationship to $PaO_2$. Pulse oxymetry is of value in long-term monitoring of oxygen therapy where the detection of hypoxia is relatively more important.

### Blood gases

These should be measured 4- to 6-hourly in infants during acute illness, preferably using arterial samples. Arterial gas tension should be correlated with monitoring values and adjustable monitors calibrated regularly. Capillary samples may be used to monitor trends in the infant without an indwelling arterial line but remember that, although arterialized capillary samples will give an accurate pH value, $PCO_2$ may be overestimated and $PO_2$ underestimated.

Any alteration in ventilation parameters should be followed after 20–30 min by a repeat blood gas evaluation unless continuous monitoring is being used.

### Oxygen concentration

This should be monitored continuously in all infants receiving additional oxygen and adjusted to keep the $PaO_2$ in the range 50–70 mm Hg (6.5–9.5 kPa) in the very preterm infant. Higher $PaO_2$ values (70–90 mm Hg; 9.5–12 kPa) would be accepted in term infants, particularly if there is pulmonary hypertension.

### Routine blood tests

On admission, haematological parameters should be measured. Thereafter, daily monitoring of electrolytes, creatinine and haematological parameters is useful until the infant is stable. Serum sodium is an excellent guide to hydration in the sick small infant over the first few days, and may be measured more frequently. Bilirubin should be measured if the infant appears jaundiced, and repeated as appropriate (see Chapter 18). Infants requiring parenteral nutrition will need further investigations (see Chapter 13).

### Weighing

Although weight is the ideal and best measure of fluid balance, it is not always practical. Sick infants should be weighed when appropriate and when care will not be compromised. An overhead warmer should be placed above the scales to minimize cold stress.

### Urine testing

Urine should be tested 2–4 times per day for the presence of blood, protein, glucose (dipstix and further clinitest if glucose is apparent), and its specific gravity measured regularly. A cotton-wool ball placed within the nappy will allow collection of adequate urine samples for these purposes.

Urine output should be monitored in all sick infants. It is usually adequate to calculate output from increases in nappy weight.

### Minimal handling

Sick babies tolerate handling poorly and may be stressed further by exposure to light and high sound levels. The environment within the NICU does not always lend itself to a reduction in these stressors.

Minor procedures will cause hypoxaemia; therefore use monitors to carry out observations and do not disturb the baby. Allow rest periods with no handling when possible, and keep painful procedures to a minimum, e.g. heel pricks, endotracheal and pharyngeal suction, X-rays.

Monitor the infant's condition throughout any procedure and stop if hypoxaemia, apnoea or bradycardia become apparent. Extraneous noise should be kept to a minimum:

- switch off alarms immediately;
- avoid slamming incubator doors and bin tops;
- avoid placing objects on the incubator top;
- respect the 'quiet periods' in your nursery;
- try not to disturb diurnal variations in lighting (dimmer switches are now widely available).

### Positioning

Developmental delay may occur if the baby is inappropriately positioned. Frequent changes of position of the infant's head, and improved management of nutrition and metabolic bone disease will help to reduce the once common flattened, elongated, asymmetrical head shape. The preterm infant lacks muscle tone and is therefore at risk of developing abnormal movement patterns and skeletal deformation. The following simple procedures will help to achieve normal posture in the preterm infant:

***Prone lying (in incubators)*** Encourage flexion and adduction of the hips and knees by placing a roll under the hips and, if necessary, under the feet. If the baby is hypotonic a 'U'-shaped folded sheet around the legs and feet will give extra support.

***Side lying*** Place a small nappy under the supporting hip, allowing the upper leg to rotate internally and lie on the mattress, thus rotating the pelvis slightly. The flexed side lying posture can be maintained by placing a folded sheet over the hips and knees, tucking it under the mattress to secure it.

***Supine lying*** Maintain the flexed adducted posture by placing a long roll on either side of the baby, plus a role under the knees to help to flex the hips.

***Wakeful playtime in the prone lying*** A small roll placed under the chest will encourage head lifting and forearm support. This is important at term as it encourages the baby's sequence of development.

## PREVENTION OF INFECTION

Unless there has been prolonged rupture of membranes or intra-uterine instrumentation, the infant is virtually clear of bacteria before delivery. Thereafter colonization occurs:

- during passage through the birth canal (mostly vaginal and perineal commensals or occasionally pathogenic organisms);
- by direct contact with the mother;
- from contact with hospital staff and equipment – this may be the major route following Caesarean delivery and immediate admission to an intensive care nursery.

### Staff and visitors

*Thorough hand washing is the single most important factor in prevention of cross-infection.* There is no evidence that routine use of gowns or masks reduces the risks of infection, or that contact with healthy adults or siblings increases it.

- Everyone should wash their hands and arms to the elbow before entering any nursery.
- Long sleeves should be rolled to the elbows before washing.
- Watches, bracelets, and rings other than simple wedding rings should be removed.
- After initial hand washing, hands may be disinfected before and after handling patients by the use of an alcohol-based rub (e.g. Hibisol). If hands become dirty or contaminated with blood, urine or faeces, they must be thoroughly washed as described above.
- Whilst handling an infant, care should be taken not to touch one's face, hair, nose or mouth – hand cleansing must be repeated if this occurs.
- Parents and staff with acute respiratory, gastrointestinal or wound infections, or with active herpes simplex infections should not be allowed to come into direct contact with babies.

### Equipment

- Use individual stethoscopes for each baby.
- Use disposables as far as possible (e.g. suction jars, ventilation tubing).
- Thoroughly clean and dry all equipment between babies (including incubators, ventilators, ultrasound probes).

**Babies**

- Use aseptic technique to care for all long lines.
- Keep sites of entry of all indwelling peripheral lines clean and dry – spray 12-hourly with 0.5% providine-iodine spray.
- Keep the umbilical cord stump clean and dry – use an alcohol preparation when needed, paying particular attention to the base.
- Dust skinfolds (axillae and groin) daily with 0.3% hexachlorophene powder.
- Isolate any infant with a potentially contagious infection (e.g. herpes).
- Take weekly swabs (nose, umbilicus and rectum) from babies on the intensive care nursery to monitor the pattern of colonization within the unit.

**The infant with a contagious infection**

- Isolate, where possible, in a single room.
- Keep the door closed.
- Wash hands thoroughly on entry to the room.
- Only place essential equipment in the cubicle.
- All equipment needed for the care of the child should be left inside the room, including charts, linen, etc.
- Notes and X-rays should be kept outside the room.
- Wash hands thoroughly after leaving the cubicle.
- Wash and disinfect equipment and instruments prior to and after removal from the cubicle.
- The nurse caring for the infant should have as few other assignments as possible.
- The parents of the isolated infant should be discouraged from visiting other babies on the unit.

Parents may find the isolation of their baby frightening and, as a result, feel isolated themselves. Staff need to support parents whilst also emphasizing the importance of prevention of cross-infection.

## THE SMALL-FOR-GESTATIONAL-AGE (SGA) INFANT

Traditionally defined as an infant whose birthweight falls below the 10th percentile for gestational age as a means of identifying children at risk of neonatal complications (see below). However, children with intrauterine growth restriction (IUGR) may have normal birth-weights, appear wasted (see Table 16.1) and be at similar risk. In contrast, many children who are SGA are small normal individuals (10% of the normal population, by definition). Serial antenatal measures are helpful for identifying fetuses with IUGR and those with worsening placental insufficiency (see Chapter 1). Where pre-term delivery is contemplated for deteriorating fetal condition, maternal steroids are indicated.

### Babies with IUGR may be:

**Symmetrically small** With low birthweight, length and head size for gestation, this suggests that there has been early onset of IUGR. Common causes include:

- early intrauterine infection, e.g. CMV, rubella, toxoplasmosis;
- severe placental insufficiency;
- chromosomal abnormalities (particularly in the presence of dysmorphism);
- severe maternal disease, e.g. renal disease, hypertension.

**Asymmetrically small** With low birthweight but relative sparing of length and head size, indicating less severe fetal malnutrition and onset of IUGR within the last few weeks of pregnancy. Causes include:

- placental insufficiency;
- pre-eclampsia;
- less severe maternal disease;
- smoking.

### Neonatal problems following IUGR

**Perinatal hypoxia** Relatively mild intrapartum asphyxia may be poorly tolerated because the low fat and glycogen stores restrict the ability to maintain anaerobic metabolism. Meconium aspiration is a particular risk (see Chapter 10).

**Hypoglycaemia** SGA infants have low glycogen stores due to de-creased availability of substrate *in utero*. Early feeding and monitor-ing are discussed in Chapter 13.

**Thermal care** The lack of subcutaneous fat (which serves both as an insulation and as an energy-source) makes SGA infants particularly vulnerable to cold stress, which may cause or exacerbate hypoglycaemia.

*Polycythaemia* Secondary to intrauterine hypoxia this may exacerbate respiratory problems and hypoglycaemia.

*Necrotizing enterocolitis* Children found to have placental insufficiency and abnormal umbilical artery Doppler studies may be at particular risk of developing NEC (see Chapter 13). There may be an advantage in delaying the commencement of enteral feeds in this group, although some sources suggest that early non-nutritive feeding may be of benefit.

*Outcome* Other perinatal problems relate to the gestational age of the infant rather than birthweight. Studies of SGA populations confirm that this is also true for long-term outcomes. Somatic growth may be impaired in symmetrically small infants, but lack of catch-up growth is difficult to predict on an individual basis.

## THE LARGE-FOR-GESTATIONAL-AGE INFANT

Infants whose birthweights lie above the 90th centile represent a particular risk group. Causes include:

- constitutional large size (top 10% of population – often familial);
- maternal diabetes – both gestational and insulin dependent;
- Beckwith-Wiedermann syndrome (see Chapter 8);
- hyperinsulism (see Chapter 16).

**Neonatal problems in the infant of a diabetic mother (see Chapter 1)**
Good diabetic control during pregnancy will reduce the risk of most neonatal problems, but has not been shown to reduce the risk of malformations.

*Hypoglycaemia* (see Chapter 16).

*Birth injury* (see Chapter 3).

*Respiratory distress syndrome (RDS)* The relative deficiency of phosphatidyl glycerol in the surfactant of infants of diabetic mothers predisposes to RDS, particularly after Caesarean section, even in relatively mature infants.

*Jaundice* (see Chapter 18).

*Hypocalcaemia* (see Chapter 16).

**Immaturity of sucking and swallowing** Even in mature infants, this may necessitate tube feeding (see Chapter 13).

**Polycythaemia** (see Chapter 19).

**Cardiovascular malformations** These are found in up to 5% of infants of diabetic mothers, particularly transposition of the great arteries, ventricular septal defects or co-arctation of the aorta.

**Cardiomyopathy** This is associated with maternal diabetes and may lead to congestive cardiac failure, with or without left ventricular outflow obstruction; echocardiogram shows marked thickening of the interventricular septum.

**Small left colon syndrome** This leads to temporary bowel obstruction (± meconium plug), possibly due to immaturity of the myenteric plexus. Clinical and radiological features are similar to those of Hirschsprung's disease (see Chapter 9), but it resolves spontaneously.

**Congenital malformations** These are found in up to 13% of infants of diabetic mothers, particularly neural tube defects, CVS anomalies (see above), vertebral, sacral and anorectal anomalies.

**Renal vein thrombosis** This is a rare complication in these children, and it may lead to transient or permanent renal impairment with haematuria (see Chapter 15).

## THE PRETERM INFANT

**Definition** Gestational age less than 37 completed weeks of gestation.
Common causes for preterm delivery include:

- intervention by the obstetrician in the interests of fetal or maternal health:
  maternal illness – pre-eclampsia, renal disease, malignancy;
  fetal compromise – fetal distress, growth retardation;
- ante-partum haemorrhage;
- cervical incompetence;
- spontaneous onset of preterm labour;
- uterine abnormalities.

**Problems of the preterm infant**

*Thermal care*

*Respiratory difficulties:*

- respiratory distress syndrome (see Chapter 10);
- apnoea (see Chapter 10);
- aspiration pneumonia – more likely to be due to immature pharyngeal co-ordination and protective reflexes.

*Retinopathy of prematurity* (see Chapter 20).

*Neurological problems:*

- immaturity of sucking and swallowing;
- immaturity of control of respiration leading to apnoea (see Chapter 10);
- periventricular haemorrhage and leucomalacia (see Chapter 12).

*Gastrointestinal problems:*

- reduced gut motility may cause abdominal distension, which may in turn compromise respiration;
- poor absorption of fat and thus fat-soluble vitamins;
- poor nutritional reserves (fat, glycogen, iron, fat-soluble vitamins) (see Chapter 13);
- risk of necrotizing enterocolitis (see Chapter 13).

*Jaundice* Hepatic immaturity leads to increased jaundice; immaturity of the blood–brain barrier may increase the risk of kernicterus at lower bilirubin levels than in term infants (see Chapter 18).

*Anaemia* (see Chapter 19).

*Renal problems* Lower glomerular filtration rate (GFR) and poor tubular function lead to an inability to excrete large water or solute load, and a poor ability to conserve water or sodium (see Chapter 15).

*Metabolic problems:*

- hypocalcaemia (see Chapter 16).
- hypoglycaemia (see Chapter 16).
- metabolic bone disease (see Chapter 13).

*Infections* The risk of infection is particularly high in infants of VLBW and/or gestation < 34 weeks; the most common pathogens include Group B streptococci, *Escherichia coli*, *Staphylococcus epidermidis*, *Pseudomonas aeruginosa* and *Serratia marcescens*.

**Patent ductus arteriosus** (see Chapter 11).

**Psychosocial problems** Consequent on the separation of the baby from his or her mother and father (see Chapter 23).

## NEONATAL ABSTINENCE SYNDROME

Addiction to any drug during pregnancy may lead to neglect of diet and self-care. The fetus will be at increased risk and may be growth retarded. In addition, there are a number of specific problems associated with particular drugs.

### Alcohol

Alcohol is best avoided in early pregnancy. Consuming an excess of alcohol during pregnancy may inconsistently result in fetal alcohol syndrome ($> 4$–$6$ units/day ; $40$–$60$ mg alcohol), often in association with binge drinking. Fetal alcohol syndrome comprises severe IUGR, learning difficulties and a characteristic facies (broad base to the nose, long upper lip and small lower jaw, epicanthic folds). Other effects (e.g. withdrawal) may occur with high intakes ($> 100$ mg alcohol/week), manifested as neonatal fits or irritability.

### Drug abuse

#### Cocaine

Cocaine or amphetamine use in pregnancy is associated with a high rate of placental haemorrhage and stillbirth, prematurity, IUGR, fetal distress and perinatal hypoxia. Cocaine is a sympathomimetic, with direct cardiovascular effects causing hypertension and vasoconstriction. Fetal effects may be mediated by placental vasoconstriction. Symptoms of withdrawal may be manifested as tremors, irritability, abnormal sleep patterns, and poor feeding for a few days. Microcephaly and cardiac malformations have been described in infants of cocaine-abusing mothers.

#### Opiates

Opiate addiction (usually heroin, morphine or methadone) has complex effects on the pregnancy and the baby.

*During pregnancy* Antenatal attendance may be haphazard, and there may be repeated maternal infections from the use of 'dirty' needles. Management is best achieved in conjunction with a specialist in drug abuse. Counselling and testing for viral infections should be considered. The advantages of switching to methadone must be weighed against the delayed and often prolonged withdrawal in the baby. If the woman and fetus can be adequately monitored, gradual withdrawal of the opiate during pregnancy may be successful.

*Following birth* The child may show signs of withdrawal within 24–48 hours, but these may be delayed for up to 14 days if the mother was using methadone. *Early signs* include irritability, high-pitched cry, sneezing, sweating and tachycardia with loose stools. *Later signs* are diarrhoea and vomiting, dehydration and seizures.

The baby should be nursed in a quiet environment and wrapped securely in blankets for comfort. Regular feeding and observation are necessary, but this can safely be carried out on the postnatal ward. If withdrawal is considered clinically significant, a single dose of oral morphine (25–50 mcg) may be all that is required to settle the child. Repeat doses are sometimes necessary. Seizures should be treated with intravenous morphine (10 mcg/kg) in the first instance and oral morphine (25–50 mcg/dose) continued on a 4-to 6-hourly basis for 24 hours, the dose and frequency gradually being reduced over the next few days.

The decision to facilitate breast feeding is a subject for individual assessment and planning, which will depend upon the lifestyle of and regular estimated dose used by the mother. This should be decided antenatally wherever possible. Note that excretion of drugs in breast milk is inconsistent and may lead to late withdrawal in the infant.

Babies of intravenous users should be immunized with hepatitis B vaccine, and BCG vaccine should be considered.

Such children are at high risk. One in 10 may die, and half will be the subject of care proceedings by the age of 2 years. Social support (where acceptable) and close community surveillance using a 'key worker' are mandatory if discharge home is planned.

### Withdrawal from other drugs
Withdrawal after exposure to other drugs of abuse (e.g. amphetamine) may present within the first 24 hours. Significant withdrawal symptoms may respond to chlorpromazine (1–3 mg/kg/day in four divided doses); seizures should be managed appropriately.

**Marijuana**
There is little evidence of harmful effects in pregnancy.

**LSD**
Reports of fetal abnormalities associated with its use in pregnancy may be related to contamination in illegally prepared LSD.

## Cigarette smoking

The risks of preterm delivery, IUGR and perinatal mortality are increased significantly (by about 30%). No anomalies have been associated with tobacco, but closure of the ductus arteriosis may be delayed. There is some evidence that the children of mothers who smoked during pregnancy are at greater risk from respiratory disease in the first years of life, even if mothers gave up smoking after pregnancy. Smoking 20 cigarettes per day during pregnancy increases the risk of cot death fourfold.

Every effort should be made to dissuade mothers from smoking.

## BIBLIOGRAPHY

British Association of Perinatal Medicine (1996) *Standards for hospitals providing neonatal intensive care.* London: British Association of Perinatal Medicine.

Pym, S. (1992) *Positioning the preterm infant.* Bristol Royal Hospital for Sick Children Pamphlet 1–2. Bristol: Bristol Royal Hospital for Sick Children.

Redshaw, M.E., Harris. A. and Ingram, J.C. (1994) *The neonatal unit as a working environment: a survey of neonatal nursing – executive summary.* London: HMSO.

World Health Organization (1993) *Thermal control of the newborn – a practical guide.* Geneva: World Health Organization.

Young, J. (1996) *Development care of the premature baby.* London: Ballière Tindall.

# Transport of the sick newborn infant

Organization of a neonatal transport service
Stabilization of the infant prior to transport
Care of the infant during transport
Transport of infants with special problems

The commonest reasons for transporting newborn infants are for management of the complications of preterm delivery or for surgical procedures. All hospitals where babies are delivered should have facilities for resuscitation of newborn infants and initial stabilization of those who are critically ill, including those born preterm. Avoidance of the need to transport critically ill infants may be achieved by arranging deliveries with known or foreseeable problems in a hospital with neonatal intensive care facilities, or by transfer of the mother with the fetus *in utero*. However, transport of mothers who are ill, bleeding or in preterm labour carries potential risks for the mother and infant, and should be avoided.

## ORGANIZATION OF A NEONATAL TRANSPORT SERVICE

### Communication

Requests for transfer of sick newborn infants should be made as early as possible in the infant's clinical course. Referring centres should have clear guidelines about whom to contact. This can be either:

- a regional 'Hot-Line' where the individual receiving the call will co-ordinate with all neonatal intensive care units in the region to identify an available cot; **OR**
- a clear roster of potentially available units with a contact number in each unit.

The individual accepting a request for transport should be in a position to:

- accept a transfer with knowledge of the local availability of intensive care cots;
- organize a transport team to collect the patient;
- give advice to local staff regarding care needed before the arrival of the transport team. This should include general advice regarding avoidance of thermal stress, hypoxaemia and hypoglycaemia, as well as specific advice relevant to the clinical condition of the infant or special problems;
- liaise with other medical staff, e.g. surgeons, regarding specific instructions prior to and during transport and organization of local facilities pending the infant's arrival.

It is desirable that the transport co-ordinator will have considerable experience of both neonatal intensive care *and* the problems of transport medicine and he or she is likely to be the most senior staff member available.

The doctor in the referring hospital should involve the baby's parents in the decision to transfer, and explain what is happening. Appropriate consent for proposed surgical procedures should be obtained and accompany the infant. Full documentation of the mother's and infant's case histories, together with radiographs and investigation results, should be available for the transport team.

A Transport Log should be kept by the receiving unit, and include:

1 demographic data regarding the infant, mother and referring physician;
2 operational data;

- *transport team personnel;*
- *times of receiving call, team departure, and arrival at referring hospital, stabilization time, departure from referring hospital and arrival at base;*

**3** clinical data

- *clinical history and examination;*
- *investigation results;*
- *procedures and medications at referring hospital;*
- *clinical condition during transport;*
- *adverse events;*
- *condition on arrival at base hospital.*

In addition to acting as a record of the transport, these data can be used for internal audit and quality assurance measures. All units which are regularly involved in the transport of sick infants should have a system of audit which includes regular assessment of the transport service.

## Personnel

Transport of sick, newborn infants is a hazardous procedure and should not be left to the most junior member of the team. The transport team should consist of:

- a transport co-ordinator (who may be either a senior doctor or nurse);
- a doctor who is experienced in neonatal intensive care and transport medicine;
- an experienced nurse.

Transport co-ordinators should have ultimate responsibility for the composition of the team. Neonatal nurse practitioners, with appropriate additional training in transport medicine, may take the place of doctors on some transport teams. If special problems are anticipated, the number of team members should be increased.

## Equipment

Transportation may take place by ground or air ambulance (either fixed or rotary wing aircraft). The mode of transport should be selected on the basis of clinical need and distance to be travelled. Except for very long distances, the disadvantages of air transport may outweigh its potential for speed.

All vehicles should have adequate space, including access for incubators and access to the infant during transport, environmental temperature control and safety equipment. Power sources should be compatible with the medical transport equipment carried by the team.

**Table 6.1** Necessary equipment for the transport of sick newborn infants

| | |
|---|---|
| *Transport incubator* | Internal and AC/DC power capability<br>Heater<br>Oxygen cylinder and air cylinder (or compressor)<br>Thermometer |
| *Transport ventilator* | Able to work on internal power supply and AC/DC supply<br>Compatible with portable gases/compressor and ambulance gas supply<br>Adjustable $FiO_2$ and integral $O_2$ analyser<br>Facilities for CPAP, IPPV, PEEP and IMV |
| *Monitors* | ECG monitor with leads<br>Thermometer (low reading) plus two thermocouple probes<br>Transcutaneous $PO_2$ (and spare membranes)<br>Pressure monitor and transducers<br>Non-invasive blood pressure monitor and cuffs<br>Stethoscopes |
| *Airway* | Self-inflating bag and masks (all sizes)<br>Endotracheal tubes (all sizes)<br>Two laryngoscopes plus spare bulbs/batteries<br>Magill forceps<br>Oxygen cylinders (take *three times* estimated requirement)<br>Suction catheters and portable suction device<br>Nasogastric tubes (all sizes)<br>Chest drains (all sizes)<br>Heimlich flutter valves for chest drains |
| *Circulation* | Intravenous syringe pumps (minimum of three)<br>i.v. catheters, tubing and connectors<br>i.v. solutions<br>Umbilical catheters<br>Central venous catheters<br>Needles/butterflies (all sizes)<br>Syringes (all sizes)<br>Three-way taps |
| *Other* | Sterile gloves, cleaning solutions<br>i.v. cut-down pack, suture materials<br>Lumbar puncture needles<br>Specimen containers (clotted blood, cultures, etc.)<br>Sterile water/saline<br>Adhesive tape, splints<br>Space blanket and spare blankets for incubator<br>Polaroid camera and spare film<br>Spare batteries<br>Travel sickness tablets for staff |

**Table 6.1** Continued

| Drugs | *Resuscitation drugs* |
|---|---|
| | Adrenaline 1:10 000 |
| | Calcium gluconate 10% solution |
| | Dextrose 10% solution (500 mL) |
| | Dextrose 50% |
| | Naloxone |
| | Phenobarbitone |
| | Phenytoin |
| | Dopamine |
| | Human albumin solution 4.5% |
| | Dried salt-poor albumin |
| | *Cardiovascular drugs* |
| | Digoxin |
| | Adenosine |
| | Lignocaine |
| | Dobutamine |
| | Frusemide |
| | Prostaglandin $E_2$ |
| | *Antibiotics* |
| | Penicillin G |
| | Gentamicin or netilmicin |
| | Cefotaxime |
| | Metronidazole |
| | *Sedatives/muscle relaxants* |
| | Morphine |
| | Midazolam |
| | Pancuronium |
| | Vecuronium |
| | *Others* |
| | Vitamin $K_1$ |
| | Heparinized saline (10 units/mL) |

Equipment should be selected on the basis of:

- portability;
- strength;
- self-contained power supply (with AC/DC compatibility);
- compatibility with other equipment and with transport vehicles' power and medical gas supplies;
- ability to be adequately secured in transit.

Equipment and drugs for transport teams should be kept in a state of readiness and should be regularly checked to ensure that electrical equipment is charged, gas supplies are adequate and drugs are not out of date. A comprehensive range of equipment and drugs should be taken to ensure that full intensive care is available to the infant during transport (Table 6.1). *Always prepare for the worst-case scenario!*

## STABILIZATION OF THE INFANT PRIOR TO TRANSPORT

There is no place in neonatal transport medicine for the '*swoop-and-scoop*' philosophy. Every effort should be made to ensure that an infant is properly stabilized before transport. This may involve the transport team at the referring hospital for up to several hours. The aim should be to deliver the infant to the intensive care unit in optimal condition, and to avoid equipment failure and physiological deterioration during transport. The commonest preventable events during transport are endotracheal tube dislodgement/blockage and loss of intravenous access.

### Respiratory care

- Anticipate physiological deterioration during transport. All infants with significant respiratory distress should be intubated before transport with a securely fixed tube (never leave an endotracheal tube open to the atmosphere; connect to CPAP $\geq 3$ cm $H_2O$ or IPPV with PEEP $\geq 2$ cm $H_2O$).
- Check for pneumothoraces. If present, insert intercostal chest tube and connect to Heimlich 'flutter' valve.
- Give adequate oxygen and respiratory support to prevent cyanosis. If possible check blood gases and, if necessary, CXR, before transport.

### Blood pressure

- If blood pressure is low (see Chapter 29) or falls during stabilization, give plasma or human albumin solution 10–15 mL/kg i.v., over 30 min to 1 hour.
- Consider use of invasive BP monitoring and inotropes (see Chapter 10) during transport.

**Thermal care**

- If rectal temperature is below 36°C then rewarm the baby rapidly before transport (check blood pressure frequently during rewarming).

**Blood sugar**

- Check heel-prick blood sugar (Dextrostix or BM stix). Commence i.v. infusion of 10–15% dextrose solution at 80–100 mL/kg/day (to give 6–10 mg/kg/min dextrose).
- Maintain infusion with syringe driver during transport.

**Empty the stomach**

- Aspiration of gastric contents is a major risk, especially after bag–and–mask resuscitation.
- Leave an open gastric tube in place for transport.

## CARE OF THE INFANT DURING TRANSPORT

Travel back to the referral unit should be smooth rather than rapid. Anticipate problems in advance (e.g. major road-works, rush hour) and request police assistance.

If major physiological deterioration occurs, be prepared to *stop* the ambulance and assess the situation. *Never* attempt major procedures such as re-intubation in a moving road vehicle.

**Thermal care**

- Minimize transfer times between hospital buildings and transport vehicle.
- Keep ambulance warm (25°C) and minimize draughts.
- Wrap baby in silver swaddler ('space blanket'), bubble plastic or cling film, and cover with a blanket.
- Avoid opening the incubator if possible, and maintain incubator temperature in the thermoneutral range (see Fig. 5.1).

**Monitor**

- Skin and axillary or rectal temperature.
- ECG.
- $FiO_2$.
- Transcutaneous $PO_2$/saturation.
- Respiration.

- Ensure adequate lighting to observe colour changes and respiratory movements of the infant.

## TRANSPORT OF INFANTS WITH SPECIAL PROBLEMS

### Gastroschisis or omphalocoele

- Minimize evaporative heat and water loss by placing the whole trunk and legs (up to axillae) in plastic bag.
- Give intravenous fluids (100–150 mL/kg/day) and colloids (plasma or human albumin solution) (see Chapter 9).

### Oesophageal atresia/tracheo-oesophageal fistula

- Nurse flat or head-up.
- Keep upper oesophagus clear by frequent suction of indwelling tube (see Chapter 9).

### Diaphragmatic hernia

- Intubate and transport on IPPV.
- Use muscle relaxants and sedation (morphine 0.05–0.1 mg/kg i.v. ± pancuronium 0.1 mg/kg i.v.) (see Table 6.2).
- Keep stomach empty by very frequent aspiration of nasogastric tube (see Chapter 9).

### Convulsions

- Check capillary blood glucose and CSF microscopy before transport.
- Treat with i.v. phenobarbitone 10–20 mg/kg.

**Table 6.2** Sedation for airway management and transport of infants (see Chapter 28)

| | |
|---|---|
| Morphine | 0.05–0.1 mg/kg i.v. or s.c.<br>Infusion 5–20 mcg/kg/hour |
| Midazolam | 150 mcg/kg i.v.<br>Infusion 60 mcg/kg/hour |
| Pancuronium | 0.1 mg/kg, i.v. bolus (may be repeated) |
| Vecuronium | 0.1 mg/kg, i.v.<br>Infusion 50–150 mcg/kg/hour |

## BIBLIOGRAPHY

Harding, J.E. and Horton, S.M. (1993) Adverse effects of neonatal transport between level III centres. *J. Paediatr. Child Health* **29**, 146–9.

Kitchen, W.H., Callanan, C., Doyle, L.W. *et al.* (1993) Improving the quality of survival for infants of birthweight < 1000 g born in non-level-III centres in Victoria. *Med. J. Aust.* **158**, 24–7.

Leslie, A.J. and Stephenson, T.J. (1994) Audit of neonatal intensive care transport. *Arch. Dis. Child.* **71**, F61–F66.

Medical Devices Agency (1995) *Transport of neonates in ambulances.* London: Medical Devices Agency.

Pon, S. and Notterman, D.A. (1993) The organization of a pediatric critical care transport program. *Pediatr. Clin. North Am.* **40**, 41–61.

# Congenital abnormalities

## INTRODUCTION

### Definitions

**Birth defect** Some imperfection, impairment or disorder of the body, intellect or personality present or arising at birth.

**Congenital anomaly** A morphological defect present at birth (and included in the chapter on congenital anomalies in the *International Classification of Disease*, (World Health Organization, 1992).

**Congenital malformation** A primary error in morphogenesis arising during the embryonic period of prenatal life.

**Congenital deformation** An alteration in the morphology of a previously normally formed part of the body arising during the fetal period.

### Incidence

This varies between different geographical areas and populations but, on average, approximately 5% of infants are found to have a congenital anomaly at birth, in the proportion of three malformed infants to two with deformation.

## Examination

Because of the high incidence of anomalies, all infants should be examined carefully using the usual methods of inspection, palpation, percussion, auscultation and manipulation (e.g. the hips). Clinical examination may be supplemented when appropriate by transillumination, ultrasound, radiological examination, chromosome analysis, and other haematological and biochemical investigations.

## Malformations

Certain history factors are associated with an increased likelihood of congenital malformation, and may help to elucidate aetiology:

- family history of genetically determined malformation;
- previous sibling malformed;
- high maternal age;
- pregnancy exposure to radiation, infection (e.g. rubella) or drugs;
- polyhydramnios or oligohydramnios;
- intrauterine growth retardation of the fetus;
- prenatal suspicion of malformation (e.g. high maternal serum AFP or ultrasound examination);
- malpresentation of the fetus;
- multiple pregnancy.

**Table 7.1** Some contrasting characteristics of congenital malformations and congenital postural deformities

|  | **Malformation** | **Deformation (postural)** |
| --- | --- | --- |
| Incidence before 20th week | Approximately 5.0% | 0.1% |
| Incidence after 28th week | Approximately 3.7% | 2.0% |
| Perinatal mortality | 41/1000 | 6/1000 |
| Structural changes | Usual | Rare |
| Spontaneous correction | Very rare | Usual |
| Correction by posture | Not possible | Usually possible |

After birth, suspicion of malformation is increased in the following circumstances:

- small-for-dates infant;
- presence of any other anomaly, including:
  - single umbilical artery (present in 1% of all babies; 4% of live-born babies have associated anomalies, but this figure increases to 20% if stillbirths are included);
  - single palmar crease (one-fifth have associated anomaly);
  - unusual facies.

## Deformations

The great majority of congenital deformations affect the musculoskeletal system and are referred to as 'congenital postural deformities'. Their incidence is increased by the following factors:

| | |
|---|---|
| First pregnancies | Maternal hypertension |
| Maternal uterine anomaly | Oligohydramnios |
| Breech presentation | Intrauterine growth retardation |
| Multiple pregnancy | |

If one deformity is present, then a most careful search should be made for others, as multiple deformities are present in a third of cases.

Deformations may also occur secondary to certain malformations, especially those that cause oligohydramnios (such as those involving the urinary tract), or those that involve the neuromuscular system (e.g. myotonia dystrophia or spina bifida).

Some of the characteristics of malformations and deformations are contrasted in Table 7.1.

## Photographic record

It is important that all congenital anomalies are well documented. Those of any significance that are visible should be photographed. This is particularly important in cases where therapy will alter appearance (as in cleft lip or talipes), or when the infant is likely to die. Apart from the medical and legal reasons for having a photographic record, parents often wish to have a photograph to keep themselves, even when the child may appear most unattractive to others.

# MALFORMATIONS

## Congenital anomalies of the skin (see also Chapter 21)

### Haemangiomata

*Naevus flammeus ('stork mark')* Fine non-raised capillary naevus, usually in midline (upper lip, forehead-upper nose, nape of neck) that tends to fade in the early months of life. No treatment is required.

*Port wine stain* Darker capillary naevus that persists and may be cosmetically disfiguring, especially on the face. When the naevus is over the distribution of the trigeminal nerve, there may be an associated intracranial haemangioma which may give rise to cerebral complications (Sturge-Weber syndrome).

*Cavernous haemangioma* Raised naevus that may extend into the subcutaneous tissues. They may be present at birth or appear as small bright red spots after 1–2 weeks ('strawberry naevi'). They often enlarge for weeks or months and then regress spontaneously. Usually they disappear within a few years. No treatment is required unless they are very large, and associated with thrombocytopenia (see Chapter 19) or on the face, leading to complications such as occlusion of an eye. In such cases a short course of high-dose prednisolone may be effective in shrinking the lesion. Recently, laser ablation has been used to reduce the size of facial lesions and α-interferon has been used for larger lesions associated with thrombocytopenia.

### Pigmented naevus
Small congenital pigmented naevi require no treatment. Large hairy 'bathing-trunk' or 'forequarter' naevi have a risk of later malignancy and may require plastic surgery.

### Epidermal naevus
A velvety or warty change, pink or yellowish brown in colour, which may be localized or extensive. Whorled and linear patterns occur. When widespread there can be associated skeletal and CNS abnormalities.

### Sebaceous naevus
Pinkish-yellow or orange plaques, usually on the scalp or hair margin. They may evolve into basal cell carcinoma later in life, and so should be removed during childhood.

### Aplasia cutis

A localized absence of skin, most commonly on the scalp, presenting as a glistening red area. Most heal spontaneously, leaving a bald patch. Injury from a fetal scalp electrode and epidermolysis bullosa are differential diagnoses. Also seen in trisomy 13.

### Cystic hygroma

These cystic lymphangiomas are usually located in the neck (where they may rarely cause respiratory embarrassment) or axilla. They transilluminate well and may grow slowly or rapidly. Treatment is usually surgical.

### Dermal sinuses

These may be found most commonly in the sacral area (pilonidal sinus), on the side of the front of the neck (branchial sinus), or in front of the ear (pre-auricular sinus). The main complication is infection. Treatment, when indicated, is by surgical excision. NB Sacral sinuses may rarely communicate with the spinal canal; an ultrasound scan is helpful in making this diagnosis.

## Anomalies of the face

### Craniostenosis

Premature closure of one or more of the cranial sutures may give rise to a variety of cranial and facial deformities, since growth is arrested in a direction perpendicular to the affected suture. The incidence is about 1 in 5000. Associated anomalies may occur, giving rise to a variety of syndromes that may be genetically determined (e.g. Crouzon, Apert, Carpenter). The diagnosis may be confirmed radiologically. Surgical treatment is usually necessary, and urgent neurosurgical opinion should be requested, as the best results are obtained from early operation (usually by 3 months of age).

### Choanal atresia

This is due to a bony or membranous obstruction between the nasal cavity and the nasopharynx. It may be unilateral or bilateral. As most newborn infants are obligatory nose breathers in the early weeks of life, the clinical presentation is that of airway obstruction and cyanosis that is relieved by crying or opening of the mouth. The diagnosis is confirmed by failing to pass a nasal catheter, or by X-ray. Initial treatment consists of inserting an oral airway. This is followed by early surgical correction. The incidence is about 1 in 10 000.

### Anomalies of the ears

Ensure the patency of the auditory meatus. If this is absent, CT or MRI scans of the middle and inner ear should be undertaken, with auditory evoked responses. An ENT opinion should be sought. Accessory auricles require surgical removal.

### Anomalies of the eyes (Chapter 20)

If microphthalmia, coloboma, glaucoma, corneal opacities, cataract, or strabismus are present, it is essential to examine the retina. Aetiology includes chromosomal and genetic factors, prenatal infection (Chapter 17) and inborn errors of metabolism (Chapter 16). An ophthalmic opinion should be sought.

### Macroglossia

Congenital macroglossia may occur in association with Down's syndrome, hypothyroidism, or as part of the Beckwith-Wiedemann syndrome (which typically includes associated omphalocele, gigantism and hypoglycaemia). It may also be due to haemangiomatous or lymphangiomatous infiltration, or simply due to muscle-fibre hypertrophy. The size of the tongue may interfere with feeding and require surgical recession for this or for cosmetic reasons.

### Tongue tie

This is caused by a congenitally short frenulum extending to the tip of the tongue, binding it to the floor of the mouth, and interfering with normal sustained sucking (and later speech). The tongue presents a V-shaped conformation. The incidence is about 1 in 1000. Surgical treatment may be necessary.

### Ranula

This is a mucus gland retention cyst under the tongue. It has a bluish appearance. Often it will rupture and disappear spontaneously. Surgical resection may rarely be necessary. The incidence is about 1 in 5000.

### Congenital teeth

Teeth, usually lower incisors, may be present at birth. The incidence is 1 in 2000. If they are supernumerary or very loose, they should be removed to avoid possible inhalation.

## Cleft lip and cleft palate

Cleft lip may be unilateral or bilateral, occur on its own or, more usually, in association with cleft palate. The incidence is approximately 1 in 1000 births. Other malformations may be present in 1 in

7 cases. There may be a family history, in which case the chance of recurrence may be increased to about 1 in 20. Because the appearance may be very unattractive, it is important to show the parents 'before' and 'after' photographs of similar babies who have undergone repair. Early management should include plastic surgical/orthodontic collaboration. The malformation should be photographed and 'dental' impressions made. A plate may be fitted in cases of cleft palate. If breast or bottle feeding is difficult, a long, soft teat with a large hole may be used, or alternatively spoon or tube feeding may be undertaken. Early complications include middle-ear infections and aspiration pneumonia. Late complications include middle-ear hearing problems, speech difficulty and orthodontic problems. Repair of the lip is usually undertaken by 3 months and repair of the palate at 6 months so as to complete surgery before speech develops. Multidisciplinary follow-up, including plastic surgery, speech therapy, orthodontic and hearing assessment, needs to be continued throughout childhood.

### Pierre Robin anomalad

The combination of retrognathia, glossoptosis and respiratory difficulty, with or without midline posterior cleft palate, is known as the Pierre Robin anomalad. The incidence is about 1 in 3000. There is evidence to suggest that the retrognathia may be due to acute flexion of the head and chin on to the front of the chest in early fetal life. This leads to backwards and upwards displacement of the tongue, which may impede fusion of the lateral palatal arches. The condition is not infrequently found in association with other congenital anomalies, especially of the heart. In general, the complications and management are similar to that for cleft palate. The main specific problem is that of respiratory-tract obstruction by the tongue. It is essential to ensure a clear airway by nursing the infant prone or, if necessary, by using a nasopharyngeal airway or other device. Pulse oxymetry may be valuable. Occasionally endotracheal intubation is required. The retrognathia tends to disappear over the first 2–3 years.

## Anomalies of the gastrointestinal tract (see Chapter 9)

## Anomalies of the CNS (see Chapter 12)

## Anomalies of the CVS (see Chapter 11)

## Anomalies of the respiratory system (see Chapter 10)

## Anomalies associated with chronic fetal infection
(see Chapter 17)

## Urogenital tract anomalies (see Chapter 15)

### Potter's syndrome
This syndrome is caused by oligohydramnios due to fetal anuria or oliguria (due to renal agenesis or malformation, or to obstructive uropathy), or may occur after prolonged leakage of amniotic fluid (see below). The incidence is around 1 in 2000 births, and usually involves male infants. The baby has a compressed appearance, with multiple postural deformities affecting all parts of the body, and a typical facies including a squashed nose, pouches under the eyes and low-set abnormal ears flattened against the side of the head. Amnion nodosum may be found on the fetal surface of the placenta. Resuscitation problems and respiratory insufficiency due to pulmonary hypoplasia and secondary pneumothorax are the rule and usually lead to death within hours of birth. Genetic advice varies according to the cause of oligohydramnios.

### Warning
When the syndrome follows premature rupture of the membranes and prolonged leakage of amniotic fluid, the urinary tract is normal and such infants may be potentially viable (see Chapter 1).

### Hypospadias (see Chapter 15)

### Ambiguous genitalia (see Chapter 16)

### Epispadias (see Chapter 15)

### Imperforate hymen
This may be readily diagnosed at birth if, on examination, the labia are separated. Hormone-induced secretions cause the hymen to bulge outwards. The condition should be differentiated from the more common mucus-retention cysts. These are rounded and white and usually more laterally placed. They disappear after spontaneous or artificial rupture. Occasionally, an imperforate hymen may lead to congenital hydrometrocolpos, with enormous distension of the uterus by retained secretions. Treatment is surgical.

### Cryptorchidism (see Chapter 15)

### Hydrocele
This is not a congenital anomaly, but will be discussed briefly here. Usually hydroceles are bilateral, of little significance unless associated

with inguinal herniae, and disappear spontaneously over a period of weeks or months. Occasionally they may form part of a more general condition such as hydrops fetalis, or Milroy's oedema. If unilateral, consider associated pathology such as torsion of the testis. If the hydrocele is very large, tense and persistent, a surgical opinion should be sought.

**Inguinal hernia** (see Chapter 9)

## Malformations of the musculoskeletal system

### Limb malformations

The limb(s) may be absent ('amelia'), hypoplastic, or show various deficiencies affecting the proximal segment of the limb ('phoco-melia'), the distal segment ('hemimelia'), or a lateral segment (e.g. radial hypoplasia). The latter may be associated with thrombocyto-penia. Management usually includes orthopaedic or plastic surgery, and may require the fitting of prostheses. Photographic and radio-logical records should be made.

### Malformation of the digits

Extra digits (polydactyly) are especially common among Afro-Caribbean babies (dominant inheritance). Usually a tiny finger is attached to the ulnar side of the hand by a fine pedicle. It should be removed surgically. Fused digits (syndactyly) may require plastic surgery and may be associated with other malformations (e.g. Apert's syndrome: cranio-synostosis and syndactyly).

### Arthrogryposis multiplex congenita

This condition of multiple contractures of the joints may be due to primary disease of the neuromuscular system, or to severe prolonged prenatal constraint or paralysis of the fetus. In the former case there is usually a history of polyhydramnios and the prognosis is poor. When the cause is oligohydramnios due to premature rupture of the membranes or to other non-renal causes, steady improvement may occur. Management usually involves orthopaedic surgery and physio-therapy. The incidence is about 1 in 5000.

### Small stature or dwarfism

This may be 'constitutional'. The infant is normally formed but of small size and grows more slowly than normal. Some cases are associated with severe, prolonged intrauterine growth retardation. A second group is made up of the *primordial* dwarfs, of which there are a great variety, including the Russel-Silver, Cornelia de Lange,

Seckel's bird-head dwarf, etc. There is no special shortening of the limbs. The third group consists of the *chondrodystrophic* dwarfs, who have disproportionately short limbs. The most common subgroups are achondroplasia, thanatophoric dwarfism and osteogenesis imperfecta. Late pregnancy in this group is often complicated by polyhydramnios. For further details concerning the latter two groups, consult Jones (1997).

## Chromosomal syndromes

Perhaps 1 in 300 liveborn infants has a chromosomal anomaly. Only four of the most common syndromes will be considered here (see Chapter 8 on Clinical Genetics).

### Trisomy 21 (Down's syndrome)
The incidence rises from 1 in 1500 among young mothers to 1 in 110 at 40 years. The overall incidence is 1 in 650.

*Features* include small-for-dates, characteristic facies with upward slanting eyes, Brushfield's spots, small ears, protruding tongue, flat occiput, open third fontanelle, general hypotonia, stubby hands with short incurving fifth finger, single palmar creases, distal palmar triradius, gap between first and second toes, congenital heart disease (50%) and duodenal atresia (10%). Mental development is delayed. Infants prone to infection. Longevity depends on associated malformations.

Ninety-five per cent are due to non-dysjunction (low recurrence) and 5% are due to translocation (high recurrence). Clinical diagnosis should be confirmed with urgent chromosome studies. Management of parents (breaking news and support) demands great skill and sensitivity. Families need continued support (see Chapter 23).

### Trisomy 18 (Edward's syndrome)
The incidence is 1 in 8000.

*Features* include small-for-dates, prominent occiput, narrow bi-frontal diameter, microcephaly, metopic suture, low-set malformed auricles, short palpebral fissures, small mouth, narrow palatal arch, micrognathia, clenched hands with inner fingers overlapped by outer ones, short hallux, rocker-bottom feet, hypertonia, congenital heart disease, cryptorchidism, renal and many other malformations, single umbilical artery and mental retardation. Almost all die soon after birth.

### Trisomy 13–15 (Patau's syndrome)
The incidence is 1 in 14 000.

*Features* include small-for-dates, large 'onion' nose, cleft lip/palate, microphthalmia, colobomata, abnormal ears, capillary haemangiomata, scalp skin defects, microcephaly, polydactyly, cryptorchidism, single umbilical artery, congenital heart disease and severe mental retardation. Almost all die in the neonatal period.

### XO syndrome (Turner's syndrome)
The incidence is 1 in 2500 girls.

*Features* include small-for-dates, 'shield-like' chest, webbed neck, cubitus valgus, lymphoedema of feet and coarctation of the aorta. Survival is normal except when there are severe associated anomalies. Intelligence is usually normal.

## DEFORMATIONS

The various congenital postural deformities are listed in Table 7.2. Only a few of the main ones will be considered here. Their

**Table 7.2** Musculoskeletal deformations of mechanical origin present at birth

| Site | Deformation |
| --- | --- |
| Skull | Dolichocephaly; plagiocephaly; depressions in skull |
| Face | Potter's facies; nasal and oral deformities; mandibular asymmetry; retrognathia; midline cleft palate; facial-nerve neurapraxia |
| Neck | Sternomastoid contracture, 'tumour' and torticollis |
| Upper limbs | Dislocation of the shoulder; club-hand; compressed arm and hand (in Potter's syndrome); radial-nerve neurapraxia |
| Body | Pigeon chest; pectus excavatum; postural scoliosis |
| Lower limbs | Dislocation of the hips; bowing of the long bones; genu recurvatum; various deformities of the feet includiing talipes equinovarus, calcaneovalgus, and metatarsus varus; sciatic and obturator-nerve neurapraxias |
| Whole body | Arthrogryposis multiplex congenita, general body compression (as in Potter's syndrome) |

*Note:* Not all cases of some of the conditions noted here are due to mechanical factors (e.g. cleft palate and arthrogryposis).

importance stems from the fact that they are common and, with early treatment, they are usually easily correctable, because growth is proceeding rapidly and the tissues are still relatively plastic.

## Congenital sternomastoid torticollis

This occurs in approximately 1 in 300 births. The condition is unilateral. Often there is associated plagiocephaly, and the jaw is tilted away from the affected side. Contracture of the sternomastoid is present at birth and may be demonstrated by turning the chin towards the shoulder on the affected side. Normally the head may be rotated so that the chin points over the back of the shoulder. When significant contracture is present the chin will not turn as far as the front of the shoulder. As granulation forms in the damaged muscle, a tumour develops. This is usually first palpable at about 2 weeks of age. As stretching of the damaged muscle is painful and may cause further haemorrhage, treatment, by passive gentle stretchings which the mother may be taught, should not be commenced until 6 weeks of age. Very occasionally a tenotomy and neck collar may be required later in the first 1–2 years.

## Congenital postural scoliosis

The incidence is approximately 1 in 1000 births. There is a single, gentle curve, which is not to be confused with the usually more angular scoliosis due to malformation of the spine. If the spine is not examined routinely for lateral flexion, the condition is easily missed until the infant sits. Examination is best carried out by lifting the laterally lying infant from the bed with a hand under the baby's side just under the rib-cage. This is then repeated on the other side. In suspected cases an X-ray should be taken in full lateral flexion to the right and to the left. Nurse prone. Orthopaedic advice and careful follow-up are required.

## Congenital dislocation of the hip (CDH)

Approximately 1.5% of all newborn infants have either dislocation of the hip (10%) or dislocatable hips (90%) at birth. While many of these hips will stabilize without treatment, some will not, and others may destabilize or become dysplastic later in infancy. Early diagnosis and treatment of all cases offers the most satisfactory outcome. Therefore it is most important that the hips are examined on the first day of life and again before discharge from hospital (or on the 10th day). Thereafter, the hips should be carefully examined at 6–12 weeks and at regular intervals until the child has a stable gait at 18–24 months. Examination should be carefully documented. If the initial screening for CDH is being undertaken by a relatively inexperienced examiner, it is essential that suspect hips be checked again on the same day by a more experienced colleague. Note that CDH is four times more common in girls than in boys, and 10 times more common in association with breech presentation. Examination should also be particularly careful if there is a family history of CDH, or if other deformities such as talipes are apparent.

### Examination

This should be gentle. The baby is placed supine with its legs towards the examiner.

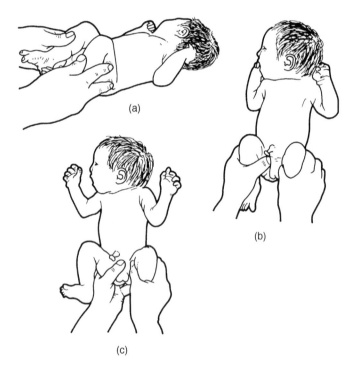

**Fig. 7.1** Examination for CDH (see text).

*First*, examine for asymmetry, wide spacing of the thighs, and limited abduction of the hips. These signs are rare at birth, but are increasingly common after the first 2–3 months.

*Secondly*, manipulate the hips to determine whether they are unstable using Ortolani and Barlow's manoeuvres as follows. The examiner grasps the baby's legs as shows in Fig. 7.1a, placing the middle finger of each hand over the greater trochanter; the flexed leg is contained in the palm of the hand, with the thumb on the inner side of the thigh opposite the lesser trochanter (Fig. 7.1b). Alternatively, the pelvis may be held and steadied by one hand, while the other hand manipulates one hip at a time (Fig. 7.1c). With the thighs in flexion and slight abduction an attempt is now made to move each femoral head in turn gently forward into or backwards out of the acetabulum. If the head of the femur is *dislocated*, then it may be felt to reduce forwards into the joint with anteriorly directed pressure. If, on applying backwards pressure, the hip is felt to displace out of the acetabulum but returns spontaneously when the pressure is released, then it is *dislocatable*. These movements are of the order of 0.5 cm in extent and are termed 'clunks'. Ligamentous 'clicks' *without* movement out of or into the acetabulum may be elicited in 5–10% of hip joints, and are usually of no significance. Experience in hip examination may be acquired through use of a teaching simulator such as the 'Baby Hippy' produced by Medical Plastics Laboratory (PO Box 38, Gatesville, Texas 76528, USA).

### Ultrasound

Static and dynamic ultrasound examination of the hips offers a useful adjunct to diagnosis and follow-up surveillance during the first 6 months. It may also be used for back-up screening of infants at high risk of CDH. With further experience it may prove safe to observe without splinting a proportion of newborn infants with hip instability whose static ultrasound morphology falls within normal limits. Radiological examination is of limited value in the first 3 months of life, but then becomes progressively more useful.

### Management

*Dislocatable* hips usually become stable after 6 weeks' treatment in a plastic over-nappy abduction splint (the Aberdeen splint), which may be removed by the mother when changing the nappies (Fig.7.2a). If the hip is still unstable at 6 weeks, continue treatment until 12 weeks.

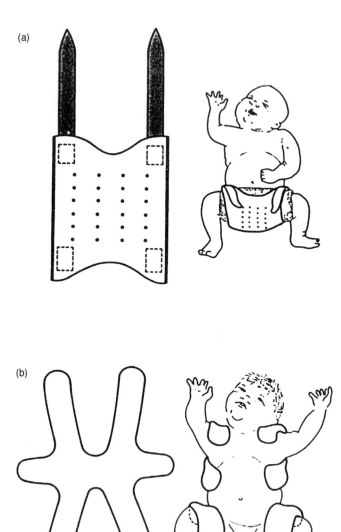

**Fig. 7.2** (a) The Aberdeen splint. (b) The von Rosen splint (see text).

*Dislocated* hips should be treated for 6 weeks in a metal abduction splint such as a von Rosen splint (Fig. 7.2b), followed by a similar period in an Aberdeen splint. Pressure should never be used to achieve abduction because tension of the adductor muscle may lead to ischaemic necrosis of the femoral head. Abduction should not exceed 80°. If there is a limitation of abduction, seek orthopaedic advice. If the hip is still unstable at 3 months, X-ray (single adducted A-P film of hips) and seek orthopaedic advice. All cases should be followed up with clinical and radiological examination at 6 months and 1 year. Occasional cases will require a longer period of surveillance.

### Informing the parents

Explain that the hip joint is lax because the baby has been tightly curled up in the womb, and the ligaments have been softened by pregnancy hormones. Explain that this is quite a common finding, that the baby is *not* abnormally formed in any way, is not in pain, and that, with early treatment with the legs kept wide for a few weeks, full recovery is the rule; and that there will be no reason why the child should not be an athlete in due course. It is essential to ensure that the parents are not unnecessarily worried or distressed, and also that they know how to handle the baby and splint.

## Congenital talipes

Deformities of the feet affect approximately 1 in 250 babies. The commonest variety is *talipes calcaneovalgus*, which is not uncommonly associated with CDH. Next comes *talipes equinovarus* or 'club-foot', followed by *metatarsus varus*. (This last deformity may also be acquired during the early weeks of life if the infant is nursed prone with the weight of the leg resting on the forefoot. This must be avoided, as the deformity is often difficult to treat and tends to give rise to problems when shoes are worn.) If the deformity is mild, the infant can move his or her foot into the neutral position, and the deformity can be over-corrected by gentle manipulation; treatment is then unlikely to be required. In more serious cases treatment should be instituted *at once*. This may range from passive exercises, to strapping or splinting in over-correction, to the need for surgical correction. All severe cases should be photographed and referred *at once* to an orthopaedic surgeon, as the ligaments of the feet tend to tighten up within a day or two of birth, making correction more difficult.

## Neurapraxias

These are temporary lower motor neurone paralyses due to pressure on a peripheral nerve *in utero* (in contrast to trauma as in Erb's palsy). The most common neurapraxias affect the facial nerve causing unilateral facial palsy (which may be associated with tilted mandible and contracture of the sternomastoid muscle), the radial nerve causing wrist drop (which may be bilateral), and the sciatic and obturator nerves (usually associated with breech presentation). The muscle weakness seldom lasts more than days or weeks. Treatment, if any, is confined to physiotherapy.

## BIBLIOGRAPHY

Brock, D.J.C., Rodeck, C.H. and Ferguson-Smith, M.A. (eds) (1992) *Prenatal diagnosis and screening.* Edinburgh: Churchill Livingstone.

Jones, K.L. (1997) *Recognisable patterns of human malformation,* 5th edn. Philadelphia, PA: W.B. Saunders & Co.

McKusick, V.A. (1972) *Heritable disorders of connective tissue,* 4th edn. St Louis, MO: CV Mosby Co.

Rosendahl, K., Markestad, T. and Lie, R.J. (1994) Ultrasound screening for developmental dysplasia of the hip in the neonate: the effect on treatment rate and prevalence of late cases. *Pediatrics* **94**, 47–52.

Sharrard, W.J.W. (1979) *Paediatric orthopaedics and fractures,* 2nd edn. Oxford: Blackwell Scientific Publications.

Smith, D.W. (1981) *Recognisable patterns of human deformation.* Philadelphia, PA: W.B. Saunders & Co.

Standing Medical Advisory Committee/Standing Nursing and Midwifery Advisory Committee (SMAC/SNMAC) (1986) Working Party Report. Screening for the detection of congenital dislocation of the hip. *Arch. Dis. Child.* **61**, 921–6.

Warkany, J. (1971) *Congenital malformations.* Chicago: Year Book Medical Publishers Inc.

Williams, P.J. (1982) *Orthopaedic management in childhood.* Oxford: Blackwell Scientific Publications.

World Health Organization (1992) Chapter 17. In *International Classification of Diseases. Vol. 1, 10th revision.* Geneva: World Health Organization, 795–851.

# 8

# Clinical genetics in the neonatal period

## THE ROLE OF THE CLINICAL GENETICIST

The clinical geneticist provides expertise in recognition of neonatal syndrome patterns, particularly involving combinations of major and minor birth defects or other dysmorphic features. He or she can advise on the appropriateness and availability of specific genetic tests for diagnosis, recurrence risk assessment and future avoidance measures, for which a close interface with current research is often required. Ascertainment and counselling of the wider family at risk is an integral part of this role.

## PARENTAL INVOLVEMENT IN THE INVESTIGATION OF DYSMORPHISM

In contrast to infants who have a major birth defect, the suggestion of genetic investigation, particularly chromosomal analysis, in infants with only minor anomalies or a dysmorphic appearance may come as an unforeseen anxiety to the parents. Prior exploration with the parents as to whether they have any concerns for their baby, and whether he or she shows similarities or differences to other family members as infants, may provide a lead into this. It would be usual to counsel parents about the implications of a chromosome test if one is proposed. Postponement of investigation of a suspected genetic problem until developmental delay or some other problem declares itself would have to be balanced against the possible consequence of delay in detecting other potential risk situations in the wider family, and possible resentment by the parents that a diagnosis was not made earlier.

## DIAGNOSIS OF MALFORMATION OR DYSMORPHISM

An infant, fetus or stillbirth may appear dysmorphic because of:

- **malformation:** due to a developmental planning problem, often genetic, e.g. polydactyly, craniostenosis, congenital heart disease;
- **deformation:** due to abnormal intrauterine forces on a normal baby, e.g. talipes in oligohydramnios, or due to normal forces on an abnormal baby, e.g. arthrogryposis in congenital spinal muscular atrophy;
- **disruption:** due to interruption or destruction of a normal developmental sequence, e.g. amniotic bands.

Diagnosis is usually made from:

- **history:** pregnancy factors to note include liquor volume, reduced fetal movement, early twin loss, maternal illness or contact, smoking, alcohol, and prescribed or recreational drugs. Any family history of fetal or congenital abnormality or retardation should be sought. Parental or family history of infertility or recurrent miscarriage may suggest a chromosomal translocation or X-linked dominant condition: parental consanguinity may point to recessive inheritance;
- **'Gestalt':** the overall appearance of the infant matched by the observer's past experience;
- **'good handles':** definite dysmorphic features (e.g. coloboma, mid-line cleft lip, polydactyly, imperforate anus) provide a differential diagnosis (see Table 8.1);
- **measurements:** to recognize whether quantitative traits are outside the limits of normality, e.g. eye spacing, head circumference;

- **minor congenital anomalies:** (e.g. ear-lobe creases) can provide confirmatory features. Multiple minor anomalies may be an indicator of a major internal structural anomaly;
- **X-rays:** these are essential for diagnosis of skeletal dysplasia. Also, in dysmorphic infants, the spine and long bone epiphyses and metaphyses often show additional dysmorphic features (e.g. epiphyseal stippling) which can assist in diagnosis;
- **photographs:** these are invaluable as a record for comparison with literature reports, for consultation with colleagues, and for education;

**Table 8.1** Some commoner syndromes by neonatal abnormality/dysmorphism

| Presenting feature | Syndrome (t = trisomy) |
|---|---|
| Arthrogryposis/talipes/ camptodactyly | Amyoplasia congenita, spinal muscular atrophy, t18, Pena-Shokeir, renal agenesis, distal arthrogryposes, Freeman-Sheldon, maternal antifetal AcCh receptor antibody, myotonic dystrophy |
| Radial ray defects | Fanconi anaemia, Holt-Oram, thrombocytopenia – absent radus, t18, Roberts, VATER |
| Polydactyly: postaxial preaxial | Dominant polydactyly, Bardet Biedl, t13, short-ribbed polydactylies (Ellis van Crefeld, Jeune, etc.), Greig, Townes Brock, oro-facio-digital, Pfeiffer |
| Hypotonia (severe) | Spinal muscular atrophy, myotonic dystrophy, congenital myopathies, Prader-Willi, osteogenesis imperfecta, Zellweger, Coffin-Lowry, t-21, other chromosomal |
| Pierre-Robin sequence | Stickler, spondyloepiphyseal dysplasia, 22q11-, Treacher-Collins, Nager, rib-gap |
| Short limbs | Many skeletal dysplasias (e.g. achondroplasia, spondyloepiphysial dysplasia) |
| Terminal limb defects | Mostly sporadic (e.g. Poland, amnion rupture) |
| Multiple organ anomaly | t13, t18, t21, other chromosomal, axial mesodermal dysplasia VATER, CHARGE, Smith-Lemli-Opitz, Fryns |
| Large fontanelles | Triploidy, other chromosomal, osteogenesis imperfecta, cleidocranial dysostosis, Coffin-Lowry |
| Overgrowth | Beckwith-Widemann, Simpson Golabi, Soto, Weaver, maternal diabetes |
| Severe IUGR | Triploidy, other chromosomal, Silver-Russell |

- **chromosomes:** the majority of infants with chromosomal abnormalities (apart from some sex chromosome aneuploidies) are dysmorphic, and often have multiple malformations. Any infant with a definite malformation, and showing other significant dysmorphism, should be karyotyped. Certain syndromes may result from sub-microscopic deletion at a specific chromosomal site, and require a request for specific fluorescent *in-situ* hybridization study (FISH) for diagnosis (see Table 8.2; e.g. a combination of heart defect and cleft palate in 22q11 microdeletion, or typical features of 4p- or 5p- but with normal standard karyotype). Some chromosome abnormalities (e.g. 12p tetrasomy in Pallister-Killian syndrome) are only ever seen as mosaics, demonstration of which may require skin biopsy for fibroblast culture rather than peripheral blood leukocyte cultures;
- **metabolic investigations:** e.g. in Smith-Lemli-Opitz syndrome, or in peroxisomal disorders;
- **DNA:** in those conditions with a common specific mutation (see Table 8.2);
- **review at a later age:** it may be easier to recognize a particular syndrome diagnosis in a young child than in a newborn infant;
- **comparison with parents and siblings:** this may give clues to a dominantly inherited condition (e.g. myotonic dystrophy). Some minor dysmorphic features may be normal familial variants.

A specific syndrome diagnosis dictates prognosis, inheritance and management; a diagnostic label should be applied only if it is certain. Diagnosis in dysmorphology is assisted by:

- **reference texts** (see Bibliography);
- **computerized databases:** these can provide differential diagnoses for combinations of 'good handles', plus syndrome reviews and references;
- **access to relevant past medical literature:** e.g. *American Journal of Medical Genetics, Journal of Medical Genetics, Clinical Genetics, Clinical Dysmorphology*;
- **discussion with colleagues:** photographs are essential.

## GENETIC COUNSELLING

Genetic counselling for conditions presenting in the neonatal period involves discussion with parents of diagnosis, prognosis, inheritance

**Table 8.2** Conditions presenting in neonates where diagnosis is primarily from a genetic test*

| Presentation | Genetic condition | Inheritance | Genetic diagnostic test |
|---|---|---|---|
| **Neurological** | | | |
| Lissencephaly | Miller Dieker | Microdeletion | FISH: 17p11 |
| Hydrocephalus | X-linked aqueduct stenosis | X-Rec | *(mutation in LICAM gene)* |
| Hypotonia | Prader Willi | Microdeletion | DNA methylation/FISH 15q11 |
| | Coffin Lowry | X-Rec | *(mutation in cloned gene)* |
| | Smith-Lemli-Opitz | Aut Rec | ↑ 7-dehydrocholesterol |
| | Fragile-X | X-Rec | DNA trinucleotide expansion (Xq28) (also in mother) |
| | Myotonic dystrophy | Aut Dom | DNA trinucleotide expansion (19q) |
| | Spinal muscular atrophy | Aut Rec | DNA deletion in SMN gene (5q) |
| | Myotubular myopathy | X-Rec | *(mutation in cloned gene)* |
| | Zellweger | Aut Rec | Very-long-chain fatty acids |
| Encephalopathy | Leigh's disease | Mitochondrial | Mutation in mitochondrial DNA |
| **Ophthalmic** | | | |
| Aniridia | WAGR (Wilm's tumour) | Microdeletion | FISH 11p13 |
| Polycoria | Rieger | Microdeletion | FISH: 4q |
| Cataract | Cockayne | Aut Rec | Fibroblasts (UV sensitivity) |
| | Lowe's | X-Rec | *(mutation in cloned gene)* |
| Pseudoglioma | Norrie | X-Rec | Esterase D for deletion |
| Retinoblastoma | Bilateral retinoblastoma | Aut Dom | *(mutation in cloned gene)* |

**Table 8.2** Continued

| Presentation | Genetic condition | Inheritance | Genetic diagnostic test |
|---|---|---|---|
| **Cardiac** | | | |
| Congenital heart disease | Shprintzen/DiGeorge | Microdeletion | FISH: 22q11 |
| | Williams | Microdeletion | FISH: 7q11 |
| Cardiomyopathy | Barth | X-Rec | 3-methylglutaconic aciduria |
| | | | (mutation in cloned gene) |
| | Noonan | Aut Dom | (mutation in cloned gene) |
| **Skeletal** | | | |
| Short limbs | Achondroplasia | Aut Dom | DNA:specific FGFR3 mutation |
| | Camptomelic dysplasia | Aut Dom | (mutation in SOX9 gene) |
| | Spond.epiphys.dysplasia | Aut Dom | (mutation in collagen gene) |
| | Thanatophoric dysplasia | Aut Dom | (mutation in FGFR3 gene) |
| Craniostenosis | Apert | Aut Dom | DNA:specific FGFR2 mutation |
| | Crouzon | Aut Dom | (mutation in FGFR genes) |
| | Pfeiffer | Aut Dom | (mutation in FGFR genes) |
| Fractures | Osteogenesis imperfecta | Aut Dom | Skin fibroblasts: collagen |
| Limb ray defects | Roberts | Aut Rec | Chromosome centromere puffs |
| | Fanconi anaemia | Aut Rec | Chromosome breakage studies |
| | Holt Oram | Aut Dom | (mutation in cloned gene) |
| | Synpolydactyly | Aut Dom | DNA trinucl expansion |

**Table 8.2** Continued

| Presentation | Genetic condition | Inheritance | Genetic diagnostic test |
|---|---|---|---|
| **Oral** | | | |
| Cleft palate | Stickler | Aut Dom | *(mutation in collagen gene)* |
| **GI** | | | |
| Meconium ileus | Cystic fibrosis | Aut Rec | DNA for CF gene mutations |
| Constipation | Hirschsprung | Aut Dom | *(mutation in cloned RET gene)* |
| **Skin** | | | |
| Icthyosis | Steriod sulphatase deficiency | X-Rec | FISH: Xp22 (some cases) |
| Streaked depigmentation | Chrom. mosaicism | Sporadic | Skin fibroblast karyotype |
| **Growth** | | | |
| Overgrowth | Beckwith syndrome | Aut Dom/sporadic | DNA for disomy at 11p |
| | Neonatal Marfan | Aut Dom | *(mutation in fibrillin gene)* |
| Growth retardation | Silver-Russell | Sporadic | DNA for disomy 7 |

\* Tests marked in *italics* are currently available only on a research basis, i.e. individual mutation testing in a cloned gene.
Aut Dom = dominant, Aut Rec = recessive, X-Rec = X-linked recessive.

and recurrence risk, often in relation to the relevance and possibilities for future avoidance strategies, particularly through prenatal testing. Counselling is invariably non-directive, aiming to facilitate informed individual decisions. Ascertainment and the offer of discussion for the wider family at risk, or reassurance to dissipate unnecessary anxiety, are also important. Genetic counselling relies on:

- accuracy of diagnosis, particularly for genetic prediction or in single cases;
- assessment of inheritance pattern, particularly if alternatives could apply;
- parents' own attitudes – the perception of risk may depend on:
  1 chance of recurrence (high, low or negligible);
  2 seriousness of the condition (quality of life, survival, and degree of burden to parents, family or society).

## INHERITANCE PATTERNS AND RECURRENCE RISKS

Possible patterns of inheritance are:

- autosomal dominant;
- autosomal recessive;
- X-linked recessive;
- X-linked dominant;
- multifactorial;
- chromosomal;
- mitochondrial and other extranuclear;
- non-genetic.

### Autosomal dominant inheritance

Fault in one copy of autosomal gene pair; 50% risk to offspring; expression may be variable, even within a family, and could include asymptomatic carriers (non-penetrance). Increasing severity with successive generations (anticipation), is observed in trinucleotide repeat disorders (e.g. myotonic dystrophy, or synpolydactyly), but depends on sex of transmitting parent.

In an apparently isolated case consider new mutation (possibly with raised paternal age), parental non-penetrance, parental germinal mosaicism, non-paternity (recurrence risk usually at least 1%).

Certain tumour suppressor genes (e.g. retinoblastoma) may exhibit dominant inheritance in a family, but recessive inheritance at cellular level (Knudson 2-hit hypothesis). Other dominant gene defects (e.g. in cell growth, growth factors, or oncogenes) may indicate a link between malformation and increased susceptibility to cancer (e.g. Beckwith-Weidemann syndrome, neurofibromatosis, Hirschsprung's disease).

### Autosomal recessive inheritance
Fault in both copies of an autosomal gene pair (one from each parent); 25% risk to future full sibs; consanguinity more likely in rare conditions; low risk to offspring of affected subject, to parent with new partner or to wider family (unless partner is related or mutant gene is endemic in population, e.g. sickle cell Hb). Recessive phenotypes usually 'breed true' in a sibship, an exception being DNA repair enzyme defects, which also demonstrate a link between malformation and cancer susceptibility.

### X-linked recessive inheritance
Faulty recessive gene on X-chromosome; males affected, connected through female line; two-thirds or more of mothers of isolated cases will be carriers (some others may be germinal mosaics); 50% risk in sons of carrier females, 50% risk in daughters of being carriers; no risk to sons of affected males, all daughters are obligate carriers.

Females can occasionally be affected through XO karyotype (Turner's syndrome); homozygosity for mutant gene; skewed X-chromosome inactivation in carrier (especially if monozygotic twin in embryogenesis); X-autosome translocation with breakpoint through the gene and inactivation of normal X.

### X-linked dominant inheritance (e.g. incontinentia pigmenti, Goltz syndrome)
Rare; usually only females affected, since usually lethal to affected XY males; 50% risk to daughters of affected female.

### Polygenic inheritance
Involves several genes, or genetic susceptibility to environmental triggers; recurrence risk is typically 3–5% in first-degree relatives and typically 1% in second-degree relatives; higher recurrence risk if index case is less commonly affected sex, or if the index is more severely affected.

### Chromosomal inheritance
Autosomal simple trisomies (i.e. t21, t18, t13) not due to transloca-tions, and sex chromosome aneuploidies (i.e. XO, XXY, XXX, XYY)

**Table 8.3** Birth incidence of chromosomal anomalies by maternal age

| Maternal age (years) | t21 | t18 | t13 | XO | All chromosome anomalies |
|---|---|---|---|---|---|
| ≤ 30 | ≤ 1/900 | | | | |
| 35 | 1/380 | 1/2000 | 1/5000 | ⎫ 1/2500 | 1/150 at any age |
| 38 | 1/190 | 1/700 | 1/2000 | ⎬ females at | |
| 40 | 1/110 | 1/360 | 1/900 | ⎭ any age | |
| 42 | 1/65 | 1/180 | 1/480 | | |

are invariably sporadic; parental chromosome analysis is not indicated. For these:

- incidence increases with rising maternal age (see Table 8.3);
- recurrence risk, which can be for any trisomy, is usually around 1%, but if maternal age is ≥ 38 years it becomes double the prior age-dependent risk.

Unbalanced chromosome abnormalities may arise *de novo* or from one of the parents carrying a balanced rearrangement, then necessitating study of the wider family.

Mosaic chromosomal abnormalities arise post-zygotically during mitosis and, with the exception of certain unstable rearrangements, are invariably sporadic. Body asymmetry or striped depigmentation may be clues.

Most cases of chromosomal microdeletion, diagnosed by specific *in-situ* hybridization, occur *de novo*, but in some cases (e.g. 22q11-) might also be detected in one parent, then conferring a 50% recurrence risk. Parental germinal mosaicism is also recorded, and recurrence risk for a *de-novo* case may never be less than 1%.

Uniparental disomy, where both chromosomes of a pair have originated from the same parent (e.g. in some babies with Prader-Willi syndrome), unless associated with parental balanced translocation, is invariably sporadic. However, since this may originate from reduction of a zygotic trisomy, there could potentially be a 1% risk of other simple trisomy in subsequent siblings.

### Mitochondrial inheritance

Since mitochondria are self-replicating organelles with their own DNA, and are present in the cytoplasm of the oocyte, mitochondrially inherited conditions show matrilineal inheritance with a high proportion of affected offspring from an affected female.

### Non-genetic abnormalities

Malformation or dysmorphism can also result from fetal exposure to maternal drugs or other adverse fetal environment (e.g. anticonvulsants, warfarin, alcohol, cigarette smoke, maternal diabetes). Some mothers or fetuses may be genetically more susceptible, and recurrence risks for problems will be very high in a further pregnancy exposed to the same agent.

Any of these inheritance patterns could result in an apparently isolated case. Clues to increased likelihood of a particular pattern may be:

- multiple congenital abnormality – consider chromosomal inheritance;
- male affected – consider X-linked recessive inheritance;
- consanguinity – consider autosomal recessive inheritance;
- recurrent miscarriage – consider chromosomal inheritance;
- raised paternal age – consider new dominant mutation;
- raised maternal age – consider chromosomal trisomy;
- 'striped' pigmentation in female – consider X-linked dominant or chromosome mosaic.

## GENETIC TESTS FOR RISK ASSESSMENT AND SUBSEQUENT PRENATAL TESTING

### For conditions where the gene has been cloned

A uniform mutation mechanism as the cause of a condition usually enables a simple specific diagnostic test (see Table 8.2). Otherwise, identification of the family specific mutation is required, which currently would usually only be undertaken by an interested laboratory on a research basis.

### For conditions where the gene is mapped but not cloned

Linkage analysis using DNA samples from other affected (and unaffected) family members may enable tracking of the section of DNA adjacent to or containing the faulty gene through a family.

Family or prenatal molecular genetic studies rely on a stored DNA sample from one or more affected members of a family. Consider requesting a blood sample (or skin fibroblast culture) for DNA extraction from all infants, stillbirths or fetuses which have serious single-gene disorders, especially if expectation of survival is low, particularly infantile polycystic kidney disease, thanatophoric dysplasia, lethal osteogenesis imperfecta, lethal epidermolysis bullosa, osteopetrosis, short-ribbed polydactylies, camptomelic dysplasia, spinal muscular atrophy and lethal metabolic disorders.

## OTHER FAMILY MEMBERS AT RISK

Following identification of an index case with a serious genetic disorder, clinicians have a responsibility (through the Clinical Genetic Service) to identify, inform and counsel other relatives who may be at risk. This is of particular importance in X-linked, autosomal dominant and familial chromosomal disorders, and in families with multiple consanguinity if at risk of a recessive disorder.

## PREDICTION OF INHERITED DISEASE IN THE NEWBORN

Testing of infants at risk of genetic conditions is important if treatment is available (e.g. phenylketonuria (PKU), hypothyroidism, galactosaemia), and if not, can be helpful if this may relieve parental anxiety through resolution of uncertainty (e.g. by creatine kinase assay in Duchenne muscular dystrophy (DMD)). Genetic testing of newborn infants or children for adult-onset disorders (e.g. Huntington's disease or Li Fraumeni syndrome) should *not be undertaken* even if there is parental pressure to do so, since the future young adult must be able to exercise their own choice in this matter.

## COLLECTION AND STORAGE OF SAMPLES

### Chromosomal analysis

- 1–5 mL blood in lithium heparin.
- Can be sent by routine daily laboratory transport, or by first-class post.
- Store (avoiding direct sunlight) at (a cool) room temperature if delayed by 24–48 hours.
- Specific FISH or chromosome breakage tests must be specifically requested. The more detailed the clinical information on the request form, the better able the laboratory will be to offer appropriate tests.

## DNA analysis

- 2–5 mL blood in EDTA (preferably 10–20 ml from adults).
- Samples will keep for 24 hours at room temperature or for 5 days at 4°C.
- Extracted DNA will store at – 70°C for many years.
  Fresh (same-day) samples are required for mRNA or high-molecular-weight DNA.
- Discuss with the laboratory if only a small blood or tissue sample is available; for certain tests, amplification of DNA by polymerase chain reaction may allow analysis, provided that any contamination is avoided.

## Skin biopsy

Skin biopsy for establishing a long-term fibroblast culture should be considered if:

- blood is not available;
- chromosome mosaicism is suspected;
- a source of mRNA is required for mutation detection;
- ongoing metabolic investigation or molecular research is anticipated.

This must be performed as a sterile procedure, preferably into specific culture medium or into sterile normal saline. Fibroblasts will usually still grow if taken up to 3 days post-mortem, and should certainly be taken for chromosome analysis from all stillbirths or fetuses with multiple malformations. Liaise with the laboratory for further details.

**The storing of blood or tissue specimens as described above should be considered from all fetuses, stillbirths or infants that may have genetically based congenital anomalies or other genetic conditions, and whose expectation of survival is low.**

## BIBLIOGRAPHY

Buyse, M.L. (1990) *Birth defects encyclopedia*. Cambridge, MA: Blackwell Scientific Publications.

Gorlin, R.J., Cohen, M.M. and Levin, L.S. (1990) *Syndromes of the head and neck*. New York: Oxford University Press.

Harper, P.S. (1993) *Practical genetic counselling*, 4th edn. Oxford: Butterworth-Heinmann.

Jones, K.L. (1997) *Smith's recognisable patterns of human malformation*, 5th edn. Philadelphia, PA: W.B. Saunders.

McKusick, V.A. (1996) *Mendelian inheritance in man*, 12th edn. Baltimore, MD: Johns Hopkins University Press.

Stevenson, R.E., Hall, J.G. and Goodman, R.M. (1993) *Human malformations and related anomalies*. New York: Oxford University Press.

Winter, R.M., Knowles, S.A.S., Bieber, S.R., and Baraitser, M. (1988) *The malformed fetus and stillbirth: a diagnostic approach*. Chichester: John Wiley.

## Computer databases

Bankier, A. (1991) *P.O.S.S.U.M.* Purley: C.P. Export.

Schinzel, A. (1994) *Human cytogenetics database*. Oxford: Oxford University Press Electronic Publications.

Winter, R., Baraitser, M. (1993) *London Dysmorphology Database*. Oxford: Oxford University Press Electronic Publications.

**9**

# Neonatal surgical problems

## ANTENATAL DIAGNOSIS (see Chapter 1)

Many surgically treated abnormalities (e.g. diaphragmatic hernia, gastroschisis, exomphalos, small bowel obstruction) are suspected from antenatal ultrasound scans. Such infants, particularly those with diaphragmatic hernia, should if possible be delivered in a referral centre with surgical and intensive-care facilities, rather than being transferred after birth. There is no evidence of benefit from elective Caesarean section for infants with abdominal wall defects, diaphragmatic hernia or oesophageal atresia, but it may be necessary with large tumours which can cause dystocia (e.g. sacrococcygeal teratoma).

## CONGENITAL DIAPHRAGMATIC HERNIA

### Description

Usually diaphragmatic hernia presenting in the newborn period is posterolateral (foramen of Bochdalek) or complete agenesis of the diaphragm. Herniae are more common on the left.

The incidence is 1 in 2000 live births.

### Diagnosis

Suspect in any baby who fails to respond satisfactorily to intubation or bag-and-mask resuscitation at birth. Confirmatory clinical signs such as displaced apex beat and scaphoid abdomen with unequal air entry should then be sought.

Definitive diagnosis is by X-ray of chest and abdomen, which shows loops of bowel in the chest and contralateral displacement of the mediastinum.

### Management (see also Chapter 10)

#### In delivery suite

- Immediate endotracheal intubation (bag-and-mask ventilation may cause visceral distension and worsen respiratory embarrassment).
- Muscle relaxants.
- Insert nasogastric tube (8F or Replogle tube*) to avoid distension of intrathoracic viscera.
- Continue intermittent positive-pressure ventilation (IPPV) during transfer to Intensive Care Nursery.

#### Preoperative management

Aim to achieve cardiorespiratory stability and minimize right-to-left shunting due to pulmonary hypertension.

- Ventilator-induced respiratory alkalosis is not necessary. High positive pressure may be required, but this increases the danger of pneumothorax. PEEP of greater than 3–4 cm $H_2O$ should be avoided. High respiratory rates or occasionally HFOV may be helpful.
- Muscle relaxation and sedation with opiates.
- Inotropes (dopamine or dobutamine) may be required for hypotension. Addition of vasodilators (epoprostenol or inhaled nitric oxide) may be helpful if right-to-left shunting persists.

- Crystalloid infusions are restricted to 60 ml/kg/day and hypovolaemia corrected with colloid boluses as required.
- Intensive monitoring (respiratory, haemodynamic and fluid balance) and minimal handling are important to avoid cardiorespiratory instability.
- Continuous suction (5–10 cm $H_2O$) applied to the gastric tube is required to decompress the intrathoracic viscera; preferably use a Replogle tube*, otherwise use an 8F nasogastric tube on free drainage and with intermittent aspiration.
- Arterial blood gases should be checked as soon as possible after IPPV is established.
- Other investigations include combined X-ray of chest and abdomen, full blood count and blood culture. Blood group and cross-match mother's and baby's blood for one unit of blood for the operation.
- Prophylactic antibiotics are given immediately prior to the operation.

### Operation

Usually between the ages of 24 hours and 72 hours. Recent evidence suggests that aggressive initial medical support, delaying operative treatment until a stable satisfactory state has been achieved, may improve results. Operation on a grossly acidotic and hypoxaemic baby is contraindicated; babies with severe pulmonary hypoplasia incompatible with long-term survival may be identified within 24 hours.

The hernia is usually repaired through an abdominal incision, either by direct suture of the defect or by patching with prosthetic material (Gortex) or rarely abdominal muscle graft. Intrapleural drains are not generally inserted postoperatively. It is essential to remember that 'pneumothorax' is inevitable postoperatively. Only if a tension pneumothorax develops (mediastinal shift to contralateral side) should a chest drain be inserted.

### Postoperative stabilization

- Aim to keep the preductal arterial oxygen around 100 mm Hg (13.3 kPa) in term babies. (70–90 mm Hg (9.3–12 kPa) in babies of < 35 weeks' gestation).
- Continue muscle relaxants and sedation for 2–3 days to avoid sudden swings in oxygenation.

* Argyle Replogle Suction Catheter. Catalogue No. 888/256504. Sherwood Medical Industries Ltd, London Road, County Oak, Crawley RH11 7YQ, Surrey.

- Moderate fluid restriction for the first 48 hours (60–80 mL/kg/24 hours). Give 10–15 mL/kg colloid boluses as required.
- Gentle physiotherapy and endotracheal toilet are particularly important in a paralysed baby.
- When stable, muscle relaxants are stopped and the patient weaned off the ventilator.
- Intravenous alimentation should be started 24–48 hours postoperatively, and enteral feeding (via gastric tube) can usually be started by 5–7 days postoperatively. Transition from tube to oral feeding may be slow. Remember that the caloric requirement may be increased.

A persistent patent ductus arteriosus is a common finding; it may be associated with significant left-to-right shunting, but rarely requires surgical ligation.

### Subsequent management

Infants who require minimal ventilatory support have a good outlook and may be out of hospital in 2–3 weeks depending on their gestational age. Those with the more severe defects are difficult to wean from ventilatory support, and some develop bronchopulmonary dysplasia with oxygen dependence which may persist for many weeks or months (see Chapter 10). In infants still being ventilated at 7–10 days after the operation, the duration of positive pressure ventilation and chronic lung disease may be reduced by nursing in a continuous negative extrathoracic pressure chamber (CNEP).

### Follow-up

Pulmonary reserve is significantly reduced in the first 1–2 years, and minor respiratory infections may lead to severe respiratory symptoms, occasionally requiring ventilatory support. A small proportion of children with the most severe diaphragmatic herniae and secondary bronchopulmonary dysplasia develop cor pulmonale and die in later infancy. The majority of surviving children achieve virtually normal lung function later in childhood.

## EXOMPHALOS (OMPHALOCELE)

### Description

This may be major (large abdominal wall defect covered by a sac of amnion and peritoneum) or minor (hernia of abdominal contents into umbilical cord). Up to 50% are associated with abnormalities of cardiovascular, genito-urinary or gastrointestinal systems and chromosomal anomalies or Beckwith-Wiedemann syndrome (exomphalos, visceromegaly, macroglossia and hypoglycaemia).

The incidence is 1 in 10 000 live births.

## Management

### In the labour suite
Place the whole body up to the axillae in a plastic bag or cover the lesion with a plastic bag or cling-film to minimize evaporative heat and water loss. Pass a large nasogastric tube (8F) and connect to low suction to prevent stomach or bowel distension. Site an intravenous infusion, and monitor perfusion, blood pressure and blood sugar.

### Subsequent management
The object is to return the gut to the abdominal cavity in order to reduce the risk of rupture of the sac and of infection. This is a relatively simple procedure in exomphalos minor. In exomphalos major, the abdominal cavity is often very small, and the lungs may be hypoplastic (because of lack of effective diaphragmatic contraction and breathing movements *in utero*). It may be possible to return the sac contents to the abdomen as a primary procedure, but large lesions, particularly those containing liver, may be managed conservatively if the sac is intact. Antiseptics are applied and natural reduction of the sac by cicatrization is awaited. By 4–6 weeks it is usually possible to achieve delayed primary closure. If the sac is ruptured and skin cover cannot be achieved at the first operation, a silastic silo may be used, and the sac size reduced by progressive plication with later closure of the defect.

Raised abdominal pressure after the operation may lead to respiratory embarrassment, inferior vena cava obstruction or renal vein thrombosis (see Chapter 15).

Pre- and postoperatively, sepsis is a major risk and broad-spectrum antibiotics (penicillin and aminoglycoside ± metronidazole) should be started preoperatively (after taking blood cultures) and continued for 5–7 days postoperatively in exomphalos major with ruptured sac.

Blood pressure, blood gases, blood electrolytes, fluid balance (including frequent urinalysis) and urine microscopy must be carefully monitored.

Intravenous feeding (see Chapter 13) should be started 24–48 hours postoperatively. Enteral feeding can be started when the infant has passed meconium and gastric aspirate is minimal (usually 5–7 days postoperatively).

## GASTROSCHISIS

### Description

Coils of intestine herniate through a defect in the anterior abdominal wall, to the right of the umbilical cord. A covering of peritoneal membrane is absent and gangrene or perforation may occur in the prolapsed bowel, due to ischaemia. It is not associated with other abnormalities apart from intestinal atresia. Babies are usually small for their gestational age and hypoproteinaemic.

The incidence has been increasing in recent years, and is now approximately 1 in 5000 deliveries, but the incidence is even higher in young mothers (< 20 years).

### Management

#### In the labour suite
As for exomphalos.

#### Subsequent management
General management is similar to that for exomphalos. Volume replacement with plasma or albumin solution is usually required during stabilization prior to surgery because extensive protein losses occur into the bowel and peritoneal cavity. Blood pressure and perfusion must therefore be closely monitored. Surgical management may be either by primary closure or by a two-stage procedure using a silastic silo and reduction of the contents gradually over a period of 7–10 days. Bowel resection (for ischaemic damage) is occasionally necessary in gastroschisis.

The bowel may take several weeks to work well and i.v. nutrition (usually through a long line) is important during this period. The average length of stay is 6 weeks.

Associated atresias occur in approximately 10% of cases, may necessitate temporary stomas, and further delay the introduction of enteral feeding.

The mortality of gastroschisis is currently 5–10%, and is usually due to an extremely short gut or the complications of long-term intravenous feeding (liver damage and central line-associated sepsis). In survivors the long-term outlook for health and nutrition is excellent.

# TRACHEO-OESOPHAGEAL FISTULA (TOF) AND OESOPHAGEAL ATRESIA

## Description

Five main types exist (see Fig. 9.1).

The most common type (87%) is oesophageal atresia with distal tracheo-oesophageal fistula, followed by oesophageal atresia without fistula (8%). Around 50% are associated with other abnormalities which can be conveniently remembered using the acronymic VATER or VACTERL association: Vertebral, Anal, Cardiac, Tracheal, Esophageal, Renal, Limb (radial aplasia or abnormalities of thumb).

Occasionally there is a family history.

The incidence is 1 in 3000 live births.

## Diagnosis

This should be made before feeding, otherwise there is a high risk of aspiration. There is usually a history of maternal polyhydramnios, and the condition may rarely be suspected antenatally if prenatal ultrasound shows a small or absent stomach.

All babies born to mothers with polyhydramnios and all 'mucusy' babies (apparent hypersalivation) should have a gastric tube passed (10F) as soon as possible after birth. In the delivery suite the distal end of a mucus trap may be used. If oesophageal atresia is present the catheter will usually not pass more than 8–10 cm from the gum margin.

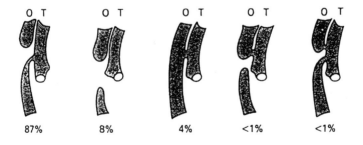

**Fig. 9.1** Diagrams of the five most common types of tracheo-oesophageal fistula and oesophageal atresia, in order of frequency (T, trachea; O, oesophagus).

The diagnosis should be confirmed by combined chest and abdominal X-ray with a radio-opaque tube pushed down the oesophageal pouch to show its level. X-ray may reveal pulmonary consolidation due to aspiration; a complete absence of bowel gas shadows in the absence of a fistula, or vertebral anomalies. Cardiac echo is performed to demonstrate cardiac anatomy and the side of the aortic arch. Renal ultrasound is necessary if other features of the VATER association are present.

## Management

A Replogle tube should be passed into the oesophageal pouch and kept on low suction (5 cm $H_2O$). The baby may be nursed head up to avoid aspiration of stomach secretions and to maximize the effect of the Replogle tube. Surgery is performed as soon as the baby's condition is stable. It may be delayed in order to improve pulmonary function with physiotherapy and antibiotics if aspiration has occurred.

Preterm infants with RDS pose particular problems, since ventilatory gases may be diverted down the fistulae. Conventional management has been emergency ligation of the fistula, but this may carry a significant mortality, and the Bristol approach has preferred an initial gastrostomy, meticulous ventilatory management using low pressures or HFOV and delayed surgical repair.

A primary end-to-end anastomosis of the oesophagus and division of the tracho-oesophageal fistula is possible in over 90% of cases, and is performed via a right posterolateral extrapleural thoracotomy. Some surgeons perform a gastrostomy. Feeding may be started via a transanastomotic tube within 48 hours of operation. An extrapleural drain is usually inserted at operation and removed on day 5 if there is no anastomotic leakage. A barium swallow is usually performed 5–7 days postoperatively to ensure integrity of the anastomosis before starting oral feeds.

## Complications

- Pneumonia or anastomotic breakdown may occur.
- Strictures requiring dilatation occur in up to 20% of cases.
- Coughing during feeds or recurrent chest infections may indicate either recurrence of the TOF or that a second fistula has been missed at operation.
- Gastro-oesophageal reflux commonly occurs and requires medical (or rarely surgical) treatment.

- A brassy cough ('TOF cough'), probably due to tracheomalacia, is very common and may persist for years. It needs no treatment.
- Mortality should be less than 10% and is usually due to associated congenital heart disease.

## The 'H' type tracheo-oesophageal fistula

This will not be diagnosed by failure to pass a nasogastric tube and usually presents later with episodes of cyanosis after feeds, or recurrent pneumonia.

### Diagnosis
Suspected clinically with a positive 'bubble test'. A large nasogastric tube (Jacques No. 12) is passed and then gradually withdrawn up the oesophagus with the proximal end under water. Bubbling should occur when the tip has reached the level of the fistula unless the tube or fistula is full of mucus. The diagnosis should be confirmed by bronchoscopy or fluoroscopy, when a small amount of contrast is trickled down the oesophagus from a fine catheter. The fistula is usually seen at level $C_7$ or $T_1$, and usually fills by reflux ('Tube oesophagogram').

### Operation
Division of the fistula is usually possible through a cervical approach.

## ANORECTAL ANOMALIES

## Description

For practical purposes rectal anomalies can be divided into high and low categories.

If the bowel has passed through the sphincter complex, prospects for long-term faecal continence are excellent with relatively minor surgery. If not, then the bowel has to be brought through the sphincter without damaging it, but only 50% of cases achieve reasonable continence. Associated abnormalities include upper urinary tract (15%), cardiovascular (10%), high gut atresias (12%), and also sacral anomalies and oesophageal atresia.

The incidence is 1 in 2000 live births.

## Diagnosis

**Low lesions** In both boys and girls may present with evidence of an anocutaneous fistula, or in girls as an ectopic, anteriorly situated, stenotic anus.

**High lesions** In boys are frequently associated with a recto-urethral fistula; in girls a rectovestibular, fistula rectovaginal fistula or cloaca may be present.

A lateral X-ray with the infant prone and slightly head down and a smear of barium over the skin dimple at 24 hours of age may help to distinguish the level of obstruction. Earlier X-rays are not usually helpful. Sacral anomalies will also be shown on this X-ray, and further spinal anatomical detail is obtained by ultrasound scan.

## Management

In low lesions the ectopic stenotic anal opening or covered anus is treated by an anoplasty.

If a high lesion is present, a divided defunctioning high sigmoid colostomy is performed, followed by a posterior sagittal anorecto plasty operation at several months of age. The colostomy is usually closed 6–12 weeks after the second operation.

Prognosis in low lesions is excellent, over 90% achieving normal faecal continence, but less good in the high lesions where continence may never be achieved. In these cases some form of long-term enema management may be the only way of avoiding unacceptable soiling.

## Complications

Urinary tract infection, especially if associated upper renal tract anomalies are present (see Chapter 15).

## BOWEL OBSTRUCTION

### Atresia and stenosis of the intestine

#### Description

Atresia may be of four types:

- type I – lumen completely obstructed by septum or septa;
- type II – two ends of gut joined by fibrous cord;
- type IIIa – ends completely separated with a V-shaped gap in the mesentery;

- type IIIb – 'apple peel' atresia, with reduced total bowel length;
- type IV – multiple atresia.

All jejunal and ileal atresias are caused by antenatal vascular accidents, whereas duodenal atresia is a true developmental malformation.

Stenotic lesions may be due to localized narrowing of the gut or a perforated septum, and may be single or multiple.

The incidence is 1 in 10 000 live births.

Duodenal atresia is associated with Down's syndrome in a third of cases. It is the commonest site of atresia (1 in 6000 live births). Small-bowel atresia may be associated with cystic fibrosis.

### Diagnosis

Approximately one-third of cases are suspected antenatally by ultrasound demonstration of dilated bowel. All except duodenal atresia above the ampulla of Vater present with bilious vomiting. In general, the lower down the small intestine the defect, the later the presentation after birth (usually 24–48 hours). All may be associated with maternal polyhydramnios, fetal growth retardation and prematurity.

An X-ray will show a 'double bubble' appearance in duodenal atresia which is pathognomonic of duodenal obstruction. Otherwise, multiple fluid levels will be seen, sometimes with flecks of calcification, indicating intrauterine perforation. A contrast enema should be performed to exclude large-bowel obstruction.

### Management

Correct any fluid and electrolyte disturbances (see Chapter 14). Duodeno-duodenostomy is the treatment of choice for duodenal atresia. In small-bowel lesions, excision of an atretic segment is followed by end-to-end anastomosis if the proximal gut is not too distended. Otherwise, either a double-barrelled enterostomy is formed to allow decompression of the gut with delayed anastomosis, or a tapering enteroplasty with primary anastomosis.

A gastric tube should be passed and connected to low suction preoperatively and for several days postoperatively. Enteral feeding should not be started until meconium has been passed and gastric aspirate is minimal. Intravenous feeding should be commenced 24–48 hours postoperatively and continued until enteral feeding is established (see Chapter 13).

Commence broad-spectrum antibiotics (penicillin, aminoglycoside and metronidazole) preoperatively (after blood culture) and continue for 48 hours postoperatively.

The prognosis is largely dependent on the percentage of small bowel infarcted in the formation of the atresia:

- 250 cm – normal length in full-term neonate;
- 70 cm – definition of short gut;
- < 50 cm – significant mortality;
- < 20 cm – survival unlikely.

Preterm babies have a correspondingly shorter natural bowel length and a greater capacity for growth and adaptation.

In short gut syndrome, the necessary use of long-term intravenous nutrition confers significant morbidity and mortality.

## Meconium ileus

### Description

- 90% of children with meconium ileus have cystic fibrosis.
- 15% of children with cystic fibrosis present in the neonatal period with bowel obstruction caused by the abnormally tenacious meconium.

### Diagnosis

This may be difficult, but the following will suggest the diagnosis.

1 Family history of cystic fibrosis or neonatal bowel obstruction.
2 Failure to pass meconium by 48 hours.
3 Clinically visible and palpable bowel loops.
4 Erect abdominal X-ray usually shows no fluid levels despite dilated loops, but may show:
  a characteristic foamy appearance of the gut contents; or
  b if there has been perforation with meconium peritonitis – flecks of calcification.
5 Blood immunoreactive trypsin level should be assayed. High levels are strongly suggestive of cystic fibrosis.

Genetic studies should be performed if diagnosis is suspected. The mutation, $\Delta$ F508 represents 78% of all CF mutations in the UK.

### Management

Contrast enema reveals a microcolon packed with meconium plugs, and gastrografin may relieve an uncomplicated obstruction by osmotic effect, increasing the water content of the stool. The level of obstruction is usually the terminal ileum.

NB During the contrast enema, loss of water from the circulation may cause hypotension. Generous intravenous fluids must be given throughout the procedure, with additional colloid boluses as required.

If this is not successful, a laparotomy is required followed by enterotomy and washout temporary double-barrelled ileostomy or primary resection and anastomosis.

A sweat test should be performed (usually at 4–6 weeks).

Pancreatic supplements should be started once full enteral feeding is established.

## Malrotation and volvulus

### Description
Failure of complete rotation of the mid-gut around the mesenteric axis. Uncommon, M:F ratio is 2:1; 75% of cases present in the first month of life.

### Diagnosis
Presents with high intestinal obstruction due to volvulus of the small intestine around the mesenteric axis or to duodenal obstruction from tight adhesions (Ladd's bands) to the overlying caecum situated in the right hypochondrium. Plain abdominal X-rays may be normal.

The clinical picture is similar to duodenal atresia except that obstruction is usually incomplete or intermittent, so that signs appear more gradually. There may be passage of blood per rectum if strangulation of the bowel occurs, but this is a late sign and diagnosis should be made earlier. Barium meal may show obstruction of the third part of the duodenum, but the most important radiological sign is malposition of the D-J flexure (to the right of the midline and below the level of the pylorus).

### Management
General management is as for atresia. *Urgent* surgery is necessary to untwist the volvulus and prevent infarction of the midgut. Bands are divided, the duodenum mobilized and the gut returned to the abdomen in the position of non-rotation, with the small bowel on the right, and the large bowel on the left.

## Hirschsprung's disease

### Description
Hirschsprung's disease is a congenital absence of ganglion cells in the myenteric and submucosal plexus of the rectum, extending proximally for a variable distance.

The incidence is 1 in 5000, the M:F ratio is 3:1, with increased family incidence.

### Diagnosis

Generally presents as large-bowel obstruction with distension and failure to pass meconium in the first week with or without vomiting. It should be considered in an asymptomatic full-term baby who has not passed meconium by 48 hours, or who passes a meconium plug. Rectal examination may reveal a narrow rectum and be followed by an explosive passage of faeces. Barium enema shows a conical 'transitional zone' where normal dilated colon cones down to the aganglionic segment. May present as enterocolitis.

Rectal suction biopsy showing absence of ganglion cells, and hyperplasia of nerve fibres is diagnostic. Acetylcholinesterase histochemistry is useful in addition to conventional histology.

### Management

General management is as for atresia, but it is important to be aware of the risk of enterocolitis. Early antibiotic cover and prompt decompression of the bowel by rectal washouts will reduce this risk.

Conventionally a divided defunctioning colostomy, in bowel shown by frozen-section biopsy to have ganglia, is performed proximal to the obstruction. Excision of the aganglionic segment and a recto-sigmoidostomy may then be performed at 3–6 months. Some surgeons now advocate a one-stage procedure avoiding colostomy. Postoperatively, enteral feeding can be commenced following action of the stomas within 48 hours.

Increased sodium losses via the colostomy should be replaced with sodium bicarbonate (a low urinary sodium level will indicate the necessity for oral sodium supplements).


## INFANTILE HYPERTROPHIC PYLORIC STENOSIS

### Description

The muscle of the pylorus is hypertrophic. The cause is unknown but the condition is not present at birth. Hereditary factors are involved; siblings of an affected baby are 25 times more likely to be affected than in the normal population.

The incidence is 3 in 1000 live births; the M:F ratio is 4:1.

## Diagnosis

Presentation is usually around 2–4 weeks with vomiting which becomes projectile but is not bile stained. There is usually constipation and commonly weight loss. The infant looks thin, alert and hungry, and may be dehydrated. There is usually a hypochloraemic alkalosis.

A test feed is performed to establish the diagnosis. Visible peristalsis may be seen, but diagnosis depends on feeling the hypertrophied pyloric muscle with the left hand just above and to the right of the umbilicus while examining the baby from the left. Projectile vomiting may occur during or after the feed. An erect plain X-ray of the abdomen usually shows an air-fluid level in the stomach with minimal distal air. Ultrasound is also helpful if the clinical diagnosis is uncertain. Barium meal is rarely necessary, but is diagnostic in cases of doubt.

### Treatment

**1** Stop feeds, nasogastric suction.

**2** Capillary blood gas (for pH and base excess) is the single most useful investigation. Serum electrolytes will usually reveal hypochloraemia, sometimes hypocalcaemia. Serum sodium is usually normal.

Correct fluid and electrolyte disturbances over 12–24 hours intravenously (see Chapter 14). The vomit, in contrast to other causes of vomiting, contains hydrogen ions and no bicarbonate. Potassium and chloride must be replaced in adequate concentrations during rehydration to enable the kidney to maintain ionic balance and correct the alkalosis.

Maintenance fluid and deficits are calculated as usual (see p. 252) and the deficit replaced over a 12-hour period. It is essential that at least 0.45% sodium chloride and dextrose containing at least 20 mmol/L of potassium chloride is used (0.18% or 0.225% saline do not contain sufficient chloride and will never correct the alkalosis).

If the alkalosis is severe (base excess > 10 mmol) or serum potassium is < 3.2 mmol/L use 0.9% ('normal') saline, to which is added 40 mmol/L potassium chloride.

**3** Surgery – extramucosal pyloromyotomy (Ramstedt operation) is performed only when the alkalosis is corrected.

**4** Postoperatively – start oral feeds after 12 hours (there is commonly some vomiting for the first few days due to reflux).

Continue i.v. fluids until the infant is tolerating oral feeds. Do not discontinue milk feeds because of vomiting, but consider anti-reflux treatment.

## INGUINAL HERNIA

The incidence is 2% in male infants.

Inguinal hernia is especially common in preterm infants.
Around 80% occur in boys and the sac usually contains small bowel. In girls the ovary may herniate into the inguinal canal.

Usually a swelling is palpable at the external inguinal ring, but as it enlarges it will extend into the scrotum or labia majora. The swelling may be constant or only noticeable on crying or straining.

There is a high risk of incarceration or strangulation of inguinal herniae in infancy, so surgical repair should be carried out before discharge from hospital. Older infants noted to have inguinal herniae should have surgical repair carried out within a few days of diagnosis.

Incarcerated hernias will usually prove to be reducible by a paediatric surgeon. Operation is delayed 24–48 hours after reduction to allow oedema to settle.

## BIBLIOGRAPHY

Freeman N.V., Burge, D.M., Griffiths, M. and Malone, P.S.J. (1994) *Surgery of the newborn.* Edinburgh: Churchill Livingstone.

Jones P.G. and Woodward, A.A. (1986) *Clinical paediatric surgery*, 3rd edn. Melbourne: Blackwell Scientific Publications.

Rickham, P.P., Lister, J. and Irving I.M. (1978) *Neonatal surgery*, 2nd edn. London: Butterworth and Co.

Spicer, R.D. (1982) Infantile hypertrophic pyloric stenosis: a review. *Br. J. Surg.* **69**, 128–35.

# 10

# Neonatal respiratory problems

Causes of respiratory disease
Care of the baby with respiratory symptoms
Continuous positive airway pressure (CPAP)
Mechanical ventilation
High-frequency oscillatory ventilation (HFOV)
The pulmonary circulation
Chronic lung disease
Recurrent apnoea

Many neonatal cardiac and respiratory disorders can present with identical clinical signs of tachypnoea, grunting, chest wall retraction and cyanosis. Although supportive care for the various disorders is similar, a definitive diagnosis is necessary to refine treatment appropriately.

## CAUSES OF RESPIRATORY DISEASE

Conditions which present with signs of 'respiratory distress' (not to be confused with respiratory distress syndrome) are listed in Table 10.1. It is usually possible to distinguish between the different conditions, based on history, clinical examination and radiological appearances.

**Table 10.1** Causes of respiratory distress

---

Disorders presenting with one or more of the physical signs of tachypnoea, grunting, retraction of the chest wall, cyanosis (some of these conditions may also present with shock, hypoventilation or apnoea)

| | |
|---|---|
| Respiratory distress syndrome (surfactant deficiency) | Diaphragmatic hernia |
| Transient tachypnoea/wet lung | Choanal atresia |
| Meconium aspiration | Congenital heart defects |
| Other aspiration syndromes (amniotic fluid, blood, milk) | Cardiac failure |
| Pneumothorax | Myocarditis |
| Pneumomediastinum | Persistent fetal circulation |
| Interstitial emphysema | Polycythaemia |
| Pneumonia (especially Group B streptococcal infection) | Anaemia |
| Pulmonary haemorrhage | Hypoglycaemia |
| Atelectasis | Hypothermia |
| Wilson-Mikity syndrome | Septicaemia/meningitis |
| Pulmonary hypoplasia (e.g. Potter's syndrome) | Drugs (e.g. diazepam, opiates, etc.) given to mother in labour |
| Lung anomalies (e.g. cysts, sequestered lobe, adenomatous malformation) | Birth asphyxia, cerebral oedema/ haemorrhage/trauma |
| | Neuromuscular disorder (myasthenia gravis, myotonic dystrophy) |

---

The relevant features of the more important differential diagnoses are given below.

## Respiratory distress syndrome (RDS)

RDS is a common disorder of preterm infants, and is associated with surfactant deficiency in the immature lung.

### Presentation

- Commoner following Caesarean section, birth asphyxia and hypothermia.
- Onset of grunting, retraction and tachypnoea within 1 hour of birth.
- There may be reduced breath sounds or bronchial breathing on auscultation.
- Signs persist beyond 24 hours of age, but the natural history is for recovery to start within 96 hours.

**Radiology**

- Chest X-ray shows a reticulogranular appearance with an air bronchogram.
- Pneumothorax and pneumonia are common complications.

**Special features/comments**

- Administration of steroids to the mother before preterm delivery can reduce the incidence of RDS by 40–60% and also reduce the incidence of PVH, NEC and neonatal death.

## Transient tachypnoea of the newborn (TTN)

Usually occurs in term infants with mature lungs but delayed clearance of lung fluid.

**Presentation**

- Often occurs after delivery by Caesarean section.
- Onset of tachypnoea and mild grunting within 2 to 3 hours of birth.

**Radiology**

- Chest X-ray shows coarse streaking and fluid in the interlobar fissures ('wet lung').

**Special features/comments**

- Usually requires 30–40% $O_2$; occasionally CPAP.
- May persist for 3 or 4 days.

## Meconium aspiration syndrome

Occurs in 5% of infants with meconium-stained liquor.

**Presentation**

- Fetal hypoxia/distress leads to passage of meconium into amniotic fluid.
- Inhalation may cause mechanical airway obstruction, chemical pneumonitis and inactivation of surfactant.
- Respiratory distress may be severe.
- Often complicated by pulmonary hypertension which exacerbates hypoxaemia.

### Radiology

- Chest X-ray shows hyperinflation of lungs with coarse streaking and patchy consolidation.
- Pneumothorax, pneumomediastinum and pneumonia are common complications.

### Special features/comments

- Immediate nasopharyngeal suction at delivery, followed by endotracheal suctioning where indicated (see Chapter 2) is an effective preventative measure.
- Apparent 'meconium staining' may occur with fetal *Listeria monocytogenes* infection.

## Air leaks (alveolar rupture)

Pneumothorax, pneumomediastinum and interstitial emphysema may be spontaneous but more often follow active resuscitation, artificial ventilation or CPAP.

### Presentation

- Occurs in babies with aspiration syndromes, RDS or pulmonary hypoplasia.
- A small air leak may be associated with minimal clinical signs, but a tension pneumothorax usually leads to cardiorespiratory collapse.
- Diagnosis may be aided by transillumination of the thorax with a cold-light source; the pneumothorax shows as increased transillumination.

### Radiology

- Diagnosis is confirmed by chest X-ray, including a lateral shoot-through view.

### Special features/comments

- In an emergency, consider needle-aspiration of air (see Chapter 27).
- Small spontaneous pneumothoraces in term infants with minimal or no symptoms will usually require no active treatment.

## Congenital pneumonia

May occur at any gestation and commonly, but not always, associated with prolonged rupture of membranes. Associated with septicaemia, usually with group B streptococcus.

### Presentation

- Mimics RDS with identical chest X-ray appearances.
- Onset of respiratory distress within 3 hours of birth; but presentation may be delayed for 24–48 hours.
- May be associated with shock and apnoea.

### Special features/comments

- Survival depends on intensive support and early use of broad-spectrum antibiotics (we use penicillin and netilmicin).
- Causal organisms may be identified in blood cultures and gastric aspirate.

## Pulmonary haemorrhage

Usually haemorrhagic pulmonary oedema presenting as frothy, blood-stained fluid coming from the trachea or endotracheal tube.
Associated with:

- asphyxia;
- hypothermia;
- infection;
- congenital heart disease;
- severe rhesus isoimmunization;
- haemorrhagic states such as DIC;
- administration of exogenous surfactant (8% in published studies).

## Pleural effusion

Uncommon.

### Presentation

- If unilateral, there may be mediastinal shift and reduced breath sounds.
- Causes include chylothorax, hydrops fetalis, pneumonia and heart failure.
- Diagnosis is confirmed by pleurocentesis (see Chapter 27).

### Radiology

- Chest X-ray shows opaque lung field with obliteration of costophrenic angle.

### Special features/comments

- May be diagnosed antenatally on ultrasound scan.

## Diaphragmatic hernia

### Presentation

- Respiratory symptoms vary from severe to none.
- May present at birth or after several hours.
- Usually left-sided with mediastinal shift to the right.
- Abdomen is commonly scaphoid.

### Radiology

- Chest X-ray shows bowel-gas pattern in thoracic cavity; absent hemidiaphragm.

### Special features/comments

- Right-sided hernias are difficult to diagnose as the mediastinal shift is not so obvious.
- Bowel sounds in the chest are late and unreliable signs.

## Cystic adenomatoid malformation

A rare malformation of the lung, presenting as a large cystic mass, predominantly in the upper and middle lobes, and nearly always unilateral.

### Presentation

- Half the babies are preterm and hydramnios or hydrops fetalis occurs in 30% of cases.
- Presents with respiratory distress from birth, and may be confused with diaphragmatic hernia.

### Radiology

- Three types depending on the size of cysts:
    - I – multiple large cysts resembling lobar emphysema;
    - II – medium cysts, often associated with other malformations, e.g. hydranencephaly, prune-belly syndrome;
    - III – small cysts appearing as a solid mass on chest X-ray.

**Special features/comments**

- Treatment is by lobectomy.

# Congenital lobar emphysema

Over-expansion of part of a lung due to external bronchial compression by cysts, tumours or aberrant vessels, or internal obstruction due to mucosal folds, plugs or stenosis.

### Presentation

- Usually involves only a single lobe (50% left upper, 28% right middle, 20% right upper).
- Half the cases are symptomatic in the neonatal period.
- 15% have coexisting cardiac abnormality.

### Radiology

- Chest X-ray may show a solid mass on day 1 due to retained lung fluid.
- It then becomes hyperexpanded with emphysema and mediastinal shift.

### Special features/comments

- Bronchoscopy may aid diagnosis and clear mucous plugs, but treatment is usually surgical.
- Insertion of a chest drain is dangerous.

# Acquired lobar emphysema

Localized cystic emphysema is usually associated with RDS complicated by interstitial emphysema in preterm infants.

### Presentation

- Most often affects the right lung.
- Onset may be delayed for several weeks.

### Radiology

- Chest X-ray shows large cystic area and mediastinal shift.

### Special features/comments

- Bronchoscopy and lavage may identify acquired bronchial stenosis and aid removal of mucous plugs by lavage.
- Selective bronchial intubation to collapse the hyperinflated lung for 2–3 days may be tried in severe or progressive cases.

- Acquired stenoses can be treated by endobronchial balloon dilatation.
- Surgery is rarely indicated.
- Do not insert a chest drain.

## Pulmonary hypoplasia

Associated with oligohydramnios of any cause, e.g. renal agenesis/ dysplasia, obstructive uropathy or prolonged rupture of membranes.

### Presentation

- Respiratory failure is often severe.
- Pneumothorax and persistent pulmonary hypertension are common.
- Also associated with diaphragmatic hernia, pleural effusion, thoracic skeletal dysplasias and neuromuscular disorders.

## CARE OF THE BABY WITH RESPIRATORY SYMPTOMS

### In the delivery room (see Chapter 2)

Prompt and effective resuscitation will reduce the severity of subsequent respiratory disease. Our policy is to intubate preterm infants (< 30 weeks' gestation) electively in the delivery room prior to transfer to the NICU for further assessment.

### In the neonatal intensive care unit

A suitable *supporting environment* is an essential prerequisite to more active and specific interventions

*Thermoneutral environment* The infant should be nursed in an incubator set to maintain a skin temperature of 36.5 °C (see Chapter 5).

*Oxygenation* Give humidified oxygen via a headbox and use a transcutaneous $O_2$ monitor or pulse oximeter initially to assess oxygenation. If the infant is given > 40% oxygen or the respiratory signs persist beyond the age of 4 hours, an arterial line should be inserted into an umbilical or peripheral artery (see p. 405). Continuous monitoring of $PaO_2$ using an intra-arterial electrode or

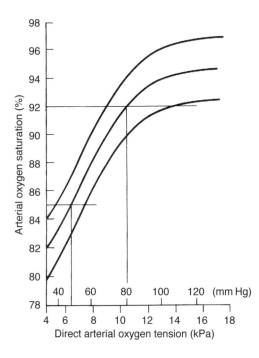

**Fig. 10.1** Comparison of 125 paired measurements of transcutaneous arterial oxygen saturation and arterial oxygen tension. The fitted mean curve ± 2 SD is shown. Adapted from Wasana, A. and Whitelaw, A.G.L. (1987) *Arch. Dis. Child.* **62**, 957–71.

$TcPO_2$ is valuable. However, no matter which technique is used, $PaO_2$, $PaCO_2$ and pH should be measured every 4–6 hours and 30 min after any change in management. The measurement of $SaO_2$ using a pulse oximeter is now a routine adjunct to the above, but may lead to unrecognized hyperoxaemia or hypoxaemia (see Fig. 10.1). Aim to keep $SaO_2$ in the range 85–92%.

***Blood pressure and perfusion*** Measure blood pressure regularly and assess perfusion by clinical assessment (core-peripheral temperature, capillary filling, skin colour) and measuring acid-base status. Avoid hypotension (see Fig. 29.1; as a working guide, mean arterial BP (mm Hg) = gestational age in weeks). Oscillometric blood pressure monitors consistently over-read in sick, very-low-birthweight infants and hypotension may be missed; continuous intra-arterial monitoring is more reliable. If the blood pressure is low, give a plasma expander (10–15 mL/kg) over 1 hour.

**Fluids** Delay enteral feeding. Start a peripheral intravenous infusion of 10% dextrose at 60–80 mL/kg/day.

**Minimal handling** Any disturbance of a sick baby may cause apnoea or a fall in $PaO_2$ or blood pressure. Use electronic monitors to record heart rate, respiration, and temperature and non-invasive oxygen monitors ($TcPO_2$ or $SaO_2$). Nurse in the prone position.

### Investigations

- Send blood for culture and start i.v. broad-spectrum antibiotics.
- Measure blood sugar 4- to 6- hourly (BMstix).
- Arrange A-P supine chest X-ray (and abdominal X-ray if umbilical arterial catheter inserted).
- Do a full blood count every 2–3 days.
- Measure urea, electrolytes and creatinine daily.

**Monitoring** Keep a flow chart at the cotside on which are recorded observations of vital signs, $FiO_2$, ventilator settings and blood gas results. Keep a cumulative record of all blood taken from the baby for investigations.

### Respiratory management

See the flowchart in Fig. 10.2. Start at the top with the baby in 40% oxygen and manage according to blood gas results.

## CONTINUOUS POSITIVE AIRWAY PRESSURE (CPAP)

### Indications

We use CPAP for the following indications.

- **RDS** CPAP should be started if the $PaO_2$ is below 50 mm Hg (6.5 kPa) in $FiO_2 \geqslant 0.40$. Early use of CPAP, preferably within 4 hours of birth, may reduce the severity of subsequent respiratory disease.
- **Recurrent apnoeas** By increasing respiratory drive, CPAP is an effective way to reduce or abolish apnoeic attacks.
- **Weaning from ventilation** By reducing post-extubation atelactasis, nasal CPAP may reduce the need for re-intubation.

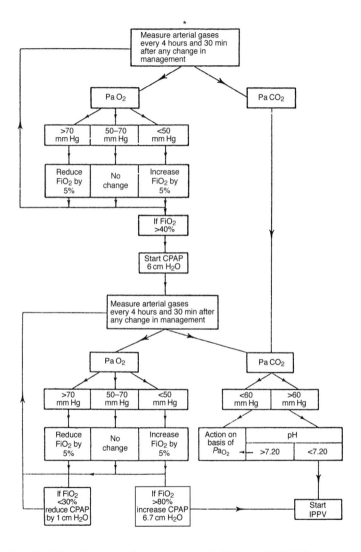

**Fig. 10.2** Flow chart for respiratory management of infants with RDS. Start at point marked*, with infant in 40% oxygen by headbox. To convert blood gas tensions in mm Hg to kPa, multiply by 0.13.

### Methods of applying CPAP

CPAP is usually administered via nasal prongs, either single or double, or sometimes by face mask. Endotracheal CPAP increases the work of breathing by increasing dead space, and prevents the infant from using upper airway closure to maintain lung volume at end-expiration. Hence, especially for small infants, we use low-rate IMV (2–5 bpm) to provide reflation of the lungs. For the same reasons, never leave an open endotracheal tube in place without CPAP/IMV.

Figure 10.3 shows the circuit diagram of a system for delivering CPAP using nasal cannulae, endotracheal tube or face mask. CPAP can also be given using any ventilator with an IMV circuit.

Figure 10.4 shows the EME Infant Flow Driver circuit for double nasal prong CPAP. This system provides a more stable pressure directly down the nostrils with low added work of breathing, and is well tolerated by infants.

### Nasal CPAP for treating RDS

- Use the EME Infant Flow Driver system with double nasal prongs (three sizes available). If this is not available, use Portex or INCA twin prongs – all are available in a variety of sizes.

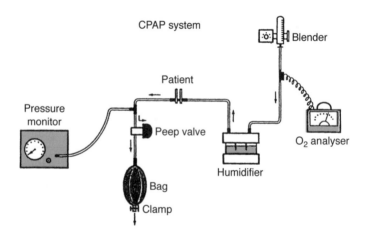

**Fig. 10.3** Diagrammatic representation of CPAP circuit. Suitable for applying CPAP by nasal prong, endotracheal tube or face mask. (NB The pressure monitor should be attached to the flow circuit as close as possible to the baby).

- Start with $FiO_2$ 0.50; CPAP 5–6 cm $H_2O$ (for the Infant Flow Driver, the pressure is regulated by the gas flow).
- Insert a 6FG orogastric tube to reduce gastric distension. Leave the end open *and* aspirate 2-hourly.
- Measure arterial blood gases within 30 min of starting CPAP and 4-to 6-hourly thereafter as shown in Fig. 10.2.
- If the $PaO_2$ is too low, $FiO_2$ can be increased gradually to 0.80 and CPAP increased up to 7–8 cm $H_2O$. If the $PaO_2$ falls below 45 mm Hg (5.8 kPa) on these settings or the $PaCO_2$ rises above 60 mm Hg (7.8 kPa), then the baby should be intubated and ventilated.
- Tension pneumothorax may complicate CPAP, and should always be suspected if the baby's condition deteriorates.

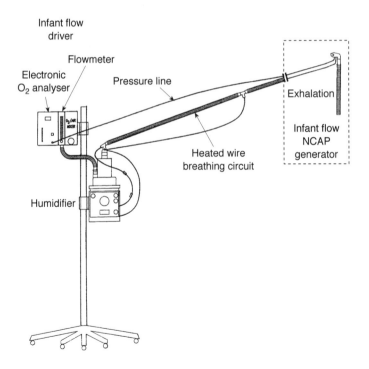

**Fig. 10.4** Infant Flow Driver System for Nasal CPAP (Reproduced with permission from Electro Medical Equipment Ltd, 60 Gladstone Place, Brighton BN2 3QD, UK).

- When the baby's condition improves, gradually reduce the $FiO_2$ and pressure (we suggest decrements of 5–10% in $FiO_2$ and 1–2 cm $H_2O$ in CPAP). Stop treatment when CPAP is 3 cm $H_2O$ and $FiO_2$ is 0.30.

## MECHANICAL VENTILATION

### Indications

Try to anticipate the need for ventilation rather than let the baby deteriorate to the state where it becomes an emergency. The indications will usually be obvious, e.g. apnoea. In the management of respiratory distress syndrome or recurrent apnoea, CPAP should be tried first. If the $PaO_2$ is < 40 mm Hg (5.2 kPa) despite CPAP 7–8 cm $H_2O$ and $FiO_2$ 0.8, or the $PaCO_2$ is 60 mm Hg (7.8 kPa) and the pH is < 7.20, the infant should be ventilated.

### General principles of neonatal ventilation

The aim of ventilation is to establish adequate gas exchange – oxygenation and $CO_2$ removal – whilst minimizing the risks of adverse effects, such as air leaks (pneumothorax, interstitial emphysema), chronic lung disease and the risks of hyperoxaemia (retinopathy of prematurity). Although many different ventilators are available, the fundamental principles of mechanical ventilation relate to the mechanical and physiological properties of the respiratory system and the pulmonary circulation.

#### Elastic properties of the respiratory system

The compliance (or stiffness) of the lungs can be described by a static pressure-volume curve (see Fig. 10.5) which has a characteristic sigmoid shape. The slope of this curve is equivalent to pulmonary compliance. The following points should be noted.

- The increment in pressure ($\Delta P$) required to inflate the lungs by a set volume ($\Delta V$) is greatest when the lungs are collapsed (at low lung volumes) or stretched (at high lung volumes).
- The pressure required to maintain a given lung volume is less during expiration than during inspiration (hysteresis).
- The slope of the pressure-volume relationship changes with lung disease, becoming flatter as the lungs become stiff, i.e. as compliance falls.

Ventilation should therefore aim to maintain lung volumes on the linear (central) part of the pressure-volume curve, thereby minimizing the ΔP required to maintain tidal volume exchanges. Once optimal lung volumes have been achieved, it may be possible to reduce ventilator pressures due to hysteresis, although this effect is generally reduced in lung disease with low pulmonary compliance.

### Distribution of ventilation

Resting lung volume is determined by the equilibrium between the elastic recoil of the lungs (the lungs' tendency to collapse) and the outward recoil, of the chest wall. Infants have compliant chest walls which offer less outward recoil and there is a tendency for air spaces in the dependent portions of the lung to collapse at end-expiration. As their volume falls, these parts of the lung become stiff and require high opening pressures.

Spontaneously breathing infants can use upper airways closure to maintain lung volumes during expiration (which may be manifested as 'grunting'), but intubated infants lose this ability and positive

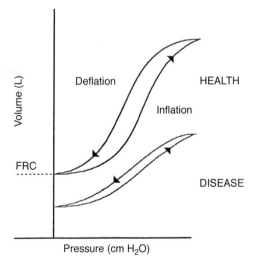

**Fig. 10.5** Typical pressure–volume relationships of the respiratory system in health and disease. With progressive lung disease, lung volume falls at a given inflation pressure, the slope (compliance) of the curve decreases, and there is less difference in inflation and deflation pressures for any given lung volume.

airway pressure (PEEP) must be applied to prevent airway closure in the lungs.

The rate at which the lungs or parts of the lung fill and empty is dependent on both pulmonary compliance and resistance to gas flow. The product of compliance (C) and resistance (R) is referred to as the time constant (which is the unit of time taken for a 63% change in volume to occur). In health this is relatively constant for all lung areas, but in lung disease there are likely to be considerable regional differences in time constants. This leads to abnormal distribution of ventilation. During mechanical ventilation:

- sufficient inspiratory time should be allowed for gas to be distributed to areas of lung with long time constants;
- expiratory time constants will increase in conditions associated with high airway resistance, e.g. meconium aspiration, bronchopulmonary dysplasia, and also as compliance increases during recovery from RDS. At fast ventilator rates, expiratory time may be insufficient for complete emptying of some lung areas. This leads to *inadvertent PEEP* as inspiration commences before expiration is complete and gas trapping occurs.

### Setting up the ventilator

Initial ventilation settings will depend on a number of factors, including the type of ventilator used, the baby's size and gestation, and the clinical diagnosis. The initial settings will almost certainly need to be adjusted to those which best suit the individual baby, and will need to be modified further as the baby's condition changes, particularly if complications such as emphysema or pneumothorax develop. However, there are certain basic principles to be considered. The following apply to time-cycled, pressure-limited ventilators which are capable of applying a positive end-expiratory pressure (PEEP) and intermittent mandatory ventilation (IMV).

***Mean airway pressure (MAP)*** Oxygenation is closely related to MAP which is calculated from the equation:

$$MAP = ([PIP - PEEP] \times [T_i/(T_i + T_e)]) + PEEP$$

MAP can therefore be altered by changes in the applied pressures during inspiration (PIP) and expiration (PEEP), and also by changes in the I:E ratio (which determines the fraction of the respiratory

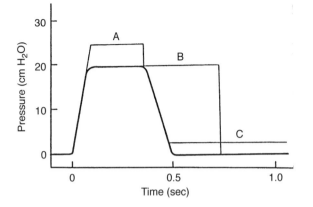

**Fig. 10.6** Airway pressure wave-form generated by a time-cycled, pressure-limited constant-flow generating ventilator (see text). Mean airway pressure (and hence oxygenation) may be increased by (A) increasing peak inspiratory pressure, (B) prolonging inspiratory time or (C) increasing PEEP. Adapted from Reynolds, E.O.R. (1974) in Keuskamp, D.H. (ed.) *Neonatal and Pediatric Ventilation*. Boston, MA: Little, Brown and Co.

cycle spent at the higher pressure). When making adjustments to ventilator settings, it is important to stop and think about how these changes will affect MAP (see Fig. 10.6).

*Peak inspiratory pressure (PIP)* An increase in PIP will improve oxygenation by increasing MAP. It will also increase tidal volume by increasing $\Delta P$, and lead to increased $CO_2$ removal. However, high $\Delta P$ applied to the alveoli leads to greater shearing forces on the epithelium, contributing to the development of chronic lung disease, and may cause air leaks. As a rule, try to keep PIP < 25 cm $H_2O$ if possible and rarely exceed PIP > 30 cm $H_2O$ unless absolutely necessary.

*Positive end-expiratory pressure (PEEP)* An increase in PEEP will improve oxygenation by increasing MAP. Its effect on tidal volume may be a reduction due to decreased $\Delta P$ but, by maintaining alveolar patency at end-expiration, lung volumes may be kept on a more advantageous part of the pressure-volume relationship and $V_T$ may increase. The optimal PEEP for infants with RDS is usually 5–6 cm $H_2O$. Higher settings may lead to reductions in ventilation and $CO_2$

retention, and may also compromise venous return to the heart by the rise in intrathoracic positive pressure.

**I:E ratio** A prolonged inspiratory time $(T_i)$ will improve oxygenation by its effect on MAP, and in some circumstances may improve the regional distribution of ventilation. The usual ratio used in RDS is 1:1 to 1:2, but *inverse* ratios of 1.5:1 or even 2:1 may be used in severe RDS with slow ventilator rates ($< 40$ bpm). It is better to consider actual inspiratory time rather than I:E ratio, and the $T_i$ is usually kept within the range 0.3–1.0 sec.

**Frequency** (ventilator rate) At conventional frequencies, minute ventilation is the product of tidal volume $(V_T)$ minus dead space $(V_D)$ and ventilator frequency $(f)$.

$$V_A = (V_T - V_D) \cdot f$$

Increasing the frequency of ventilation will increase minute ventilation and lead to increased $CO_2$ removal. If the I:E ratio remains unchanged, increases in ventilator frequency should have no effect on MAP. However, the above equation assumes *square wave* pressure generation which may not be achieved at higher rates, leading to a reduction of MAP. Moreover, at high frequencies with no reduction in I:E ratio, $T_e$ may become insufficient for complete expiration and gas trapping will occur.

Ventilator rates of 60–120 bpm may reduce the incidence of pneumothorax, possibly by inducing the baby to breathe in synchrony with the ventilator. This may be achieved more readily by the use of trigger ventilation modes (*q.v.*). Higher rates may also be associated with improved oxygenation, particularly in the presence of severe pulmonary interstitial emphysema (PIE), but there is little evidence that rates over 60 bpm are beneficial.

**Oxygen** High $FiO_2 > 0.8$ causes resorption atelectasis by displacing nitrogen from alveoli. Because nitrogen is poorly taken up across the alveolar capillary membrane, it acts to *splint* the airway. Atelectasis will lead to an increased shunt fraction $(Q_p/Q_s)$ due to perfusion of non-ventilated lung units, causing a fall in oxygenation and loss of lung volume. Higher pressures are then required to maintain minute ventilation. There is some evidence that high $FiO_2$ causes impaired mucociliary clearance, reduced antiprotease concentrations potentiating lung inflammatory damage, and increased microvascular leakage in the air spaces. Try to improve oxygenation by better

ventilation, including optimization of ventilation/perfusion matching, rather than by turning up the $FiO_2$ to > 0.8, although sometimes
this is unavoidable.

*Patient-triggered ventilation* Spontaneously breathing infants are
often observed to breathe out of synchrony with imposed, time-
cycled ventilator breaths. This reduces the efficiency of ventilation by
varying the tidal volume delivered by preset inspiratory pressures,
and may lead to transient high pulmonary pressures with the
consequent risk of alveolar rupture. The problem of ventilatory
asynchrony may be addressed by increasing ventilator frequency or
by sedating the infant. The alternative approach is to trigger the
ventilated breath to the onset of the infant's spontaneous
inspiration.

Ventilator breaths may be initiated by detection of:

- inspiratory flow;
- a predetermined inspired volume;
- a pressure drop within the airway.

In practice, most infant ventilators are flow-triggered, which has
been demonstrated to achieve better ventilatory response than
pressure-triggering. Ventilators vary in their trigger delay times and
trigger work, and these measurements may also be affected by the
ventilatory demand of the baby. Suboptimal conditions for patient
flow-triggering may be met when ventilatory demand is high,
particularly in the presence of a small ET tube diameter (e.g.
2.5 mm). The infant should be carefully observed when patient-
triggered ventilation is started to ensure that adequate triggering is
occurring, ventilatory asynchrony is reduced or abolished, and there
are no adverse effects on oxygenation, heart rate or blood pressure.

Patient-triggered ventilation (PTV) has been demonstrated to
reduce significantly the proportion of asynchronous breaths in
spontaneously breathing ventilated infants, and is associated with
improved minute ventilation and oxygenation compared to conventional ventilation. Reductions in blood pressure variability during
PTV may have implications for the risk of periventricular haemorrhage (see p. 203).

Patient-triggered ventilation can be set up using similar pressure
and $FiO_2$ settings to conventional, pressure-limited ventilation. During the acute phase of respiratory distress, when the lungs are stiff
and ventilatory demand is high, the trigger is usually set to maximum sensitivity and the $T_i$ is set to 0.3–0.45 sec, depending on the

baby's respiratory rate. During the recovery phase, weaning may be achieved by:

- switching to synchronous intermittent mandatory ventilation (SIMV);
- decreasing PIP and continuing to support each breath.

There is no evidence that weaning is achieved more rapidly or more successfully by progressive reduction of PIP compared with weaning the rate of SIMV.

**Exogenous surfactant** Several preparations of replacement surfactant are available. They fall into two broad groups; artificial surfactants (e.g. Exosurf, ALEC) and natural surfactants from either porcine (e.g. Curosurf) or bovine (e.g. Survanta) sources. There is clear evidence that the use of exogenous surfactant in infants with RDS is associated with reductions in mortality and morbidity. Surfactant is associated with short-term improvements in pulmonary mechanics and oxygenation and with a reduction in the incidence of alveolar leaks resulting in pneumothorax or PIE. However, there is little evidence that the use of exogenous surfactant in RDS has resulted in a decreased incidence of chronic lung disease.

Standard two-dose surfactant regimens at 12-hour intervals have been compared with 3–4 dose regimens for both natural and synthetic surfactants. No differences in major outcomes such as mortality, pneumothorax or BPD rates have been demonstrated. There is some evidence that natural surfactant is associated with improved short-term outcomes, including oxygen requirement, mortality and retinopathy of prematurity. There is also a difference in the time-course of changes in respiratory mechanics following surfactant treatment, with natural surfactant significantly improving compliance in the 12 hours following administration.

**Surfactant dosage and administration** All are given down the endotracheal tube using a syringe and catheter.

- **ALEC** (Pumactant) – 100 mg (1.2 mL) repeated after 1 and 24 hours.
- **Curosurf** (Poractant) – 100 mg/kg (1.25 mL/kg). Two further doses of 100 mg/kg may be given after 12 and 24 hours.
- **Exosurf** (Colfosceril) – 67.5 mg/kg (5 mL/kg) repeated after 12 and 24 hours.
- **Survanta** (Beractant) – 100 mg/kg (4 mL/kg) repeated 6-hourly for up to 4 doses.

*Timing* The earlier the first dose is given the better. Prophylactic surfactant given immediately after birth has advantages, but results in some babies being treated unnecessarily. Try to give the first dose by 2 hours of age (early rescue). Beware of acute deterioration in the first few minutes after administration.

Monitor blood gases frequently and be prepared to adjust $FiO_2$ and ventilator settings rapidly as the baby's condition often improves rapidly.

## Initial ventilator settings

These will depend on the disorder for which the baby is to be ventilated and the gestation. Settings should be individualized for each baby. For example, a high PEEP and prolonged inspiratory time would be detrimental to a baby with normal lung compliance who is ventilated for apnoea, meconium aspiration or alveolar rupture. A suggested range of initial settings is given below.

**1** $FiO_2$ 0.4–0.5

**2** Inspiratory time 0.4–0.6 sec $\qquad$ Frequency (rate) 50–75/min

I:E ratio 1:1

**3** Expiratory time 0.4–0.6 sec

**4** Inspiratory pressure (PIP) 18–20 cm $H_2O$

**5** Expiratory pressure (PEEP) 4 cm $H_2O$

**Example**
Pressure 20/4 cm $H_2O$
Rate 50/min
$T_i = T_e = 0.6$ sec
$MAP = ((20 - 4) \times (0.6/1.2)) + 4$
$= 12$ cm $H_2O$

Measure blood gases 30 min after starting ventilation and adjust the settings to manipulate MAP and minute ventilation so that you keep $PaO_2$ in the range 50–80 mm Hg (6.5–10.4 kPa) and $PaCO_2$ in the range 35–50 mm Hg (4.5–6.5 kPa), respectively. It is not necessary to have perfect blood gases and there is evidence that vigorous ventilation to keep $PaCO_2$ in the normal range is associated with an increased risk of chronic lung disease (BPD).

### Troubleshooting

**Sudden clinical deterioration** Usually accompanied by a fall in $PaO_2$ ± a rise in $PaCO_2$.

**Action:** disconnect ventilator and use a manual inflation bag.

(1) *Baby's condition improves*: presume deterioration due to a ventilator problem.

> Possible causes:
> mechanical or electrical failure;
> disconnected tube or leaking connection;
> excess condensation in patient circuit;
> fall in $FiO_2$.

**Action:** correct fault or replace ventilator.

(2) *Baby's condition remains poor*: presume a problem with the baby.

> Possible causes:
> ET tube blocked or displaced;
> pneumothorax.

**Action:** suck ET tube; check breath sounds and chest movement bilaterally. If no improvement, reintubate immediately.

- Transilluminate chest; urgent AP and lateral chest X-ray.
- If condition is critical, needle pleural spaces to relieve possible pneumothorax (see Chapter 27).

**Gradual deterioration** Usually accompanied by a slow rise in $PaCO_2$. This may also be due to a blocked tube or alveolar leak, and these should be excluded first.

Other possible causes:

*Inappropriate ventilator settings*

1 Due to progressive deterioration in disease state: consider increasing peak inspiratory pressure, inspiratory time, rate or $FiO_2$.
2 Due to improvement in disease state: consider reduction in peak inspiratory pressure, PEEP or inspiratory time.

*Ventilator asynchrony (baby 'fighting' ventilator)*

Reconsider the need for ventilation. If IPPV is essential, then consider the following:

**1** patient-triggered ventilation (*see above.*)
**2** raising the ventilator rate to 80–100 bpm may cause the baby's breathing efforts to synchronize with the ventilator breaths, thus avoiding the need for sedation or muscle relaxants;
**3** sedation with or without muscle relaxants. NB The ventilator settings may need to be significantly increased when the baby is sedated or given muscle relaxants, as its own efforts are no longer contributing to ventilation or maintenance of lung volume.

*Periventricular haemorrhage* Check PCV for sudden fall and ultrasound brain scan.

*Patent ductus arteriosus* (see Chapter 11).

*Infection* Do a full septic screen and X-ray chest. Consider antibiotic therapy (see Chapter 17).

*Hypotension* Check BP, and if low (see p.465) give colloid (10–15 mL/kg).

*Anaemia* Check PCV and haemoglobin concentration. If PCV < 40% or Hb < 10 g/dL, transfuse.

*Metabolic imbalance* Check blood urea, electrolytes, calcium, glucose and bilirubin.

*Poor environmental support* Avoid excessive handling. Ensure that the baby is in a thermoneutral environment (see Chapter 5).

**Refractory hypoxaemia** If the $PaO_2$ remains below 40 mm Hg (5.2 kPa) despite apparently adequate ventilation and $FiO_2 > 0.8$, this may be due to the baby 'fighting' or breathing asynchronously with the ventilator, increased shunt fraction due to lung collapse, or pulmonary arterial hypertension with right-to-left shunting at the level of the foramen ovale and/or ductus arteriosus.

Consider the following:

**1** increasing the ventilator rate to 60–80/min;
**2** sedation and/or muscle relaxation (see Table 10.2)

| Possible benefits: | Possible dangers: |
|---|---|
| • improved gas exchange; | • worse gas exchange; |
| • less barotrauma; | • increased ventilator requirements; |
| • more stable $PaO_2$; | • tachycardia/hypotension; |
| • less risk of IVH; | • jaundice; |
| | • drug interaction (pancuronium + gentamicin). |

**Table 10.2** Drugs used for (a) sedation and (b) muscle relaxation in ventilated infants

(a) Sedatives

| Drug | Dose (range) | |
|------|------|------|
| | i.v. bolus | i.v. infusion |
| Morphine | 100 mcg/kg | 5–20 mcg/kg/hour |
| Diamorphine | 180 mcg/kg | 10–40 mcg/kg/hour |
| Fentanyl* | 15 mcg/kg | 2–8 mcg/kg/hour |
| Midazolam | 100 mcg/kg | 50–100 mcg/kg/hour |

(b) Muscle relaxants

| Drug | Dose (range) |
|------|------|
| Pancuronium | 50–100 mcg/kg i.v. bolus |
| Vecuronium | 100 mcg/kg i.v. bolus |
| | 50–150 mcg/kg/hour i.v. infusion |
| Atracurium | 0.5 mg/kg i.v. bolus |
| | 5–10 mcg/kg/min i.v. infusion |

Short-acting drugs, when given by infusion over long periods, may accumulate and cause withdrawal symptoms or prolonged neuromuscular blockade.

* Fentanyl is the least likely of opioids to cause systemic hypotension. Higher doses have been associated with chest wall rigidity.

**3** patient-triggered ventilation (see above, p.149);
**4** high frequency oscillation (see below, p.155);
**5** pulmonary vasodilators (see below, p.162).

## Nursing care of the intubated infant

### Initial assessment

- All infants who are receiving mechanical ventilation will initially require analgesia/sedation (see Table 10.2).
- Check that the ETT is secure.
- Cut spare ETT to the appropriate length and leave taped to the incubator, remaining within the packet. This will facilitate earlier re-intubation should accidental extubation occur.
- Check that suction units are in working order and appropriate sized catheters are available.

### Routine observations and activities

- Check and record ventilator settings hourly.
- Check humidity, temperature and water level hourly.
- Listen to breath sounds (usually 2- to 4- hourly).
- Perform ETT suction as appropriate. The frequency will be determined by the baby's condition and type of ventilatory support. For children with RDS it is usually unnecessary to suction ETT for 24–48 hours after birth, and then only as required. Use a tape measure attached to the incubator to determine the suction distance (pass suction catheter no more than 1 cm beyond the end of the ETT to avoid damage to bronchial mucosa.
- At routine care (usually 6- to 8-hourly):
  change the baby's position and perform all care – positioning may be important to optimize ventilation; infants can be nursed prone if this improves oxygenation or ventilation; the head should be positioned to prevent movement of the ETT; aspirate gastric tube;
  empty excess water from tubing;
  ensure that tubing connections are secure and not kinked.

### Weaning from ventilation

When the baby's condition has improved as demonstrated by a consistent $PaO_2$ over 70 mm Hg (9.1 kPa) and $PaCO_2$ below 45–50 mm Hg (5.9–6.5 kPa), start to reduce the PIP and $FiO_2$ gradually in alternate steps. When the $FiO_2$ is < 0.5 and PIP is < 20 cm $H_2O$, stop giving sedation and muscle relaxants and allow their effects to wear off.

For weaning via synchronous (patient-triggered) ventilator modes, see p.149.

Weaning using conventional modes:

- Reduce $T_i$ gradually to 0.3 sec, and at the same time maintain or decrease the frequency by prolonging $T_e$.
- Maintain $T_i$ at 0.3 sec, reduce PIP to 12–14 cm $H_2O$, and reduce $FiO_2$. Consider the use of aminophylline or caffeine.
- When the rate is 5/min, $FiO_2$ < 0.35 and pressure 12–14/3–4, extubate to either headbox oxygen or nasal CPAP.

## HIGH FREQUENCY OSCILLATORY VENTILATION (HFOV)

Because conventional ventilation relies on the production of large pressure changes to induce mass flow of gas in and out of the lungs, it may be associated with deleterious consequences of volume and pressure changes at alveolar level. These include air leaks, such as PIE and pneumothorax, and bronchiolo-alveolar injury leading to chronic lung disease. The use of high-frequency ventilation at low tidal volumes ($V_T < V_D$) allows the primary goals of ventilation, oxygenation and $CO_2$ removal to be achieved without the costs of pressure-induced lung injury.

The strategy of high-frequency oscillatory ventilation (HFOV) depends on:

- inflation of the lungs and recruitment of lung volume by the application of distending pressure (mean airway pressure (MAP));
- alveolar ventilation and $CO_2$ removal by the imposition of an oscillating pressure waveform on the MAP.

By recruitment of 'lung units' which are not contributing to gas exchange, oxygenation will be improved by increasing the surface area available for gas exchange through increased ventilated lung volume, and optimizing ventilation perfusion matching by the effects of optimal lung inflation on pulmonary vascular resistance (PVR). At low lung volumes, intrapulmonary vessels have a small cross-sectional area and PVR is high. Lung inflation results in radial traction on pulmonary vessels, leading to a reduction in PVR. However, overdistension of the lungs will compress alveolar vessels, thereby increasing PVR. Overdistension will also compromise venous return and lead to reductions in cardiac output.

Optimal oxygenation is achieved by gradual increments in MAP to recruit lung volume, and monitoring of the effects on arterial oxygenation. The aim is to achieve maximum alveolar recruitment without causing overdistension of the lungs.

During HFOV, alveolar ventilation is determined by the equation:

$$V_A = (V_T)^2 \cdot f.$$

Therefore, $CO_2$ elimination is more dependent on tidal volume than it is during conventional ventilation. Furthermore, with increasing ventilator frequency, lung impedance and airway resistance increase, so the tidal volume delivered to the alveoli *decreases*. This leads to the apparent paradox that increasing ventilator frequency may reduce $CO_2$ elimination, leading to raised $PaCO_2$.

## Clinical applications of HFOV

The principal applications of HFOV are in diffuse lung diseases with refractory hypoxaemia, or where the risks of high-pressure conventional ventilation and lung injury are unacceptably high, and in persistent pulmonary hypertension of the newborn (PPHN), due to the beneficial effect on PVR. Conditions which have been successfully treated by HFOV include:

- respiratory distress syndrome;
- pneumonia;
- air leak/PIE;
- persistent pulmonary hypertension (PPHN).

In severe RDS, there is evidence that HFOV is associated with a reduced incidence of air leaks and improved oxygenation. There is also evidence from studies in animals that HFOV causes less epithelial disruption and lung inflammation compared to conventional ventilation, despite the higher MAP used during HFOV. As yet, studies indicate only weak evidence of a reduction in the incidence of BPD in human infants.

In non-homogenous lung disease, such as bronchopulmonary dysplasia (BPD) or meconium aspiration syndrome (MAS), the role of HFOV is less clear. As high MAP is applied to recruit lung volume, overdistension of areas of lung with normal compliance may occur. This may contribute to air leaks and ventilation/perfusion mismatching.

The presence of congenital diaphragmatic hernia and associated lung hypoplasia in infants with severe respiratory failure is likely to be predictive of non-responsiveness to HFOV. In these cases, extracorporeal membrane oxygenation (ECMO) may be considered when conventional ventilation is inadequate to maintain adequate gas exchange.

Some ventilators allow the use of oscillation on top of a conventional pressure waveform, either as a continuous feature or during part of the respiratory cycle only, usually expiration. This strategy has no physiological basis, and there is no evidence to suggest that it has any place in the ventilation of newborn infants.

## Setting up the ventilator for HFOV

As with conventional ventilator settings, there is no ideal for every situation, and settings will vary according to the clinical diagnosis, the baby's size and gestation, and the progression of the underlying respiratory disease.

There are three variables to be considered when initiating HFOV:

- mean airway pressure (MAP);
- frequency (f)
- amplitude ($\Delta$P)

of the oscillating pressure wave.

For an infant with RDS who is being ventilated on a conventional time-cycled pressure limited ventilator, the following procedure should be used.

- Work out the current MAP; set the MAP on the oscillator 2 cm $H_2O$ above this value.
- Set the frequency to 10 Hz (NB oscillator frequencies are expressed in Hertz (cycles per second,) not breaths per minute: 10 Hz = 600 bpm); consider high frequencies (15 Hz) in tiny infants.
- Connect the patient to the ventilator circuit and gradually increase the amplitude until the chest is observed to 'bounce'.
- The MAP should be increased gradually by increments of 2 cm $H_2O$ to achieve optimal oxygenation; the $FiO_2$ will need to be reduced as lung recruitment and improved ventilation/perfusion matching occur.
- Continuous monitoring of oxygenation (see p.138) and frequent blood gas analysis are necessary during the establishment of HFOV.
- Frequent chest X-rays are taken to ensure optimal lung expansion. We aim to maintain lung volumes so that the diaphragm rests at around T8/9 on plain frontal chest X-ray.
- The patient circuit should be opened as little as possible, e.g. for ET tube suctioning; loss of pressure will result in alveolar volume loss and the need for subsequent volume recruitment by increasing MAP.
- Blood pressure may fall as high intrathoracic pressure impedes venous return. Intravenous plasma expanders (e.g. human albumin solution, 4.5%) may be necessary. Give 10 mL/kg boluses and observe the responses of blood pressure and heart rate.

## Adjustments/troubleshooting

### Low PaO$_2$

Consider:
*ET tube patency*

- check for chest movement and breath sounds;

*Air leak/pneumothorax*

- chest moving symmetrically?
- transilluminate;
- urgent chest X-ray;

*Suboptimal lung volume recruitment*

- increase MAP;
- consider chest X-ray;

*Overdistension*

- check blood pressure (and CVP if available); give colloid 10–15 mL/kg if BP is low (see p.465);
- reduce MAP; does oxygenation improve?
- consider chest X-ray.

### High PaCO$_2$

Consider:
*ET tube patency and air leaks*
*Insufficient alveolar ventilation*

- increase $\Delta$P; does chest wall movement increase?
- increased airway resistance (meconium aspiration syndrome; BPD); non-homogenous lung disease; is HFOV appropriate?
- suboptimal volume recruitment; distending pressure delivered on non-compliant part of pressure-volume curve; increase MAP;
- overdistension; lungs 'stretched' and non-compliant; reduce MAP;
- reduce oscillator frequency; lung impedance and airway resistance fall, leading to increased $V_T$.

## Potential complications of HFOV

The following have been reported as complications of HFOV:

- necrotizing tracheobronchitis;
- focal obstruction due to mucus impaction;
- hypotension due to obstructed venous return;
- intraventricular haemorrhage;

Tracheal injury is a potential complication of any form of ventilation requiring endotracheal intubation. Recent evidence suggests that high pressures and lack of humidity are more important factors than the mode of ventilation.

There is conflicting evidence regarding the risk of IVH with HFOV compared to conventional ventilation. It has been suggested that high intrathoracic pressures during HFOV obstruct cerebral venous return and cause raised cerebral venous pressure. Studies using the strategies outlined above have not demonstrated a difference in the incidence of IVH between HFOV and conventionally ventilated newborn infants.

## Weaning from HFOV

As the baby's condition improves, the MAP can be slowly reduced, usually in decrements of 0.5–1 cm $H_2O$. As lung compliance increases, the amplitude of oscillation can also be reduced to maintain constant alveolar ventilation.

Weaning from HFOV to extubation can be achieved via progressively lower mean airway pressures. The criteria for extubation are similar to those for conventional ventilation, i.e. $FiO_2 < 0.35$; MAP < 6–8 cm $H_2O$. The baby may be extubated to headbox oxygen or to nasal CPAP.

An alternative strategy is to switch the infant to conventional CMV or PTV during the weaning phase, usually when MAP < 10 cm $H_2O$, and to reduce the ventilation according to the guidelines given (see p.155). This may be particularly advantageous when there are significant chest secretions and vigorous physiotherapy and ET tube suctioning is required.

## Extracorporeal membrane oxygenation (ECMO)

ECMO has been demonstrated to be an effective treatment for severe respiratory failure associated with a number of neonatal conditions including meconium aspiration syndrome and severe RDS, and possibly in congenital diaphragmatic hernia/pulmonary hypoplasia.

Much of the current literature evaluating ECMO in neonatal diseases pre-dates the introduction of HFOV and effective pulmonary vasodilator treatment, such as inhaled nitric oxide. ECMO requires considerable technical expertise and support from a multidisciplinary team including neonatal physicians, surgeons, nurses and perfusionists. It is available in a number of specialist centres in the UK.

## THE PULMONARY CIRCULATION

Pulmonary vascular resistance (PVR) is high *in utero* and falls after birth. Persistence of raised PVR leads to pulmonary artery hypertension, which results in right-to-left shunting across the ductus arteriosus and foramen ovale, and contributes to ventilation/perfusion mismatching. Persistent pulmonary hypertension of the newborn (PPHN) may be:

1 *Primary*; or
2 *Secondary* to:
- RDS;
- perinatal asphyxia;
- meconium aspiration;
- polycythaemia;
- Pulmonary hypoplasia ($\pm$ diaphragmatic hernia).

In primary PPHN the chest X-ray will usually show a normal-sized heart and oligaemic lung fields. The condition should be differentiated from cyanotic congenital heart disease (see Chapter 11), and the major difficulty arises with obstructed totally anomalous pulmonary venous connection. Echocardiography should be performed, including a careful examination of the pulmonary veins.

### Management of PPHN

Remember that hypoxaemia, hypercapnoea and acidosis will exacerbate pulmonary hypertension. Autonomic activity due to pain or discomfort during care may also contribute to increased PVR. Therefore, before considering the use of vasodilators, the following points should be addressed.

- Ensure that the infant is optimally ventilated and receiving high $FiO_2$. Consider the use of patient-triggered ventilation to reduce asynchronous respiratory efforts. Also consider HFOV, which has been demonstrated to be effective in PPHN due to the effects of lung inflation on PVR (see p.155). Increase minute ventilation to reduce $PaCO_2$ and respiratory acidosis. Consider correction of metabolic acidosis (see p.182, *but* remember that giving intravenous bicarbonate will increase $PaCO_2$).
- Invasive blood pressure monitoring via an arterial catheter (see Chapter 27) is essential; non-invasive monitoring with an inflatable cuff is sub-optimal in this situation.

- Consider the use of sedation with or without muscle relaxants (see Table 10.2). Remember that opioids and muscle relaxants can also have profound effects on cardiac output and systemic vascular resistance, leading to severe hypotension.
- Consider insertion of a central venous catheter (see Chapter 27) for delivery of vasodilators, emergency administration of intravenous fluids and possible requirement for inotropes to support the systemic circulation.
- Have colloid available (10–20 mL/kg) for rapid intravenous infusion if BP falls precipitously, and consider inotropic support.

## Treatment of systemic hypotension

The use of intravenous 'pulmonary' vasodilators is associated with systemic hypotension due to a reduction in systemic vascular resistance. In the event of systemic hypotension, start by giving 10–20 mL/kg of colloid intravenously. However, the effect of repeated boluses of volume expanders is likely to be limited and the use of inotropes should be considered.

**Dopamine** 1–20 mcg/kg/min i.v. infusion. At higher doses, dopamine has a vasoconstrictive effect and may exacerbate pulmonary hypertension. It also causes renal vasoconstriction and possible oliguria at doses of > 5–10 mcg/kg/min.

**Dobutamine** 1–20 mcg/kg/min i.v. infusion. It has less vasoconstrictive effects than dopamine, but there is evidence that it may be less effective in newborn infants. Often used in combination with dopamine.

**Adrenaline** 0.05–2 mcg/kg/min i.v. infusion. It may be used in severe hypotension. Has potent vasoconstrictor activity in addition to positive inotropic and chronotropic effects.

Start with low-dose dopamine infusion (2–4 mcg/kg/min) and, depending on the response, consider increasing dopamine to 5–10 mcg/kg/min and add dobutamine, e.g. dopamine 5 mcg/kg/min + dobutamine 10 mcg/kg/min.

## Drugs used to treat PPHN

**Tolazoline** Tolazoline is a histamine antagonist which acts directly on smooth-muscle receptors. It has been suggested as a specific pulmonary vasodilator due to its selective effects depending on the initial degree of vasoconstriction.

However, it also acts on gastric histamine receptors, increasing gastric acid secretion, and it is associated with gastric bleeding. Other adverse effects include systemic hypotension, oliguria and, rarely, thrombocytopenia.

Tolazoline is given as an initial i.v. bolus of 1 mg/kg over 1–2 min to assess the response. This may be accompanied by a rapid fall in systemic blood pressure. If there is a response to tolazoline, as evidenced by a rapid improvement in $PaO_2$, an infusion may be commenced at 0.1 mg/kg/hour.

**Prostaglandins** Epoprostenol ($PGI_2$; formerly called prostacyclin) is the most commonly used and most potent of the prostaglandins which have been used for the treatment of pulmonary hypertension. It is produced naturally from the vascular endothelium and causes vasodilatation through its effect on cGMP. There is evidence that its effects are potentiated by hypoxaemia, and this may give it a degree of pulmonary selectivity in PPHN. However, as with other intravenous vasodilators, its effects are limited by systemic vasodilatation and hypotension. Epoprostenol is also a very potent inhibitor of platelet aggregation and may potentiate haemorrhage.

Intravenous epoprostenol is administered as an infusion, preferably through a central venous catheter, at a rate of 5–40 ng/kg/min depending on the response (larger doses have been used). Start at 5 ng/kg/min and increase in increments of 5–10 ng/kg/min every 30 min. Epoprostenol has a short half-life (2–3 min) and its effects disappear within 30 min of discontinuing the infusion.

Inhaled prostaglandins have been reported to increase the pulmonary selectivity of vasodilatation, but their use may be superseded by the availability of inhaled nitric oxide.

**Nitric oxide** Nitric oxide (NO) has a biological activity identical to that of endothelium-dependent relaxing factor (EDRF), which is produced in endothelial cells and causes vasodilatation by increasing cGMP in smooth muscle. When NO diffuses into the intravascular space it is rapidly bound to haemoglobin, forming methaemoglobin. NO thus has a very short half-life and, when given by inhalation, its effects are confined to the pulmonary circulation. Because NO is not available to the systemic circulation, its use is not limited by systemic hypotension. It therefore acts as a **selective** pulmonary vasodilator.

Nitric oxide gas (1000 ppm in $N_2$) is delivered into the ventilator circuit via a low-flow rotameter to achieve a final dilution of 3–80 ppm in the inhaled gas. An oxygen analyser should be incorporated within the circuit to measure $FiO_2$ after the addition of $NO/N_2$ gas mixture. NO and $NO_2$ concentrations must be measured continuously by sidestream sampling from the y-connector of the inspiratory and expiratory limbs of the ventilator circuit. The expired $NO_2$ concentration should not be allowed to exceed 2–3 ppm.

Treatment with NO is started at a low concentration of 3–5 ppm and increased in incremental steps until no further increment in oxygenation is observed. The onset of effect is usually rapid and, because of the short half-life of NO, the effect disappears immediately on withdrawal of NO from inspired gas. This should be borne in mind when disconnecting the baby from the ventilator circuit, e.g. for bag-and-mask ventilation during procedures, etc.

Because NO is a free radical, it is highly reactive and forms nitrates and nitrites on decomposition. The key practical concerns are formation of methaemoglobin and $NO_2$, which has potent toxic effects on the lung. Studies of the use of NO in infants with pulmonary hypertension have demonstrated blood methaemoglobin concentrations rarely exceeding 5% and expired $NO_2$ concentrations below 3 ppm. Long-term effects on the lungs and other organs have yet to be determined.

**Magnesium sulphate** Magnesium antagonizes calcium ion entry into smooth-muscle cells and causes vasodilatation. An intravenous infusion of magnesium sulphate, 200 mg/kg, over 20–30 min has been demonstrated to improve oxygenation in infants with PPHN. However, there is evidence that a significant degree of reversible PVR persists after magnesium infusion, and deleterious effects on systemic vascular resistance may limit its usefulness.

## CHRONIC LUNG DISEASE

Causes of chronic ventilator dependency and/or the need for prolonged supplemental $FiO_2$ include the following:

1 bronchopulmonary dysplasia (BPD);
2 chronic pulmonary insufficiency of prematurity – secondary atelectasis probably due to chronic hypoventilation in the very immature baby;
3 congenital pulmonary hypoplasia – may be primary or secondary; associated with congenital diaphragmatic hernia, Potter's sequence and other causes of oligohydramnios;

**4 Wilson-Mikity syndrome** – prolonged respiratory distress associated with characteristic chest X-ray appearances; cause unknown and usually associated with minimal mechanical ventilation and $FiO_2$ for RDS;

**5 pulmonary interstitial emphysema;**

**6** chronic lung disorders may also be associated with **PDA, pulmonary haemorrhage, infection, inspissated secretions, recurrent aspiration** (± gastroesophageal reflux) and **osteopenia of prematurity.**

There is considerable overlap in the clinical and radiological features of these conditions, particularly between BPD and Wilson-Mikity syndrome. These babies may need prolonged IPPV or IMV, and are usually difficult to wean from ventilation. They may have a dependency on increased $FiO_2$ for several weeks to months.

## Bronchopulmonary dysplasia

BPD is a chronic sequela of lung injury associated with mechanical ventilation and high $FiO_2$ for RDS. It is more common in extremely preterm and low-birthweight infants in whom increases in prevalence may be due to improved survival. Infants may have associated problems of prematurity. Particular management considerations in infants with BPD include the following.

*Nutrition* Although poor growth and weight gain in infants with BPD are often related to persistent hypoxaemia, vigorous attention should be paid to optimal nutritional care. Poor growth may occur despite high caloric intake as the resting metabolic rate is raised. The advice of a dietician should be sought to ensure adequate nutrition (> 120 kcal/kg/day) without excessive water intake. Optimal caloric intake may be limited by poor appetite, aversion to oral feeding and gastro-oesophageal reflux. Gastrostomy feeding ± fundoplication is occasionally necessary.

### Infection

- Intercurrent infections of the lower respiratory tract occur with increased frequency in infants with BPD.
- Most infections are probably due to viral organisms.
- RSV infection may be treated with inhaled ribavirin.
- Pertussis vaccine should be given to all infants with BPD unless contraindicated.

The drug treatment of BPD includes the following.

*Oxygen* Chronic hypoxaemia and pulmonary hypertension are significant contributors to morbidity and mortality in infants with BPD. Low-flow oxygen can be given by nasal cannulae to maintain $SaO_2 > 94\%$. This should be regularly assessed during wakefulness, sleep and feeding (see Chapter 24).

*Aminophylline* May be used as an adjunct during weaning from ventilation and to prevent apnoea of prematurity. There is theoretical evidence for increasing diaphragmatic efficiency, but little clinical evidence of alterations in the natural history of BPD.

*Diuretics* Short-term improvements in pulmonary function have been demonstrated with diuretics, including frusemide, chlorothiazide and spironolactone. Long-term use of frusemide is associated with electrolyte disturbance, metabolic alkalosis and nephrocalcinosis. We use chlorothiazide (10 mg/kg twice daily) and spironolactone (1 mg/kg twice daily).

*Steroids* Persistent pulmonary inflammation has been demonstrated in infants with BPD. Treatment with steroids leads to more rapid weaning from ventilation and improved lung function. There is some evidence that early treatment with steroids may improve the outcome for infants with BPD by a direct effect on inflammation and the fibroproliferative responses of the lungs.

There is still uncertainty about the optimal steroid regimen. Start with dexamethasone (0.2 mg/kg every 8 hours). If no improvement occurs within 72 hours, discontinue. If improvement occurs, halve the dosage for 3–5 days and gradually tail off over 1–2 weeks.

Adverse effects of steroid therapy include hyperglycaemia, hypertension, cardiomyopathy and gastrointestinal bleeding.

The use of inhaled steroids in the primary treatment of BPD is under evaluation. We use budesonide (200–400 mcg, twice daily by metered aerosol and spacer with mask; Aerochamber, Trudell Medical, London). This is commenced at the same time as parenteral steroid therapy and continued at least until the infant is no longer dependent on increased $FiO_2$.

*Bronchodilators* There is evidence of short-term improvements in respiratory mechanics with bronchodilator therapy, including beta-adrenergic agents (salbutamol, terbutaline) and antimuscarinic agents (ipratropium bromide). However, the effects are often transient, dose delivery to infants' lungs is variable, and paradoxical deterioration in lung function and oxygenation may occur. The need for regular bronchodilator therapy should be carefully reviewed on an individual basis.

Infants with severe BPD, poor growth and/or poor response to treatment should be re-assessed for the following.

- *Adequate oxygenation* during wakefulness, sleep and feeds.
- *Absence of evidence of airway obstruction.* Upper airway obstruction (e.g. sub-glottic stenosis, tracheomalacia) or bronchial obstruction (e.g. bronchomalacia, acquired bronchial stenosis) may complicate BPD. Consider polysomnography if available. Consider airway endoscopy.
- *Recurrent aspiration* Gastro-oesophageal reflux is common in infants with BPD. Carry out pH studies and consider the need for contrast radiographic studies. Treat GOR with feed thickeners, Gaviscon and cisapride (0.2–0.4 mg/kg, 8-hourly). Consider the need for fundoplication.
- *Congenital heart disease* Cardiologist review and echocardiography.
- *Pulmonary hypertension* Echocardiography (see Chapter 11). Cardiac catheterization and response to increased $FiO_2$.
- *Reassess drugs* Efficacy and side-effects.

For follow-up after discharge of an infant with BPD, see Chapter 24.

## RECURRENT APNOEA

Periodic breathing is normal in preterm infants. Apnoeic attacks are repeated episodes of absent respiratory movements for > 20 sec or shorter episodes associated with bradycardia and/or colour change (pallor or cyanosis). $PaO_2$ and $SaO_2$ will usually fall during an apnoea. Recurrent apnoea is extremely common in very preterm infants, and they should have continuous cardiorespiratory monitoring for the first 2 weeks at least.

### Causes

- Lung disease + hypoxaemia.
- Airway obstruction.
- Cardiac disorder (especially PDA).
- Cerebral oedema/haemorrhage (in some infants, apnoeic attacks may be the only manifestation of convulsions).

- Infection.
- Anaemia.
- Metabolic disturbance (hypogycaemia, hypocalcaemia, hyponatraemia, acidosis).
- Drugs (e.g. maternal sedation in labour, maternal substance abuse).
- Unstable environmental temperature (apnoea commonly occurs as the environmental temperature rises).
- REM sleep.
- Intolerance of enteral feeds/gastro-oesophageal reflux.
- 'Apnoea of prematurity'

## Investigations

- Review history, description and timing of apnoeas.
- Physical examination, especially cardiorespiratory system, neurobehavioural data, evidence of infection. Measure blood pressure.
- Review feeding – volume and route. Remember that a nasogastric tube obstructs 50% of the infant's airway.
- Measure:
    Hb, PCV;
    WBC count and differential, C-reactive protein (CRP);
    Blood glucose, urea, electrolytes (including calcium, magnesium) and albumin;
    Blood pH, gases and $HCO_3$.
- Infection screen.
- Chest X-ray.
- Cerebral ultrasound scan.
- Oesophageal pH study.

## Management

### Continuous monitoring of:

- Heart rate.
- Breathing.
- $TcPO_2/SaO_2$.
- Skin and environmental temperature.

### Treat underlying causes:

- Antibiotics for infection.
- Remove airway obstruction, e.g. nasogastric tube.
- Temporarily reduce volume of enteral feeds.

- Treat gastro-oesophageal reflux (see Chapter 13).
- Treat cardiac failure (diuretics and, if indicated, digoxin).
- Transfuse if Hb < 12 g/dL.
- Correct hypotension by infusion of blood or plasma.
- Correct low blood glucose, calcium, sodium or albumin.
- Stabilize thermoneutral environment.
- Consider nursing the baby prone to reduce the work of breathing.

### Treatment and prevention of attacks

Many apnoeic attacks are self-correcting or respond to tactile stimulation. Babies of < 35 weeks' gestation who have frequent apnoeas should be given methylxanthines, e.g. aminophylline (see below). If more vigorous resuscitation is required (e.g. bag-and-mask ventilation) or they occur more often than every 3–4 hours, then specific treatment should be started as follows.

1 Start nasal CPAP (see p.140) 3–4 cm $H_2O$ in air.
2 $FiO_2$ may need to be increased to prevent hypoxaemia, but may cause hyperoxia between attacks, and these babies have a high risk of ROP. Hyperoxia may also lead to less frequent but more severe apnoea. Measure blood gases and aim to keep $PaO_2$ in the range 50–70 mm Hg (6.5–9.1 kPa).
3 Start aminophylline 6 mg/kg i.v. loading dose followed by 2 mg/kg every 8–12 hours. Monitor blood concentration and aim to keep it in the range 28–55 μmol/L. Caffeine may be used as an alternative.
4 If the attacks persist, try IMV through nasopharyngeal prong with PIP 10–15 cm $H_2O$, rate 5–10 bpm.
5 If all else fails, intubate and ventilate at a rate of 10–20 bpm; PIP 16 cm $H_2O$; PEEP 3 cm $H_2O$ and $T_i$ 0.5 sec.

## BIBLIOGRAPHY

Abman, S.H. and Groothius, J.R. (1994) Pathophysiology and treatment of bronchopulmonary dysplasia: current issues. *Pediatr. Clin. North Am.* **41**, 277–315.

Clark, R.H. (1994) High frequency ventilation. *J. Pediatr.* **124**, 661–70.

Cooke, R. (1995) The current use of exogenous surfactants in the newborn. *Br. J. Obstet. Gynaecol.* **102**, 679–81.

Greenough, A. (1990) Bronchopulmonary dysplasia: early diagnosis, prophylaxis and treatment. *Arch. Dis. Child.* **65**, 1082–8.

Halliday, H.L. (1995) Overview of clinical trials comparing natural and synthetic surfactants. *Biol. Neonate.* **67**, 32–47.

Pranka, M.S., Clark, R.H., Yoder, B.A. and Null, D.M. (1995) Predictors of failure of high frequency oscillatory ventilation in term infants with severe respiratory failure. *Pediatrics* **95**, 400–4.

Roberts, J.D. and Shaul, P.W. (1993) Advances in the treatment of persistent pulmonary hypertension of the newborn. *Pediatr. Clin. North Am.* **40**, 983–1004.

Vallance, P. and Collier, J. (1994) Biology and clinical relevance of nitric oxide. *B. M. J.* **309**, 453–7.

# Cardiac problems

## INCIDENCE

Congenital heart disease (CHD) is found in approximately 7 per 1000 live births. It may occur as an isolated defect but is frequently found in association with other malformations, such as oesophageal atresia, anorectal anomalies, exomphalos and skeletal defects. CHD is particularly common in chromosomal disorders and with some maternal conditions (Table 11.1).

## ASSESSMENT OF THE INFANT WITH SUSPECTED CONGENITAL HEART DISEASE

### History

- Birth details (peripartum asphyxia?).
- Maternal illness or drug ingestion.
- Family history.

**Table 11.1** Frequency of congenital heart disease

|  | CHD frequency (%) | Common malformations |
|---|---|---|
| **Chromosomal disorders** | | |
| Trisomy 21 | 40–60 | Atrioventricular septal defect, ventricular septal defect (VSD), atrial septal defect (ASD), patent ductus arteriosus (PDA) |
| Trisomy 18 | 90 | VSD, PDA |
| Trisomy 13 | 80 | ASD, VSD |
| Turner's syndrome (XO) | 10–20 | Coarctation of aorta |
|  |  | Aortic and mitral valve abnormalities |
| 22q11 deletion | 70–90 | Aortic arch anomalies |
|  |  | Conotruncal anomalies |
| **Maternal factors** | | |
| Rubella infection | 35 | PDA, pulmonary stenosis, VSD, ASD |
| Diabetes mellitus | 3–5 | Transposition VSD |
|  |  | Coarctation |
| Phenylketonuria | 25–50 | Tetralogy of Fallot |
| Fetal alcohol syndrome | 25 | VSD, ASD |
| Phenytoin | 2–3 | Pulmonary and aortic stenosis |
| Systemic lupus erythematosus (SLE) | 30–40 | Complete heart block |

- Symptoms in baby:
  - cyanosis;
  - poor feeding;
  - breathlessness;
  - excess weight gain.

## Examination

- Colour (cyanosis or pallor).
- Respiratory rate, respiratory distress.
- Heart rate.
- Peripheral pulses:
  - inequality of volume between right and left brachial pulses?
  - weak femoral pulses?
  - pulses weak or bounding?
- Cardiac impulse (RV or LV prominence).

- Heart sounds:
  - S2 single, widely split, or loud?
  - gallop rhythm or ejection click.
- Murmur: timing, nature, duration, loudness, site and radiation.
- Hepatomegaly.
- Oedema.
- Peripheral perfusion and temperature (core-peripheral gap).
- Blood pressure in all four limbs.

## Investigations

- Chest X-ray.
- Electrocardiogram (ECG).
- Arterial blood gas.
- Hyperoxia test if hypoxaemic.
- Echocardiogram.

## Chest X-ray interpretation

- Heart size, shape and position. Do not be confused by the thymic shadow which is variable in size and shape.
- Pulmonary vascularity: oligaemic or plethoric?
- Pulmonary oedema, fluid in horizontal fissure, pleural effusions.
- Position of aortic arch: left or right sided?
- Position of gastric bubble and liver: abnormal situs?
- Skeletal abnormalities.

## ECG interpretation

**QRS axis** (see Fig. 11.1).

1 Use leads *I* and *aVF* or *I* and *II*.
2 Measure the height of *R* and subtract the depth of *S* in lead *I*, plot (*R* − *S*) along axis of lead *I*.
3 Repeat the above procedure for lead *aVF* (or *II*) and plot along the axis of *aVF* (or *II*).
4 Draw lines perpendicular to the lead axes through the plotted points. Join the intersection of the perpendicular lines to the origin; this is the *QRS* axis.

The normal neonatal *QRS* axis is 60°–160° (mean 130°). The axis moves to the left during the first months of life and is 5°–105° (mean 60°) by 6 months of age.

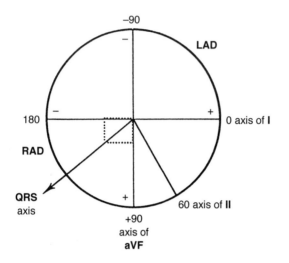

**Fig. 11.1** Calculation of **QRS** axis of ECG (see text).

Left-axis deviation (0° to –90°) in a cyanosed infant suggests tricuspid atresia, and in a non-cyanosed infant suggests an atrioventricular septal defect.

### P-wave
*P* > 3 mm in any lead = right atrial hypertrophy.
Biphasic *P* or terminal *P* inversion in lead *V1* > 1 mm = left atrial hypertrophy.

### PR interval
Normal range = 0.07–0.16 sec.
Prolonged in first-degree heart block. Shortened in Wolff-Parkinson-White syndrome and junctional rhythm.

### Q-wave
*Q* > 4 mm in *V6* > septal hypertrophy.
*Q* > 0.03 sec is pathological, e.g. in myocardial infarction associated with anomalous origin of the left coronary artery.

### T-wave
During the first 3 days after birth, the *T*-wave may be inverted in leads *I, aVL* and *V6* and upright in *V1*. After the third day, the *T*-wave axis changes and becomes upright in *I, II, aVF* and *V6* and inverted in *V1*.

### Right ventricular hypertrophy

$QR$ pattern in $V1$ (need to look carefully to exclude a small, initial, positive deflection).

$R > 30$ mm in $V1$, $S > 10$ mm in $V6$.

Upright $T$ in $V1$ after 48 hours of age.

Right ventricular hypoplasia, as seen in tricuspid atresia or pulmonary atresia with intact ventricular septum, may be suspected if there are low right-sided voltages, e.g. $R$ in $V1 < S$ in $V1$.

### Left ventricular hypertrophy

$S > 22$ mm in $V1$.

$R > 16$ mm in $V6$.

### ST segment

Elevation seen in pericarditis, myocarditis and myocardial infarction. Depression suggests myocardial ischaemia (e.g. peripartum asphyxia), 'ventricular strain' or digoxin treatment.

## Hyperoxia test

Suspected cyanosis must always be confirmed by measurement of the $PaO_2$ on blood obtained from the right radial artery. The hyperoxia test requires measurement of $PaO_2$ (or $TcPO_2$ from preductal skin; right upper quadrant of chest) in air and after breathing 100% oxygen for 10 minutes. If $PaO_2$ does not exceed 150 mm Hg (20 kPa), a right-to-left shunt due to CHD, severe respiratory disease or PPHN is present.

## Echocardiography

Cross-sectional and Doppler echocardiography has facilitated the rapid and accurate diagnosis of CHD. Many neonatal units have ultrasound scanners suitable for screening patients with suspected heart disease *but*, even in specialized units, conditions such as anomalous pulmonary venous connection may be difficult to diagnose. *It is better to seek early advice from a cardiologist.*

The normal echocardiographic views are shown in Fig. 11.2.

## Presentation of infants with heart disease

Presentation is usually with cyanosis, heart failure, heart murmur or a combination of these features.

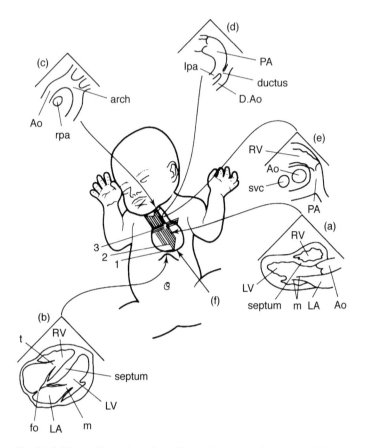

**Fig. 11.2** Diagram illustrating echocardiographic cross-sectional planes (2D). *1,* Long-axis plane (approximately sagittal); *2,* Four-chambers plane (approximately frontal); *3,* Short-axis plane (approximately transverse).

Transducer sites and planes obtainable are indicated as follows. (a) Left parasternal (long-axis plane – also short axis and parasternal four chambers, obtained by rotating and angling transducer). (b) Sub-xiphoid (four chambers – also long axis by rotating transducer). (c) High parasternal and transternal (high short-axis or long-axis parasagittal – 'ductus' cut). (f) Apex (four chambers or long axis). (d,e) Suprasternal (semi-long axis for aortic arch).

a, b, c, d, e, f. Diagrammatic representations of normal cross-sectional views.

(**a**) 'Long axis' cut as seen with transducer in left parasternal position.

(**b**) 'Four chambers' cut as seen from sub-xiphoid view.

(**c**) Semi-long axis cut of aortic arch as obtained from the suprasternal view.

# THE CYANOSED INFANT

## Common causes of cyanosis

- Transposition of the great arteries.
- Pulmonary atresia + VSD.
- Tetralogy of Fallot.
- Tricuspid atresia.
- Total anomalous pulmonary venous connection (TAPVC).
- Ebstein's malformation.
- Persistent pulmonary hypertension (PPHN; persistent fetal circulation).
- Severe lung disease.

## Transposition of the great arteries

### Clinical features

- Most frequent cyanotic defect in the neonatal period.
- Degree of cyanosis depends on mixing between pulmonary and systemic circulation via the foramen ovale, PDA or VSD when present.
- Cyanosis is present from birth and increases over 24–48 hours.
- Heart failure may develop after 2–3 weeks if there is a large PDA or VSD.
- No murmur unless VSD or pulmonary stenosis is present.

### Radiology

- Narrow pedicle.
- 'Egg-shaped' heart.
- Pulmonary plethora?

### ECG

- Right ventricular hypertrophy.
- May appear normal initially.

(**d**) High long axis parasagittal view to show ductus arteriosus.

(**e**) Short axis cut through the great arteries just above the heart.

*Abbreviations*: RV, right ventricle; LV, left ventricle; Ao, aorta; M, mitral valve leaflets; T, triscuspid valve leaflets; Fo, foramen ovale; Rpa, right pulmonary artery; Lpa, left pulmonary artery; PA, pulmonary artery; D, Ao, descending aorta; Svc, superior vena cava; LA, left atrium; RA, right atrium.

(Reproduced from Roberton, N.R.C. (1986) *Textbook of neonatology* with the permission of Churchill Livingstone.)

### Echocardiography

- Diagnostic.

### Treatment

- Maintain ductal patency with a prostaglandin infusion (see p. 182).
- Balloon atrial septostomy is performed to create a large ASD to allow intracardiac mixing.
- Corrective surgery using the arterial switch operation may be performed in the first or second week.

## Pulmonary atresia

### Clinical features

- Commonest type of pulmonary atresia occurs with VSD.
- Degree of pulmonary artery development is variable; in severe cases, pulmonary flow is dependent on collateral arteries.
- Murmurs are frequent and originate from the PDA or collaterals.
- Single S2 is present.

### Radiology

- Hollow pulmonary arc.
- Uptilted apex.
- Pulmonary oligaemia.

### ECG

- RVH initially.
- Later biventricular hypertrophy may be seen.

### Echocardiography

- VSD with overriding aorta.
- Atretic pulmonary valve.

### Treatment

- Maintain ductal patency with prostaglandin infusion (see p. 182).
- An urgent aorto-pulmonary shunt operation is usually required.

### Pulmonary atresia with intact interventricular septum

- Presentation is similar.
- In the absence of a VSD, the right ventricle is usually atretic.
- There may be a murmur due to tricuspid regurgitation.
- Radiology: right atrial dilatation.

- ECG: LV dominance with reduced RV voltages.
- Echocardiogram: small cavity RV with thickened walls; pulmonary atresia.
- Treatment: as for pulmonary atresia with VSD. In some cases transcatheter perforation of the valve is possible.

### Critical pulmonary stenosis

- Presentation similar.
- RV less hypoplastic; may even be RVH.
- Harsh pulmonary ejection murmur and ejection click.
- Echocardiogram: stenosed pulmonary valve.
- Treatment: maintain ductal patency (see p. 182). Surgical valvotomy or balloon valvuloplasty.

## Tetralogy of Fallot

### Clinical features

- Usually presents outside the neonatal period.
- May be diagnosed early due to echocardiographic screening of neonatal murmur.
- Cyanosis in the neonatal period is usually associated with severe infundibular stenosis and pulmonary artery hypoplasia.
- Less severe forms present with harsh pulmonary ejection murmur, single S2 and mild cyanosis.

### Radiology

- Pulmonary oligaemia.
- Hollow pulmonary arc?
- Uptilted apex?

### ECG

- RVH.

### Echocardiography

- Typical anatomy and side of aortic arch.

### Treatment

- Infants with hypoxaemia may require a prostaglandin infusion and subsequent systemic-to-pulmonary shunt operation.
- Typical cyanotic spells seen in older children are rare during the neonatal period.

## Tricuspid atresia

### Clinical features

- Usually associated with a VSD and RV outflow tract/pulmonary valve narrowing.
- The degree of cyanosis depends on:
    size of the VSD;
    degree of RV outflow tract obstruction.
- Associated with transposition of great arteries in 20% of cases. This group has a high pulmonary flow.
- Murmur common and single S2.

### Radiology

- 'Square' heart.
- Large right atrium.
- Pulmonary oligaemia.

### ECG

- Left axis deviation.
- Left ventricular dominance.
- Right atrial hypertrophy.

### Echocardiography

- RV hypoplasia.
- Absent or imperforate tricuspid valve.
- Size of VSD and degree of RVOTO.

### Treatment

- Prostaglandin infusion if severe cyanosis occurs.
- Severe cyanosis following ductal closure requires a systemic-to-pulmonary shunt operation.

## Total anomalous pulmonary venous connection (TAPVC)

### Clinical features

- Depends on drainage of pulmonary veins and presence of obstruction:
    - SVC via an ascending vein (supracardiac);
    - portal vein via a descending vein (infracardiac);
    - right atrium via coronary sinus (intracardiac).
- Supracardiac and infracardiac commonly associated with obstructed pulmonary venous flow.

- Severe obstruction:
  - infant ill soon after birth;
  - severe cyanosis;
  - pulmonary oedema leading to respiratory failure;
  - hepatomegaly;
- Usually no murmur (commonly confused with severe respiratory disease).

### Radiology

- Normal heart size.
- Severe pulmonary congestion and pulmonary oedema.
- May appear similar to RDS.

### ECG

- May be normal initially.
- Later shows RVH and right atrial hypertrophy (RAH).

### Echocardiography

- Can usually demonstrate the presence and site of the anomalous pulmonary venous connection.
- LV and LA appear small; RV and RA are dilated.
- Colour flow Doppler echocardiography is particularly helpful in demonstrating the site and pattern of pulmonary venous connection.

### Treatment

- Surgical repair is required (urgent if obstructed).
- *Prostaglandin infusion may be deleterious.*

## Ebstein's malformation

### Clinical features

- More severe defects present soon after birth with:
  moderate cyanosis;
  heart failure.
- Cyanosis usually improves over the first month as PVR falls.
- Large 'v'-waves and a pulsatile liver if tricuspid regurgitation is severe.

### Radiology

- Gross cardiomegaly.
- Large RA.
- Pulmonary oligaemia.

### ECG

- RAH.
- Right bundle branch block (RBBB).
- First-degree heart block.

#### Echocardiography

- Right atrial dilatation.
- Tricuspid anatomy.

#### Treatment

- Heart failure may require diuretics.
- Surgical treatment in infancy has poor results.
- Supportive therapy is the best option; spontaneous improvement occurs.

## Persistent pulmonary hypertension (see Chapter 10)

## Management of cyanotic congenital heart disease

All patients with suspected cyanotic CHD require referral for pae-diatric cardiological assessment. The major difficulties are to differentiate heart disease from PPHN, RDS or transient tachypnoea.

#### Prostaglandin E$_2$ therapy

Maintenance of ductal patency is important in the majority of cyanotic defects and in certain obstructive lesions on the left side of the heart (see p. 183). This can be achieved by i.v. or oral prosta-glandin therapy. An intravenous infusion is the preferred route for sick infants, and the usual dose is 10–20 ng/kg/min, although this can be increased up to 50 ng/kg/min (for infusion rates, see Table 11.2).

Adverse effects include apnoea and, at higher doses, pyrexia and jitteriness. It may also predispose to necrotizing enterocolitis.

#### Treatment of metabolic acidosis

Maintain a thermoneutral environment and consider IPPV, particularly if there is a respiratory component to the acidosis. If hypotensive, give plasma and/or inotropic support (see p. 162). Heart failure may need treatment with diuretics.

**Table 11.2** Cardiac drugs

| Drug | Route | Dose range |
|------|-------|------------|
| **Inotropes and chronotropes** | | |
| Adrenaline | i.v. or intraosseous bolus | 10 mcg/kg (followed by 100 mcg/kg if no response) |
| | Endotracheal bolus | 100 mcg/kg |
| | i.v. infusion | 0.05–2.0 mcg/kg/min |
| Dopamine | i.v. infusion | 1–20 mcg/kg/min |
| Dobutamine | i.v. infusion | 1–20 mcg/kg/min |
| Noradrenaline | i.v. infusion | 0.05–1.0 mcg/kg/min |
| Isoprenaline | i.v. bolus | 5 mcg/kg |
| | i.v. infusion | 0.02–1.0 mcg/kg/min |
| Atropine | i.v. bolus | 10 mcg/kg |
| **Vasodilators** | | |
| Epoprostenol | i.v. infusion | 5–20 ng/kg/min |
| Tolazoline | i.v. bolus | 1 mg/kg |
| | i.v. infusion | 0.1–0.5 mg/kg/hour |
| **Antiarrhythmics** | | |
| Adenosine | i.v. rapid bolus | 50 mcg/kg (if no response, 100 mcg/kg, then 250 mcg/kg, to a maximum dose of 500 mcg/kg) |
| Digoxin | Loading dose i.v. p.o. | 10 mcg/kg/dose, 8-hourly for three doses |
| | Maintenance p.o. | 5 mcg/kg, 12-hourly (term baby) |
| Flecainide | i.v. over 20 min | 1–2 mg/kg |
| Disopyramide | i.v. over 5–10 min | 2 mg/kg |
| **Maintenance of ductal patency** | | |
| Prostaglandin $E_2$ | i.v. infusion | 10–20 ng/kg/min (higher doses may be used, up to 50 ng/kg/min; may cause apnoea) |

## THE INFANT WITH HEART FAILURE

## Clinical signs of neonatal heart failure

- Tachycardia > 200/min at rest.
- Tachypnoea > 60/min; respiratory distress and/or apnoea in the preterm infant.
- Hepatomegaly > 1.5 cm below costal margin (most specific sign).

- Gallop rhythm.
- Peripheral oedema and excessive weight gain.
- Hypotension and poor peripheral perfusion is a later sign.

## Causes of neonatal heart failure

### Congenital heart disease

1 Left heart obstructive lesions:
   - hypoplastic left heart syndrome;
   - coarctation of aorta;
   - interrupted aortic arch;
   - aortic stenosis;
   - cor triatriatum.

2 Left-to-right shunt:
   - patent ductus arteriosus;
   - ventricular septal defect;
   - atrioventricular septal defects;
   - common arterial trunk (truncus arteriosus);
   - complex lesions with high pulmonary blood flow (e.g. double-inlet left ventricle).

3 Primary myocardial failure:
   - endocardial fibroelastosis;
   - hypertrophic cardiomyopathy
     (infant of diabetic mother, glycogen storage disease or familial);
   - myocarditis;
   - myocardial ischaemia secondary to birth asphyxia;
   - anomalous origin of left coronary artery from the pulmonary trunk.

4 Arrhythmias:
   - supraventricular tachycardia;
   - complete heart block.

### Other causes

- Anaemia.
- Polycythaemia.
- Sepsis.
- Hypoglycaemia.
- Hypocalcaemia.
- Hypo- or hyperthyroidism.

- Arterio-venous malformation (usually cerebral or hepatic).
- Fluid overload.

## Hypoplastic left heart syndrome

### Clinical features

- Infants normal initially, but rapidly become ill when the PDA starts to close (12–72 hours).
- Pale, cyanosed, with weak pulses.
- Severe heart failure.
- Soft systolic murmur at left sternal border.
- S2 loud and single.

### Radiology

- Cardiomegaly
- Pulmonary plethora and oedema.
- Occasionally the heart size is normal with intense pulmonary plethora (similar to TAPVC).

### ECG

- RVH.
- RAD.
- Reduced left ventricular voltages.

### Echocardiography

- Aortic hypoplasia (usually < 4 mm in diameter).
- LV hypoplasia.
- Aortic and mitral valve atresia.

### Treatment

- Previously this condition was not amenable to surgical repair, and compassionate treatment alone was offered.
- Options now include either the Norwood operation or neonatal heart transplantation. However, the former procedure is associated with a high perioperative and postoperative mortality. Neonatal transplant programmes are available in few centres. These options need careful discussion between parents and paediatric cardiologists.

## Coarctation and interruption of the aorta

### Clinical features

- Associated lesions are common, including aortic valve stenosis and VSD.

- Present with heart failure from 1–10 days of age.
- Femoral pulses are weak or absent when the PDA starts to close.
- Blood pressure gradient of > 20 mm Hg between the upper and lower limbs.
- Ejection murmur and gallop rhythm in many cases.

### Radiology

- Cardiomegaly.
- Pulmonary congestion.

### ECG

- RVH.
- RAD.
- May be normal.

### Echocardiography

- Anatomy of aortic arch on high parasternal views.

### Treatment

- Give diuretics for heart failure.
- In ill infants, IPPV and inotropes may be necessary.
- Prostaglandin therapy may produce dramatic improvements.
- Urgent surgical repair is required.

## Aortic valve stenosis

### Clinical features

- Severe AV stenosis causes heart failure during the first few days of life.
- Peripheral pulses are weak or impalpable.
- There is an aortic ejection murmur ± ejection click.

### Radiology

- Cardiomegaly.

### ECG

- LVH.
- Variable $T$-wave changes.

### Echocardiography

- Thickened, narrow valve.
- Hypertrophied (poorly functioning?) left ventricle.

**Treatment**
- Medical treatment as for coarctation.
- Surgical valvotomy or balloon valvuloplasty.

# Patent ductus arteriosus

This is an important cause of heart failure in the preterm infant (see p. 189).

# Ventricular septal defect

### Clinical features
- A large VSD can cause increasing heart failure starting from the second to third week, as the PVR falls and the left-to-right shunt increases.
- There is a harsh murmur at the left sternal border ± diastolic apical murmur.

### Radiology
- Cardiomegaly.
- Pulmonary plethora.

### ECG
- Biventricular hypertrophy.

### Echocardiography
- Identifies site and size of the defect.
- Doppler echocardiography can predict the degree of pulmonary hypertension.

### Treatment
- Medical therapy with diuretics and captopril.
- Surgical closure is required for:
    large defects;
    significant pulmonary hypertension;
    failure to thrive.

# Atrioventricular septal defect

### Clinical features
- Commonly associated with trisomy 21.
- Presentation is similar to that of VSD.
- There may be pan-systolic murmur of common AV valve regurgitation.

### Radiology

- Cardiomegaly.
- Pulmonary plethora.

### ECG

- LAD; **rSR** pattern in **V2R** and **V1**.
- Biventricular hypertrophy.

### Echocardiography

- Is diagnostic.
- May demonstrate associated lesions, e.g. PDA.

### Treatment

- Surgical repair is usually required before 6 months of age.

## Common arterial trunk (truncus arteriosus)

### Clinical features

- Mild cyanosis.
- High-volume peripheral pulses.
- Ejection systolic murmur, ejection click and single S2.
- Early diastolic murmur?

### Radiology

- Cardiomegaly.
- Pulmonary plethora.
- Pulmonary arteries high or not seen.

### ECG

- Biventricular hypertrophy + LV strain pattern.

### Echocardiography

- Identifies the abnormal truncal valve overriding the interventricular septum.

### Treatment

- Surgical correction in infancy.

## Anomalous origin of the left coronary artery from the pulmonary trunk

- Rare condition causing heart failure at 1–4 months of age.
- ECG is diagnostic; deep, wide **Q**-waves and inverted **T**-waves in left-sided chest leads.
- Treatment is surgical reimplantation of the left coronary artery.

## Treatment of heart failure

Supportive treatment consists of oxygen therapy, temperature maintenance in the thermoneutral range, and respiratory support. Fluid restriction to 75% of maintenance requirements and diuretic therapy (frusemide 1–2 mg/kg 12-hourly) are the mainstays of treatment. Additional benefit may be obtained by using vasodilators, e.g. captopril or hydrallazine.

Digoxin probably has little effect in conditions with a large left-to-right, shunt but may be useful if there is any left ventricular dysfunction (give 4 mcg/kg 12-hourly in preterm infants and 5 mcg/kg 12-hourly in term infants). Great caution is required in the presence of renal impairment, and frequent measurement of serum concentrations is recommended.

In the presence of systemic hypotension and peripheral hypoperfusion, give dopamine (5 mcg/kg/min).

If the above measures fail, surgical correction should be considered.

## Patent ductus arteriosus in the preterm infant

Clinically apparent PDA occurs in about 75% of infants of birthweight < 1.0 kg and in 10–15% of those of 1.5–2.0 kg. The lower the gestational age and the sicker the infant, the less likely it is that the PDA will close.

### Clinical features

- High volume peripheral pulses.
- Systolic murmur peaking towards S2, maximal upper left sternal border and radiates to the back; sometimes a continuous murmur.
- Need for prolonged or increased respiratory support without evidence of increased lung disease.
- Pulmonary plethora and cardiomegaly on chest X-ray.

### Management

1 Restrict fluids to 75% of maintenance requirements.
2 Avoid hypoxaemia, as this will tend to keep the duct open.
3 Maintain Hb > 12 g/dL by small volume blood transfusions.
4 Diuretic therapy (frusemide 1–2 mg/kg, 12-hourly).
5 If the above measures do not succeed, consider indomethacin (see below).

**6** If indomethacin fails (two courses may be used) or is contraindicated and symptoms persist, consider surgical ligation.

### Indomethacin therapy

Indomethacin is a prostaglandin synthetase inhibitor which can be used to close the duct, but which has many adverse effects, including:

- transient renal failure – oliguria, increased blood urea and creatinine;
- hyponatraemia;
- gastrointestinal and intracranial bleeding;
- decreased platelet aggregation;
- displacement of bound bilirubin.

The use of indomethacin is contraindicated in babies with bleeding disorders, including periventricular haemorrhage, thrombocytopenia, necrotizing enterocolitis, bilirubin > 200 μmol/L, or renal insufficiency (creatinine > 100 μmol/L or urea > 5 mmol/l).

**Dose** Two regimens are in use:

**1** 0.2 mg/kg i.v. or oral, once daily for a maximum of three doses;
**2** 0.1 mg/kg i.v. or oral, once daily for a maximum, of six doses.

The second regimen is associated with fewer side-effects and less frequent reopening of the duct.

Measure blood urea, creatinine, electrolytes, FBC, platelets and urine output before treatment and then daily, i.e. before the next dose, and for 3 days after treatment.

## ASYMPTOMATIC HEART MURMURS

Murmurs are common in the neonatal period and are often innocent, but the diagnosis of an innocent murmur should be made with caution. The murmur of a PDA is often present during the first 24, hours but should disappear subsequently.

The most common murmur encountered is a mid-systolic murmur at the left sternal border, often radiating to the back. This is frequently innocent, but it is difficult to differentiate from mild pulmonary or aortic stenosis.

The murmur of significant pulmonary or aortic stenosis will be present on the first day, and is usually associated with an ejection click.

Ventricular septal defects usually produce a harsh pansystolic murmur after the first 24 hours, as the pulmonary vascular resistance falls.

## Management

All babies with a murmur must have a full examination. If the murmur persists beyond the age of 36–48 hours, the following procedures should be carried out:

- chest X-ray;
- ECG;
- regular observations of heart rate, respiratory rate, feeding and daily weight.

If the infant is asymptomatic, consider early follow-up in the neonatal clinic. Cardiac referral should be considered if the clinical signs are suggestive of significant pathology or if there is a family history of congenital heart disease. *Remember that a normal ECG and chest X-ray do not exclude significant pathology.*

## NEONATAL ARRHYTHMIAS

### Supraventricular tachycardia (SVT)

Paroxysmal episodes of heart rate > 220–300/min occur. These usually start and stop abruptly. The heart is commonly structurally normal, but occasionally SVT is associated with congenital heart disease.

The infant presents with pallor, sweating, rapid breathing and difficulty with feeding. Tachycardia is often well tolerated despite a heart rate of 300/min. Diagnosis is made from an ECG where a narrow *QRS* complex tachycardia is seen. *P*-waves may be seen between *QRS* complexes (best seen in *V1*). About 30% of cases have Wolff-Parkinson-White syndrome and, following return to sinus rhythm, this should be looked for (short *PR* interval with a delta wave on the upstroke of the *R*-wave). Others may have atrial flutter with characteristic 'saw-tooth' atrial activity at a rate of 300–450/min.

#### Management
If attacks are short-lived and infrequent, then no drug treatment will be necessary. Prolonged episodes may cause heart failure, but rarely cause death.

1 Vagal manoeuvres (e.g. facial ice pack) may be used in the absence of signs of shock. Alternatively, the diving reflex may be elicited by facial immersion in cold water. Do this under ECG monitoring.

2 If these are unsuccessful, consider one of the following.

   a Intravenous *adenosine*. Start with 50 mcg/kg i.v. and increase to 100 mcg/kg after 2 min if this is not successful. If still unsuccessful, give one further bolus of 250 mcg/kg. The total dose should not exceed 500 mcg/kg. Intravenous boluses should be administered rapidly through the most central vein available.

   b *Digoxin*. A loading regimen of 10 mcg/kg, 8-hourly, followed by the standard maintenance dose. Great caution should be used in renal impairment; it is best to give a single dose and to check the serum concentration.

   c Other anti-arrhythmics:
   - **propranolol**, 1 mg/kg 8-hourly can be given orally; slow intravenous infusion of 100 mcg/kg may be used with caution, but can cause asystole;
   - **flecainide**, 1–2 mg/kg i.v. over 20 min;
   - **disopyramide**, 2 mg/kg i.v. slowly.

   *Verapamil should be avoided in infants, as it may cause cardiovascular collapse and death.*

   Flecainide and disopyramide appear to be relatively safe and are particularly effective in Wolff-Parkinson-White syndrome.

3 In acutely sick infants and/or when signs of shock are present, use synchronous DC cardioversion. Start with 0.5 J/kg and, if unsuccessful, increase to 1 J/kg and then 2 J/kg if necessary. Consider the use of anti-arrhythmics and seek cardiological advice.

## Congenital heart block

This is often diagnosed antenatally because of persistent fetal brady-cardia. The heart rate is usually < 80/min. Fifty per cent of infants have structural heart defects, usually 'congenitally corrected' trans-position of the great arteries (A-V and V-A discordance) or left atrial isomerism with atrioventricular septal defect. Many of those without structural abnormalities are associated with maternal anti-Ro anti-bodies as seen in systemic lupus erythematosus.

Presentation is usually with persistent bradycardia (40–60/min). Heart failure may occur in a small proportion.

The ECG shows dissociation between the atrial and ventricular activity (third-degree block).

### Treatment

Frequently no treatment is required. If there is a structural heart abnormality, heart failure, wide **QRS** complex, persistent bradycardia < 55/min, or frequent ventricular ectopy, cardiac pacing should be considered. In sick infants with severe bradycardia, isoprenaline infusion can be used to increase the heart rate as a short-term bridge to permanent pacemaker insertion.

## BIBLIOGRAPHY

Davignon, A., Rautaharju, P., Boiselle, E. *et al.* (1979) Normal ECG standards for infants and children. *Pediatr. Cardiol.* **1**, 123–31

Freedom, R.M., Benson, L.N. and Smallhorn, J.F. (1992) *Neonatal heart disease.* Berlin: Springer-Verlag.

Rennie, J.M. and Cooke, R.W.I. (1991) Prolonged low-dose indomethacin for persistent ductus arteriosus of infancy. *Arch. Dis. Child.* **66**, 55–8.

Stark, J. and De Leval, M. (1983) *Surgery for congenital heart defects.* London: Grune & Stratton.

# Neurological disorders

The newborn infant is susceptible to a wide range of neurological disorders, both congenitally determined and acquired during antenatal, perinatal and postnatal life. Longer term neurological integrity is perhaps the most important factor in determining the quality of life for the child and parents. Careful and appropriate medical intervention is thus essential.

## NEUROLOGICAL ASSESSMENT

Neonatal neurological assessment is particularly sensitive to external influences (see Table 12.1), which may make interpretation difficult. Always record the child's behavioural state (asleep, quiet and awake, irritable, etc.). Neurological assessment may form part of gestational

**Table 12.1**  Factors which may influence neurological assessment

---

**Drugs**

(Direct administration or via placenta or breast milk)
  Drugs of abuse/alcohol
  Antihypertensives
  Analgesics/sedatives/anaesthetics
  Anticonvulsants (especially benzodiazepines/phenobarbitone)

**Systemic illness**

  Infection, RDS, hypothermia

**Short gestation**

  See Chapter 22

**Behavioural state**

  Initially alert but somnolescence from 48 hours

**Hunger**

  Irritable before feeds

**Maternal illness**

  Diabetes, toxaemia

**Perinatal history**

**Family history**

---

assessment (see Chapter 22). A fuller protocol is found in Dubowitz and Dubowitz (1979).


## Head circumference (HC)

Measure carefully, check twice and plot on a centile chart (see Figs. 22.1 and 22.2). Hold the end of the tape over the flat temporal region for greatest reproducibility. The HC may change by 5–6 mm as moulding resolves in the first few days and subsequently increases by 5–8 mm/week. Review HC before discharge if >97th centile; early ultrasound scan will show presence or absence of hydrocephalus. The commonest cause of a large HC is constitutional or familial; check parents' HC (97th centile: adult men 58.5 cm; adult women 58 cm). If the HC is below the third centile, look for evidence of congenital infection (see Chapter 17) or dysmorphic features (see Chapter 8).

## Neurological examination

Assess posture, movement, limb and truncal tone, reflexes and neurobehaviour.

**Posture** Check the degree of limb flexion when supine.

**Movement** Note the frequency of spontaneous movement, tremors, hand clenching, thumb adduction, rhythmic mouthing, and 'cycling' or 'swimming' movements of limbs.

**Limb tone** Look for asymmetry. Use standard postures to compare limbs (e.g. scarf sign, heel-ear, popliteal, adductor and heel angles) (see Dubowitz and Dubowitz, 1979, or Amiel-Tison and Grenier, 1986, for a full description). Also assess by degree of elbow and knee flexion during arm and leg traction, respectively, noting the degree and speed of recoil on release.

**Neck and truncal tone** Assess extensor and flexor muscles separately – better extensor control suggests abnormally high extensor tone or compensation for upper airways obstruction. Head control is assessed by the ability to return the head to vertical after allowing it to fall forwards and then back when held in the sitting position. Then compare the head posture in ventral suspension with head lag during traction to sitting posture.

**Reflexes** Check tendon jerks – there should be a wide range of normal reflex activity – and primitive reflexes, e.g. palmar, plantar, rooting, Moro response (useful if asymmetrical, but otherwise only measure of degree of responsiveness).

### Neurobehaviour

- Check auditory response – startle or stilling to rattle at 10 cm, from 28 weeks' gestation.
- Check visual response – light reactive pupils, blinking to flashes, fixation on an object at 20 cm. Some babies may follow laterally and vertically.
- Also assess *alertness*, *irritability* and *consolability* when crying.

## Skin signs and neurological problems

| Signs | Association |
|---|---|
| Jaundice | Kernicterus |
| Café-au-lait spots | Neurofibromatosis |
| Depigmented patches | Tuberous sclerosis |
| Trigeminal port-wine stain | Sturge-Weber syndrome |
| Giant pigmented lesions of the head | Meningeal naevi: convulsions and hydrocephalus |

## NEONATAL CONVULSIONS

Neonatal convulsions are common and underdiagnosed because of the relative rarity of classic tonic/clonic signs.

### Categories of convulsions

**Subtle** The most common type. Look for tonic deviation of the eyes, fluttering of the eyelids, sucking and chewing, 'cycling' of the arms and legs, and apnoea (often *not* accompanied by bradycardia, but usually associated with other subtle signs).

**Clonic** May be multifocal (non-ordered migratory clonic convulsions) or focal (usually of metabolic origin, but may occasionally be localizing).

**Tonic** Especially preterm infants, often indicating cerebral damage. Extension and stiffening of the body and upward deviation of the eyes.

**Myoclonic** Least common type. Synchronized jerking of limbs; distinguish from jitteriness by grasping and gently flexing the limb, which abolishes jitters but has no effect on myoclonic jerks.

### Causes of convulsions

Neonatal seizures are usually secondary to underlying brain disturbances, in contrast to the primary epilepsies of childhood. Up to 90% may be ascribed to definite or probable aetiologies.

**Metabolic** (see Chapter 16)

- Hypoglycaemia (see Chapter 16).
- Hypocalcaemia and hypomagnesaemia (see Chapter 16).
- Hyper- and hyponatraemia (see Chapter 14).

- Inborn errors of metabolism, including:
  organic acidaemias (see Chapter 16);
  pyridoxine dependency;
  non-ketotic hyperglycinaemia (see Chapter 16);
  urea-cycle disorders (see Chapter 16).

### Haemorrhagic, hypoxic or ischaemic encephalopathy

- Perinatal hypoxia.
- Subarachnoid haemorrhage.
- Tentorial tear.
- Subdural haemorrhage.
- Periventricular brain lesions in preterm infants.
- Cerebral contusion.

### Infections

- Bacterial meningitis.
- Herpes, varicella, rubella, toxoplasmosis, cytomegalovirus, Coxsackie B and echovirus infections.
- Other CNS infections.
- May accompany severe systemic infection (e.g. septicaemia, urinary tract infection).

### Drugs and toxins

- Drug withdrawal (narcotics, barbiturates, amphetamines).
- Local anaesthetic (accidentally given into fetal scalp before delivery).
- Kernicterus.

### Others

- Idiopathic.
- Fifth day fits (? zinc deficiency).
- Benign familial neonatal seizures.
- Polycythaemia (due to either hypoglycaemia or focal ischaemia).
- Cerebral malformation or arteriovenous malformation.
- Cerebral venous thrombosis.
- Incontinentia pigmenti.

## Investigation

*Must include:*

- Blood sugar (check BM stix *immediately*).
- Serum electrolytes (calculate anion gap – normal < 15 mmol/L (see p. 45).

- Serum calcium (total or ionized).
- Blood gases and pH.
- Sepsis screen, including lumbar puncture (see Chapter 17).
- Packed cell volume (PCV), white blood cell (WBC) count and platelets.
- Cerebral ultrasound.

*May include:*

- Magnesium.
- Metabolic screen (see Chapter 16).
- Clotting screen.
- EEG.
- CT or MR scan.

NB The EEG may be useful in confirming seizure activity in the presence of subtle neurological signs, for assessing control in children treated with sedatives or muscle relaxants, and for prognosis. However, seizures may arise from deep neural structures and some (e.g. tonic) may not be associated with EEG discharges.

## Management

Treatment of a prolonged seizure is urgent, as the enormously increased oxygen consumption during a fit may outstrip its delivery.

### Correct underlying disorder

For example, hypoglycaemia, hypocalcaemia (see Chapter 16) or meningitis (see Chapter 17).

### Anticonvulsant drugs (in order of preference)

- *Phenobarbitone:* give a loading dose of 20 mg/kg as 10 mg/kg followed by a further 10 mg/kg 30–60 min later if there is no response. Maintenance treatment may be started after 3–4 days if required: half-life is 60–180 hours; therapeutic range is 20–30 mcg/mL (45–110 µmol/L).
- *Paraldehyde:* Stat dose of rectal preparation or i.v. infusion of 5% solution at 0.5–2.0 mL/kg/hour (dilute paraldehyde (100%) with 5% dextrose; protect from light; avoid prolonged contact of undiluted paraldehyde with plastics; change infusion sets 12-hourly).
- *Lignocaine:* Stat dose of 2 mg/kg by slow i.v. injection followed by 2 mg/kg/hour infusion. Monitor heart rate during loading dose, at risk of arrhythmia.

- *Other anticonvulsants:* Clonazepam, phenytoin, sodium valproate and thiopentone may be useful for rapid seizure control. *Avoid* diazepam, which has very prolonged elimination characteristics and is particularly depressant to the respiratory system, and phenytoin if lignocaine has been used.

**Prognosis**

Mortality after isolated seizures is low, but neurological sequelae, usually neuromotor and developmental impairments, may occur and are dependent on the underlying aetiology. Favourable aetiologies include primary subarachnoid haemorrhage and hypocalcaemia. Children with seizures due to symptomatic hypoglycaemia, hypoxic ischaemic encephalopathy and group B streptococcal meningitis have a better than 50% chance of normal development. Children with structural anomalies of the brain have the least favourable outcome, emphasizing the importance of an accurate aetiological diagnosis.

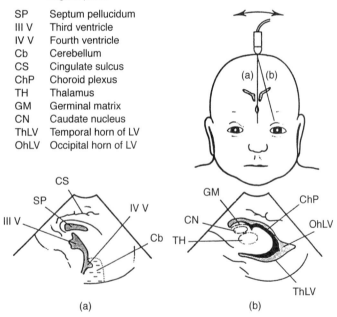

Sagittal plane

| | |
|---|---|
| SP | Septum pellucidum |
| III V | Third ventricle |
| IV V | Fourth ventricle |
| Cb | Cerebellum |
| CS | Cingulate sulcus |
| ChP | Choroid plexus |
| TH | Thalamus |
| GM | Germinal matrix |
| CN | Caudate nucleus |
| ThLV | Temporal horn of LV |
| OhLV | Occipital horn of LV |

**Fig. 12.1** Neonatal cerebral anatomy on ultrasound scan: sagittal and parasagittal planes.

Prognosis is most clearly related to abnormalities of the background EEG activity but interpretation is difficult and must take account of gestational age.

## HAEMORRHAGIC AND ISCHAEMIC BRAIN LESIONS

### Cerebral ultrasound scanning

Routine transfontanelle cerebral ultrasound scanning using a 5–10 MHz sector scanner facilitates the detection and management of perinatal brain pathology. All children of < 33 weeks' gestation should be scanned on admission to the special care baby unit (SCBU) and at intervals of a few days during the acute illness. Follow-up scans should be performed weekly in the presence of abnormalities. Even in the absence of early abnormalities, one or two

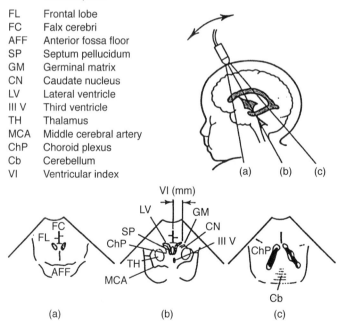

Coronal plane

FL     Frontal lobe
FC     Falx cerebri
AFF    Anterior fossa floor
SP     Septum pellucidum
GM    Germinal matrix
CN    Caudate nucleus
LV     Lateral ventricle
III V    Third ventricle
TH     Thalamus
MCA   Middle cerebral artery
ChP    Choroid plexus
Cb     Cerebellum
VI     Ventricular index

**Fig. 12.2** Neonatal cerebral anatomy on ultrasound scan: coronal plane.

later scans should be performed and will occasionally show previously unsuspected abnormality, especially periventricular leucomalacia. In the term infant, haemorrhage, ischaemic lesions and gross cerebral oedema may be observed. Most major brain malformations are also detectable.

Coronal and parasagittal scans (Figs. 12.1 and 12.2) should be performed and suspected lesions confirmed in two planes of examination. Haemorrhage and oedema appear as bright echogenic areas, clotted blood within the ventricle being particularly easy to identify (Levene *et al.*, 1995). Particular care should be taken in setting up the ultrasound machine, in order to avoid over-interpretation of echodensities, and a systematic search for abnormality of the observable brain should be made.

Early scans (< 7 days) will identify the severity of any haemorrhagic lesion by size, position and distribution. No grading scheme is perfect; it is better to describe exactly what is seen. Describe the size (small or large) of any intraventricular lesions, the size of the ventricles (normal or dilated, and measures if necessary) and any intraparenchymal echodensities (site and extent).

Later scans (> 7 days) will indicate the extent of any ventriculomegaly (measure ventricular index; Fig. 12.3) and identify the

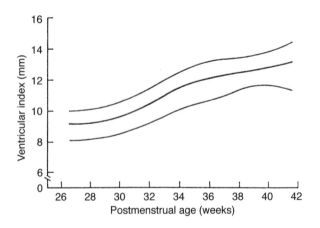

**Fig. 12.3** Ventricular index (see (b) of Fig. 12.2) and postmenstrual age: 3rd, 50th and 97th percentiles. (From Levene, M.I. (1981) *Arch. Dis. Child.* **56**, 900–904.

site, nature and extent of cortical echodensities and cysts as they evolve.

## Haemorrhagic lesions

### Classification

| Site | Comment |
|------|---------|
| Periventricular | See below |
| Subdural | Torn bridging veins (trauma) |
| (a) Supratentorial | Rarely directly fatal |
| (b) Infratentorial | Usually fatal |
| Subarachnoid | Associated with bleeding tendency and anoxia; may extend from intraventricular haemorrhage; usually venous (contrast with adults) |
| Intracerebral | Infarction associated with sepsis, asphyxia, embolism and PVH |
| Cerebellar and brain stem | Rarely detected in life |

### Diagnosis

Suspect intracranial haemorrhage after traumatic or asphyxial delivery. Symptoms may include cerebral depression, seizures, apnoea, circulatory collapse, poor temperature regulation and rapid fall in haematocrit, although subarachnoid and small periventricular haemorrhages are often asymptomatic. Microscopy of CSF is unreliable.

### Investigations

- *Cerebral ultrasound* – first choice for supratentorial lesions.
- *CT scan* – useful for posterior fossa lesions and if subdural collections are suspected.
- *MR scan* – less useful for pure haemorrhagic lesions.
- *Coagulation screen* – in children of > 34 weeks' gestation.
- *Other investigations* – for example, subdural taps, largely superseded.

## Periventricular haemorrhage (PVH)

This usually originates in the germinal matrix (26–32 weeks' gestation). It may rarely occur in term infants (usually from the choroid plexus). It is uncommon immediately after birth and appears during the first week. It may be confined to subependymal layers, rupture into ventricles or pass into the subarachnoid space, and may be associated with separate haemorrhagic lesions in the periventricular parenchyma ('extension'). It may be followed by complete resolution (usually) or posthaemorrhagic hydrocephalus (see below), and may be associated with later periventricular leucomalacia.

### Risk factors

- Infants of < 33 weeks' gestation (incidence 10–20%).
- Respiratory distress.
- Pneumothorax.
- Hypercapnia and acidosis.
- Hypotension.

### Prognosis
Outcome is best evaluated by sequential scanning and relates to the degree of ischaemic changes (see below).

### Prevention

- Vitamin E (25 mg/kg i.m. given on admission to NICU), ethamsylate (12.5 mg/kg/qds i.v. for 16 doses) and infusion of fresh frozen plasma (10 mL/kg) have been studied as potential prophylactics (among others), but despite encouraging early trials their efficacy has not been confirmed.
- Avoid acidosis, hypercapnia, pneumothorax and other situations which may lead to swings in blood gas status or perfusion (e.g. endotracheal suctioning).
- Pay close attention to the maintenance of peripheral perfusion and blood pressure using colloid and inotropic support if necessary.

### Management

- Correct bleeding tendency and transfuse if necessary.
- Avoid exacerbation by acidosis, hypotension and fluctuations in blood pressure.
- Perform serial scans to detect ventriculomegaly. (Neurosurgical intervention is unnecessary with PVH.)

## Ischaemic brain lesions

### Classification

- *Persistent ventricular enlargement* – non-progressive dilatation of lateral ventricles (> 97th percentile; Fig. 12.3). Probably represents mild cortical atrophy. Significance uncertain.

- *Cystic periventricular leucomalacia (PVL)* – cystic degeneration in periventricular tissue 10–21 days after ischaemic injury. Cysts are usually small (< 1 cm) and multiple. Significance depends upon site: fronto-parietal lesions are usually associated with few sequelae; bilateral occipital changes with neuromotor impairment.
- *Subcortical leucomalacia* – cystic changes in more superficial cortical layers, indicating a very severe injury. They are found more frequently in mature infants. Poor neuromotor outcome.
- *Porencephaly* – large (> 1 cm) cysts, usually solitary (occasionally multiple) and unilateral. May represent progression of parenchymal haemorrhage or PVL. High frequency of cerebral palsy.

### Aetiology

All are endpoints of ischaemic brain injury of uncertain pathology. May have origins in antenatal period (suspect if cystic changes occur in first week).

### Management

- See PVH above; in addition, avoid hypocarbia.
- Sequential scanning to characterize lesion.
- Careful parental counselling.
- Close neurodevelopmental follow-up.

## HYDROCEPHALUS (see Table 12.2)

Cerebrospinal fluid, produced by the choroid plexuses of the lateral ventricles, passes through the foramina of Monro into the third ventricle, from there through the aqueduct to the fourth ventricle, and then through the central foramen of Magendie and lateral foramina of Luschka to reach the subarachnoid space. In the subarachnoid space it flows over the cerebral hemispheres and out of the cranial cavity down the spinal cord, to be absorbed by the arachnoid (granulations are not present in the early postnatal period). Obstruction of this flow may cause hydrocephalus, which is defined as non-communicating (with the subarachnoid space) if it is at or proximal to the foramina of Magendie and Luschka, and communicating if it involves the arachnoid granulations or flow over the hemispheres and within the posterior fossa.

**Table 12.2** Some causes of hydrocephalus

| Cause | Level of obstruction |
| --- | --- |
| Post-haemorrhagic (following intraventricular haemorrhage) | Usually communicating but may progress to obstruction of IVth ventricle foramina. Occasionally non-communicating, obstruction proximal within ventricular system |
| Arnold-Chiari malformation of cerebellar vermis (commonly associated with meningomyelocele) | IVth ventricle foramina; occasionally cerebral aqueduct |
| Dandy-Walker malformation – cystic dilatation of IVth ventricle | IVth ventricle foramina; occasionally cerebral aqueduct |
| Congenital aqueductal stenosis | Cerebral aqueduct |
| Post-infection (toxoplasma, rubella, CMV, meningitis) | Cerebral aqueduct, IVth ventricle foramina (often also cerebral atrophy) |
| Cerebral tumours and arterio-venous malformations (rare) | Various |
| Choroid plexus papilloma (rare) | No obstruction; CSF over-production |

## Investigations

- *Ultrasound scan:* first-line investigation.
- *CT scan:* may further define posterior fossa lesions.
- *Intrauterine infection screen:* if indicated (e.g. calcification seen).
- *Queckenstedt's test:* free rise and fall of lumbar CSF pressure on jugular venous compression confirms communication.

## Management

Hydrocephalus is a dynamic condition and should be differentiated from cortical atrophy ('hydrocephalus *ex vacuo*'). Thus before treatment is started an excessive increase in ventricular size (Fig. 12.3) and head circumference (see Chapter 22) should be documented. CSF production may later fall to match resorption and the hydrocephalus 'arrest'.

After PVH, progressive ventricular dilatation may occur. Serial CSF drainage by lumbar puncture or ventricular tap has been advocated, but has little effect on the need for shunting or outcome. Cerebrospinal fluid (CSF) (10–20 mL/kg) may be removed to control symptoms (seizures, apnoea) or rapid head growth until the CSF protein level falls below 1 g/L, when shunt insertion is possible.

Other medical treatments, e.g. acetazolamide, 100 mg/kg/day, may temporarily reduce CSF production, but are of little long-term benefit. Ventriculoperitoneal shunt insertion remains the treatment of choice when hydrocephalus progresses despite more conservative measures. Third ventriculostomy has recently been used to avoid or delay shunt insertion with success.

## PERINATAL HYPOXIA IN THE TERM INFANT

Despite recent improvements in perinatal care, significant perinatal hypoxia still occurs in between 3 and 9 per 1000 births, and it remains an important cause of neurological impairment. Careful postnatal management of the asphyxiated infant may reduce further cerebral injury.

### Assessment of perinatal hypoxia

**Intrapartum** (see Chapter 1)

- *Perinatal history:* prenatal hypoxia (abnormal UA Doppler signal or antenatal cardiotocograph (CTG); reduced activity or liquor), APH, prolapsed cord.
- *Intrapartum CTG:* bradycardia, poor variability.
- *Meconium staining of liquor:* recent fresh (poor sign).
- *Fetal scalp pH:* < 7.20.

**Postnatal** (see Chapter 2)

- *Apgar scores:* 5 or 10 min score < 5.
- *Cord blood pH:* venous pH < 7.10.
- *Need for resuscitation:* > 10 min to establish spontaneous respiration.

#### Neonatal course

- *Encephalopathy:* (see below)
- *Hypoxic injury to other organs:* oliguria, elevated liver enzymes, hypotension, thrombocytopenia, pulmonary hypertension, coagulopathy.

#### Hypoxic-ischaemic encephalopathy
Signs may evolve over the first few hours. Record condition daily and note worst state for prognosis. Various classifications exist (e.g.

Sarnat and Sarnat, 1976; Levene *et al.*, 1985), broadly summarized as follows.

- *Mild encephalopathy:* 'hyperalert', awake, restless, jittery, poor feeding, resolution by 48 hours to 7 days.
- *Moderate encephalopathy:* 'lethargic', hypotonic, decreased responsiveness, poor suck, usually seizures (easy to control), some resolution by 7 days.
- *Severe encephalopathy:* 'stuporose', profound hypotonia, unresponsive, depressed/absent reflexes, seizures common and difficult to control, high mortality, survivors recover over many weeks.

## Management of the asphyxiated infant

No specific interventions have yet been shown to improve outcome following perinatal hypoxia although potential therapies are being evaluated. Careful, anticipatory, supportive management is therefore recommended.

### Fluids

- Fluid overload may exacerbate cardiac dysfunction and cerebral oedema or lead to hyponatraemia, which increases cerebral irritability and the risk of convulsions.
- Restrict fluids to 30–50 mL/kg in the first 24 hours, as oliguria (from antidiuretic hormone (ADH) secretion and renal ischaemia) is likely.
- Assess fluid balance by monitoring (see Chapter 14):
    urine output and specific gravity (± osmolality);
    urine Na, Cl, K and urea;
    plasma urea, Na, K, Cl and creatinine (± osmolality);
    weight (daily);
    blood pressure.

### Perfusion

- Poor perfusion may be due to hypovolaemia or secondary to myocardial ischaemia.
- Assess perfusion regularly using capillary refill time, toe-core gap, blood pressure and measurement of base deficit.
- Treat with inotropes if poor perfusion persists after initial dose of colloid.

**Respiration**

- Maintain good oxygenation and avoid hypoventilation or apnoea.
- Monitor blood gases 2- to 4-hourly and aim to keep $PaO_2 > 60$ mm Hg (7.8 kPa) and $PaCO_2 < 40$ mm Hg (5.2 kPa).
- Consider intermittent positive-pressure ventilation (IPPV) if there are apnoeic spells or $PaCO_2 > 60$ mm Hg (7.8 kPa), and treat pulmonary hypertension if appropriate.

**Blood glucose**

- Aim for normal blood glucose levels: hypoglycaemia may worsen CNS damage; hyperglycaemia may exacerbate acidosis.
- Check blood glucose levels 2- to 4-hourly and maintain at 4–7 mmol/L by i.v. infusion of 10–15% dextrose (NB hypertonic solutions are frequently necessary as fluid volume is restricted).

**Blood electrolytes**

- *Hyponatraemia* (Na < 130 mmol/L) without excessive urinary sodium loss is likely to be due to excess ADH secretion. Manage by further fluid restriction.
- *Hyperkalaemia* may occur during the acidotic phase (as $K^+$ leaves red cells in exchange for $H^+$ ions). Do not add potassium to i.v. fluids until good urine flow is established.
- *Hypokalaemia* may occur later as renal sodium loss leads to secondary hyperaldosteronism.

**Seizures** Should be treated as above (see p. 199); resistant seizures in the presence of ultrasound evidence of cerebral oedema may respond to the measures outlined below.

**Acidosis** We correct acidosis by improving perfusion and maintaining oxygenation. There is no evidence that correction with buffer improves the condition, although it seems prudent to attempt to correct severe acidosis (pH < 6.9) if problems with perfusion persist despite treatment.

**Coagulopathy** Careful observation for clinical signs of coagulopathy are needed, as this may accompany perinatal hypoxia – monitor platelet count and investigate clinical evidence of bleeding.

**Raised intracranial pressure (ICP)** Cerebral oedema leads to raised ICP and may worsen cerebral perfusion. Ultrasound appearances of generalized echogenicity or compressed ventricles reflect only gross changes and palpation of the anterior fontanelle or transfontanelle measurement of ICP are very inaccurate. Direct monitoring of ICP (indwelling transducer or catheter) should only be attempted in experienced units, and is without proven benefit. Aggressive clinical management of raised ICP has not improved the prognosis. Suggested additional strategies to control raised ICP have included the following.

- *Raise head of cot* 10–15 cm.
- *Frusemide*, 1–2 mg/kg, i.v.
- *Hyperventilation* to lower $PaCO_2$ to 28–35 mm Hg may help to control ICP, but lower levels are associated with a marked reduction in cerebral blood flow.
- *Mannitol*, 2 mL/kg, 20% solution over 30 min has been shown to reduce ICP temporarily.
- *Steroids* are usually considered unhelpful.

**Prognosis**

Perinatal asphyxia is associated with a mixed spastic/dystonic quadriplegic cerebral palsy, often with associated sensorineural hearing loss and central visual impairment. The best predictors of outcome are the worst grade of encephalopathy recorded and time taken to establish sucking feeds. Mild encephalopathy is not associated with neurological sequelae. Most of those with severe encephalopathy will die or develop severe neuro-impairment. Following moderate encephalopathy the outcome is less certain, and approximately 15–20% will develop neuro-impairment. Only 50% of the infants with seizures will have a poor outcome.

Early indicators of poor outcome include EEG abnormalities over the first few hours and high-velocity, low-pulsatility Doppler ultrasound signals from cerebral vessels. Later indicators are > 7 days to establish sucking feeds, and areas of attenuation on the CT scan performed in the second week. MR scan appearances are being evaluated and may prove to be good predictors of outcome.

## THE FLOPPY INFANT

### Diagnosis

- Distinguish between paralytic and non-paralytic conditions; evaluate tendon jerks carefully. The infant moving limbs against gravity or maintaining posture of a passively elevated limb is not paralysed (see Table 12.3) (Dubowitz, 1976).

**Table 12.3**   The floppy infant (Dubowitz (1976) *Clin. Dev. Med.* **79**)

### (1) Paralytic conditions with incidental hypotonia

*Hereditary infantile spinal muscular atrophy*
Werdnig-Hoffman disease
Benign variants

*Congenital myopathies*
Structural   Central core disease
             Minicore disease
             Nemaline myopathy
             Myotubular myopathy
             Myotubular myopathy, X-linked
             Mixed myopathies
             Congenital fibre-type disproportion
             Mitochondrial myopathies
             Other subcellular abnormalities
             'Minimal-change myopathy'

Metabolic   Glycogenosis types II, III, (IV)
            Lipid storage myopathy
            Periodic paralysis

*Other neuromuscular disorders*
Congenital myotonic dystrophy
Congenital muscular dystrophy
Neonatal myasthenia; congenital myasthenia
Motor neuropathies
Other neuromuscular disorders

### (2) Non-paralytic conditions: hypotonia without significant weakness

*Disorders affecting the central nervous system*
Non-specific mental deficiency
Hypotonic cerebral palsy
Birth trauma, intracranial haemorrhage, intrapartum asphyxia and hypoxia
Chromosomal disorders; Down's syndrome
Metabolic disorders; aminoacidurias; organic acidurias; sphingolipidoses
   (leucodystrophies)

*Connective tissue disorders*
Congenital laxity of ligaments
Ehlers-Danlos and Marfan syndromes
Osteogenesis imperfecta
Mucopolysaccharidoses

*Prader-Willi syndrome* (hypotonia – obesity)

*Metabolic, nutritional, endocrine*
Renal tubular acidosis, hypercalcaemia, rickets, coeliac disease, hypothyroidism

*Benign congenital hypotonia* (essential hypotonia)

- In the paralytic group exclude neonatal and congenital myasthenia (maternal history and edrophonium (Tensilon) test).
- Examine the mother for myopathic facies and non-relaxing handshake, which suggests myotonic dystrophy (also commonly a history of polyhydramnios).

### Investigations

- *Muscle biopsy:* usually quadriceps (this is the definitive investigation for paralytic causes). Electron microscopy, enzyme histochemistry and histology must be performed. Best delayed until 3 months, but infants who may die need earlier investigation.
- *Nerve condition velocity:* slow in demyelinating peripheral neuropathy and, to a lesser degree, in axonal neuropathies and spinal muscular atrophy.
- *Electromyography:* distinguishes myopathies, denervation, myotonia and myasthenia.
- *Creatine phosphokinase:* this is usually unhelpful. It is moderately raised in congenital muscular dystrophy, and very high in Duchennee's dystrophy (asymptomatic at this age).

### Management

- Establishment of feeding (may need long-term tube-feeding).
- Physiotherapy for limb and joint deformities.
- Bladder expression may be necessary.
- The diagnosis is important for prognosis and genetic counselling.

## SPINA BIFIDA AND MENINGOMYELOCELE

Spina bifida with meningomyelocele is common, although with current antenatal screening and termination the condition is rarely seen. Aggressive, non-selective surgical closure of these defects has led to the survival of many children with multiple severe handicaps. Most centres now adopt a selective approach to early surgical closure.

### Definitions

- **Spina bifida**        Failure of mid-line fusion of vertebral bodies.

- **Spina bifida occulta** — Spinal cord intact (but may be damaged by the effects of tethering). Detectable only by X-ray or dissection. Sometimes there is an overlying skin pit, hairy patch or dimple. Very common.
- **Meningocele** — Skin covered lesion usually has a good prognosis.
- **Meningomyelocele** — Cystic herniation of both meninges and cord through the bony defect, commonly a large lumbar or thoracic defect. Frequent major neurological deficit. Most common type diagnosed in the neonatal period.
- **Myeloschisis or myelocele** — Failure of closure of the neural tube. The spinal cord forms a flat disc covered by the granulation tissue. Major neurological deficit. Uncommon.

## Assessment

While awaiting preoperative assessment, cover the lesion with plastic film or place the lower half of the body in a suitable plastic bag and pay attention to temperature stability.

**General** Temperature, colour, respiration and evidence of birth injury.

**Head** Circumference, separation of sutures, anterior fontanelle size and pressure. Ultrasound scan (to detect hydrocephalus).

**Back** Level and size of lesion, width of bony defect and availability of skin for repair. Intactness of meningeal sac.

**Neurological** Especially sensory and motor levels. Beware of interpreting reflex activity in the lower limbs as spontaneous movement.

**Sphincter function** Both anal and urinary.

**Orthopaedic** Limitation of movement, muscle wasting, and fixed deformities of lower limbs; spinal deformities; dislocated hips.

**Radiological** X-ray spine with wire markers around the external lesion.

## Factors predictive of severe disability

- Gross hydrocephalus at birth.
- Kyphosis or scoliosis.
- Absence of voluntary movement below L3.
- Incontinence of urine and faeces.
- Postural abnormalities of lower limbs.
- Major associated defects.

The final decision on early surgery rests with parents and attending doctors (see Chapter 25).

*Advice for future pregnancies* Multifactorial inheritance. Preconceptional folic acid supplements are recommended.

## OTHER DEVELOPMENTAL DEFECTS OF THE CNS

### Encephalocele

A sac of meninges and cortex protruding from the skull, usually with intact skin cover, and frequently associated with intracerebral anomalies of poor prognosis. When no neurological tissue is contained within the sac it may be excised with a reasonable prognosis.

### Anencephaly

This is due to failure of closure of the anterior neuropore, just as meningomyelocele is due to failure of closure of the posterior neuropore. Fifty per cent of these pregnancies are associated with polyhydramnios. Only 25% are liveborn, and most die within a week.

### Holoprosencephaly

This is due to defective cleavage of the forebrain, and is often associated with mid-line facial abnormalities. Two-thirds of cases are associated with chromosomal anomalies, particularly trisomy 13. Most are stillborn or die early in the newborn period.

### Agenesis of corpus callosum

May be diagnosed by ultrasound scan. It may be associated with megalencephaly and hypertelorism, but generally is clinically silent.

## Microcephaly

Commonly results from cerebral damage early in pregnancy due to environmental agents or congenital infection. Many chromosomal anomalies are also associated with microcephaly. There are also autosomal recessive and X-linked forms. Developmental delay is usually evident during infancy.

## Porencephalic cysts and hydranencephaly

These are thought to be due to vascular accidents during pregnancy, sometimes associated with congenital infection. Some porencephalic cysts develop postnatally following haemorrhage or infarction. Transillumination may be of value.

## BIBLIOGRAPHY

Amiel-Tison, C. and Grenier, A. (1986) *Neurological examination of the newborn infant.* New York: Oxford University Press.

Dubowitz, L. and Dubowitz, V. (1979) The neurological assessment of the preterm and full-term newborn infants. *Clinics in developmental medicine. Number 76.* London: Spastics International Medical Publications.

Dubowitz, V. (1976) The floppy infant. *Clinics in developmental medicine. Number 79.* London: Spastics International Medical Publications.

Levene, M., Kornberg, J. and Williams, T.H.C. (1985) The incidence and severity of post-asphyxial encephalopathy in full-term infants. *Early Hum. Dev.* **11**, 21–8.

Levene, M.I., Bennett, M.J. and Punt, J. (eds) (1995) *Fetal and neonatal neurology and neurosurgery.* 2nd edn. Edinburgh: Churchill Livingstone.

Pape, K.E. and Wigglesworth, J.S. (1989) *Perinatal brain lesions.* Oxford: Blackwell Scientific Publications.

Rennie, J.M. (1997) *Neonatal cerebral ultrasound.* Cambridge: Cambridge University Press.

Sarnat, H.B. and Sarnat, M.S. (1976) Neonatal ecephalopathy following fetal distress. *Arch. Neurol.* **33**, 696–705.

Volpe, J.J. (1990) *Neurology of the newborn*, 3rd edn. Philadelphia, PA: W.B. Saunders.

# Nutrition and gastroenterology

## INTRODUCTION

The goals of appropriate nutrition are to provide fuel for activity and metabolism and to support normal growth and development. Term infants who are not growth retarded have sufficient stores of fat and glycogen to augment a relatively low milk intake in the first few days of life. Very preterm infants have virtually no fat stores and only sufficient glycogen to provide approximately 4 hours' glucose. Preterm infants also have immature renal and metabolic function, reduced gut motility and limited enzyme capacity. Growth-restricted infants have low stores of both fat and glycogen. Early establishment of an adequate energy supply, either enterally or intravenously, is thus an important priority in successful adaptation to extrauterine life.

## NUTRIENTS AND REQUIREMENTS

**Water** is one of the most important requirements, and intake is usually increased gradually over the first few days (see Chapter 14). The normal maintenance requirement is about 150 mL/kg/day for term infants and 180 mL/kg/day for preterm infants.

**Energy** is supplied by oxidation of three main classes of nutrients: fat, carbohydrate and protein. The energy produced is approximately as follows:

- carbohydrate – 3.7 kcal/g;
- protein – 5.4 kcal/g;
- fat – 9.3 kcal/g.

Normal calorie requirements are approximately 110 kcal/kg/day for term infants and 130 kcal/kg/day for healthy preterm infants. Infants with IUGR often demand a high-calorie intake. Breast milk has been shown to contain about 60–70 kcal/100 mL; standard infant formulae contain 66–68 kcal/100 mL (see Table 13.1), and formulae designed for preterm infants contain up to 82 kcal/100 mL. Ideally protein in the infant's diet is used for growth and not broken down to provide energy; thus adequate 'non-protein calories' must be provided.

**Carbohydrate** in both breast milk and infant formula is supplied as lactose (disaccharide of glucose and galactose) and as glucose in intravenous fluids and parenteral nutrition. Breast milk, and most formulae, contain about 7g carbohydrate in 100 mL (Table 13.1); 10% dextrose solution contains 10g of glucose polymer in 100 mL; 5% infusion, 5g/100 mL etc.

**Protein** includes casein and a mixture of other ('whey') proteins including lactalbumin and lactoferrin. In breast milk, whey proteins predominate and include valuable components such as immuno-globulins, a variety of peptide hormones and growth factors and free amino acids. In parenteral nutrition protein is provided as a solution of amino acids. There are nine essential amino acids for adults; cysteine, histidine and taurine are also thought to be essential dietary

**Table 13.1** Composition of breast milk and infant formulae*

(a) Feeds for mature infants – composition per 100 mL

| | Breast milk | Whey-predominant formulae | | | Casein-predominant formulae | | | | |
|---|---|---|---|---|---|---|---|---|---|
| | | C&G Premium | SMA Gold | Farley's First | Milupa Aptamil | C&G Plus | SMA White | Farley's Second | Milupa Milumil |
| Energy | | | | | | | | | |
| kcal | 65–70 | 66 | 67 | 68 | 67 | 66 | 67 | 66 | 69 |
| kJ | 275–293 | 277 | 280 | 284 | 281 | 277 | 280 | 277 | 290 |
| Protein (g) | 1.2–1.4 | 1.4 | 1.5 | 1.45 | 1.5 | 1.7 | 1.6 | 1.7 | 1.9 |
| casein/whey | | 40:60 | 40:60 | 40:60 | 40:60 | 80:20 | 80:20 | 77:23 | 80:20 |
| Carbohydrate (g) | 7–8 | 7.1 | 7.2 | 7.0 | 7.2 | 7.2 | 7.0 | 8.3 | 8.4 |
| Fat (g) | 3.5–4.5 | 3.6 | 3.6 | 3.8 | 3.6 | 3.4 | 3.6 | 2.9 | 3.1 |
| Na (mmol) | 0.5–1 | 0.8 | 0.7 | 0.74 | 0.87 | 1.1 | 0.96 | 1.1 | 1.04 |
| K (mmol) | 1.4–1.7 | 1.7 | 1.7 | 1.5 | 1.9 | 2.3 | 2.05 | 2.2 | 2.2 |
| Cl (mmol) | 1.0–1.5 | 1.1 | 1.2 | 1.3 | 1.1 | 1.6 | 1.6 | 1.6 | 1.3 |
| Ca (mmol) | 0.8 | 1.35 | 1.15 | 1.0 | 1.3 | 2.0 | 1.4 | 1.5 | 1.8 |
| P (mmol) | 0.5 | 0.9 | 0.9 | 0.9 | 1.0 | 1.5 | 1.4 | 1.5 | 1.8 |
| Ca/P ratio | 1.6 | 1.5 | 1.3 | 1.1 | 1.3 | 1.3 | 1.0 | 1.0 | 1.0 |

**Table 13.1** (a) Continued

| | Breast milk | Whey-predominant formulae | | | Casein-predominant formulae | | | | |
|---|---|---|---|---|---|---|---|---|---|
| | | C&G Premium | SMA Gold | Farley's First | Milupa Aptamil | C&G Plus | SMA White | Farley's Second | Milupa Milumil |
| Fe (mg) | 0.06–0.1 | 0.5 | 0.8 | 0.65 | 0.7 | 0.5 | 0.8 | 0.66 | 0.4 |
| Folate (mcg) | 3.1–6.2 | 10 | 8 | 3.4 | 10.1 | 10 | 8 | 3 | 5 |
| Vitamin A (mcg) | 40–76 | 76 | 75 | 100 | 60 | 80 | 75 | 97 | 57 |
| Vitamin $B_1$ (mcg) | 15 | 4 | 10 | 4 | 4 | 4 | 10 | 0.04 | 0.03 |
| Vitamin $B_{12}$ (mcg) | 0.01 | 0.2 | 0.2 | 0.14 | 0.15 | 0.2 | 0.2 | 0.13 | 0.2 |
| Vitamin C (mg) | 3.1–4.5 | 8 | 9 | 6.9 | 8.1 | 8 | 9 | 6.6 | 7.6 |
| Vitamin D (mcg) | 0.1 | 1.1 | 1.1 | 1.0 | 1.0 | 1.1 | 1.1 | 1.0 | 1.0 |
| Vitamin E (mg) | 0.3–0.4 | 0.8 | 0.74 | 0.48 | 0.6 | 0.8 | 0.74 | 0.46 | 0.8 |
| Vitamin K (mcg) | 1.7 | 5 | 6.7 | 2.7 | 3.0 | 5.0 | 6.7 | 2.6 | 4.0 |

(b) Feeds for preterm infants

| | Preterm breast milk | | Preterm formulae | | | | | |
| | 1 week | 4 weeks | +BMF C&G (3 g) | +BMF Milupa (3 g) | C&G Nutriprem | SMA LBWF | Farley's Osterprem | Milupa Prematil |
|---|---|---|---|---|---|---|---|---|
| **Energy** | | | | | | | | |
| kcal | 67 | 70 | 80 | 82 | 80 | 82 | 80 | 80 |
| kJ | 280 | 293 | 336 | 348 | 336 | 343 | 335 | 335 |
| Protein (g) | 2.4 | 1.8 | 2.5 | 1.9 | 2.4 | 2.0 | 2.0 | 2.4 |
| casein/whey | | | | | 40:60 | 40:60 | 40:60 | 40:60 |
| Carbohydrate (g) | 6.1 | 7.0 | 9.0 | 9.1 | 7.9 | 8.6 | 7.7 | 7.9 |
| Fat (g) | 3.8 | 4.0 | 4.0 | 4.0 | 4.4 | 4.4 | 4.6 | 4.4 |
| Na (mmol) | 2.2 | 1.3 | 1.5 | 1.5 | 1.8 | 1.4 | 1.8 | 1.8 |
| K (mmol) | 1.8 | 1.6 | 1.6 | 1.6 | 2.1 | 1.9 | 1.8 | 2.1 |
| Cl (mmol) | N/A† | 1.7 | 1.9 | 1.7 | 1.4 | 1.5 | 1.7 | 1.4 |
| Ca (mmol) | 0.62 | 0.54 | 2.1 | 1.8 | 2.5 | 1.9 | 2.8 | 2.5 |
| P (mmol) | 0.46 | 0.46 | 1.7 | 1.3 | 1.6 | 1.3 | 2.0 | 1.6 |
| Ca/P ratio | 1.3 | 1.2 | 1.2 | 1.4 | 1.6 | 1.5 | 1.4 | 1.6 |

**Table 13.1** (b) Continued

| | Preterm breast milk | | Preterm formulae | | | | | | |
| | 1 week | 4 weeks | +BMF C&G (3 g) | +BMF Milupa (3 g) | C&G Nutriprem | SMA LBWF | Farley's Osterprem | Milupa Prematil |
|---|---|---|---|---|---|---|---|---|
| Fe (mg) | N/A | 0.1 | N/A | | 0.9 | 0.67 | 0.04 | 0.9 |
| Folate (mcg) | N/A | 5.0 | 53.1 | | 48 | 49 | 50 | 48 |
| | | | | | | | | |
| Vitamin A (mcg) | N/A | N/A | ≥130 | 90 | 227 | 74 | 100 | 108 |
| Vitamin $B_1$ (mcg) | N/A | N/A | 140 | | 140 | 82 | 95 | 140 |
| Vitamin $B_{12}$ (mcg) | 0.24 | 0.03 | 0.22 | | 0.2 | 0.25 | 0.2 | 0.2 |
| Vitamin C (mg) | N/A | N/A | ≥12 | 19 | 16 | 7 | 28 | 16 |
| Vitamin D (mcg) | Very little | | ≥0.5 | | 5 | 1.2 | 2.4 | 2.4 |
| Vitamin E (mg) | 1.3 | 0.6 | ≥2.6 | 0.6 | 3 | 1.1 | 10 | 3 |
| Vitamin K (mcg) | N/A | <0.2 | ≥6.3 | 1.7 | 6.6 | 7.1 | 7 | 6.6 |

*Data for Tables 13.1(a) and 13.1(b) are taken from the manufacturers' product information and from *Nutritional needs of the preterm infant* (Tsang, Lucas, Uauy and Zlotkin, eds).

†N/A indicates either that data are not available, or that the normal range is very wide and therefore not generalizable. For further information the reader is referred to individual chapters of *Nutritional needs of the preterm infant*.

BMF = Breast Milk Fortifier

components for neonates. Infants require between 2 and 4 g/kg/day of protein. For protein content of various milks see Table 13.1.

**Fat** contributes about 50% of the infant's energy. Both breast milk and formula contain approximately 4 g/100 mL. Most of the fat in breast milk is triglyceride, with a mixture of saturated and unsaturated fatty acids, and there is a small amount of phospholipid and cholesterol. Fat in formula milk is provided by either modified cow's milk fat or a mixture of vegetable oils, or a mixture of the two, and is almost entirely triglyceride. Long-chain polyunsaturated fatty acids, which are derived from the two essential fatty acids (omega-3 and omega-6 families) are important in the development and function of neural membranes. They are present in breast milk and have recently been added to a number of formula milks, particularly those designed for preterm infants.

### Minerals

**Sodium** is important for maintenance of extracellular fluid volume and osmolarity, and hence blood pressure, and also for bone growth. The normal requirement is 1–2 mmol/kg/day for term infants and 2–5 mmol/kg/day for preterm, but may be greater in cases of excess loss, e.g. ileostomy, diuretics.

**Potassium** is the principal intracellular cation and is important for maintaining intracellular fluid volume. It is also important for propagation of action potentials in skeletal muscle. The normal requirement for term and preterm infants is 2–3 mmol/kg/day.

**Calcium** is mainly present in bones, which contain 99% of the total body calcium. Of the remaining circulating calcium, 40% is bound to albumin. Most of the unbound calcium is ionized, and it is this portion which is vital for neuromuscular transmission. Of the total body calcium in a term infant, 80% is accumulated in the last trimester of pregnancy, and preterm infants thus have a high dietary requirement. Intake, absorption, vitamin D and phosphate status are all important determinants of calcium balance. The normal requirement for term infants is 1–2 mmol/kg/day and for preterm infants is 3–4 mmol/kg/day.

**Phosphate** is a major component of bone and also important in energy-containing compounds such as ATP. The requirement for term infants is 1–2 mmol/kg/day and for preterm infants is 2–3 mmol/kg/day.

**Magnesium** is important as an intracellular anion and in the regulation of neural transmission. Deficiency may exacerbate fits, particularly after birth asphyxia. The requirement for newborn infants is approximately 0.25 mmol/kg/day.

**Iron** is important for the production of haemoglobin and cytochromes. The bioavailability of iron is much higher from breast milk than from formula or pharmacological preparations. The requirement for term infants is 0.5–1.5 mg/kg/day and for preterm infants is 2–4 mg/kg/day.

### Trace elements
Most of the trace elements required in the diet are involved in a variety of enzyme reactions. Deficiency syndromes tend to be quite non-specific unless extreme.

**Zinc** is involved in a wide range of enzyme reactions, including synthesis of DNA and RNA. Deficiency causes diarrhoea, impaired growth, dermatitis and alopecia. Zinc is available in breast milk and formula, and is added to parenteral nutrition. Levels should be measured in prolonged TPN treatment.

**Copper** is also involved in a wide range of enzyme reactions including fatty acid elongation and desaturation. It is present in breast milk and formula, and added to TPN. Deficiency causes psychomotor retardation, hypotonia, anaemia, neutropenia and bone changes.

**Manganese and selenium** are both important components of antioxidant enzymes, which are important for protecting preterm infants from oxygen radical-induced damage involved in the development of BPD, retinopathy, anaemia and complications of intraventricular haemorrhage, and in asphyxial brain damage.

**Iodine** is necessary for the production of thyroid hormones. It is present in breast milk (except in regions with endemic iodine deficiency), and is added to formula and TPN.

### Vitamins
Vitamins are important as enzymes and cofactors in many metabolic reactions, and often act as antioxidants. 'Classic' deficiency syndromes are described, but these are usually in cases of gross deficiency – subtle signs of depletion may be non-specific. Vitamins A, D, E and K are fat soluble; the vitamin B group, folic acid and vitamin C are water soluble. Recommended daily intake for term and preterm infants are available.

**Vitamin A** is important for synthesis of rhodopsin in the retina and as an antioxidant. It is degraded by light.

**Vitamin D** is the precursor for 25-hydroxy- and 1,25-dihydroxy-vitamin D, whose main role is in the absorption of calcium and phosphate from the gut and renal tubules, thus enhancing bone mineralization.

**Vitamin E** is important as an antioxidant in cell membranes, preventing peroxidation of polyunsaturated fatty acids. Deficiency results in haemolysis, and contributes to the anaemia of prematurity.

**Vitamin K** is a cofactor for the synthesis of clotting factors II, VII, IX and X in the liver.

**Vitamin B group** includes thiamine, riboflavin, niacin, pyridoxine, pantothenic acid and biotin, all of which are involved in intermediate metabolism as enzymes and cofactors.

**Vitamin $B_{12}$ and folic acid** are both important in RNA and DNA synthesis. Deficiency of folic acid results in anaemia, and in $B_{12}$ deficiency results in both anaemia and irreversible neurological damage.

**Vitamin C (ascorbic acid)** has a number of metabolic roles, particularly in amino acid metabolism and in optimizing the activity of folic acid.

## BREAST FEEDING

### Background

Breast feeding has evolved to provide the newborn human infant with a perfectly balanced and nutritionally complete source of food. Breast milk also provides important defences against infection and diseases of infancy, delivers biochemical triggers which modulate gut function and supplies primed enzymes to aid digestion and nutrient utilization. The natural evolution of breast feeding makes it likely that optimal orofacial development and optimal ties of affection between mother and infant are promoted.

For the mother, breast feeding completes the natural hormonal cycle initiated at conception, allows her to use the reserves of body fat accumulated during gestation, and confers a degree of lactational infertility. A well-nourished mother can meet the nutritional demands of her term infant for at least *3 or 4 months*. In addition, breast feeding is the safest form of feeding under unhygienic conditions.

Clinical staff have a duty to highlight these often intangible benefits for mothers, whilst not placing them under undue pressure or engendering any sense of guilt in those mothers who elect to bottle feed.

## Antenatal preparation

There is little evidence that any physical preparation ('nipple toughening') is necessary to prepare for the act of breast feeding, in contrast to the excellent evidence that mental and emotional preparation is highly beneficial. Antenatal education should include the opportunity to observe and discuss issues with a breast-feeding mother, simple facts on the physiology of lactation, practical advice on optimal position and fixing, and some awareness of the common problems encountered.

Although the decision as to how to feed a baby may be made before pregnancy, it is possible to encourage a large proportion of mothers to breast feed in the immediate neonatal period, irrespective of how feeding is managed in the long term. Mothers of preterm children often do so when encouraged by clinical staff, to promote early growth and health. Such mothers must be praised for their personal contribution to their baby's course.

## Postnatal considerations

### Physiology

The *initiation* of breast milk production occurs as a result of the removal of inhibition of high circulating levels of prolactin by placental steroids (mainly oestrogens) following expulsion of the placenta. However, milk production and time to achieve it are, very variable (2–5 days postpartum: initial output 200–900 mL/24 hours).

Milk production is *sustained* by three factors:

- Frequent afferent stimulation of the nipples by sucking;
- Effective removal of freshly synthesized milk from the breast;
- The milk ejection reflex, mediated by oxytocin secretion.

If milk is not removed, engorgement and milk stasis are followed by involution of mammary tissue – the natural process of events in mothers who elect for artificial feeding. In contrast adequate milk production may be sustained by the exclusive use of an electric breast pump (e.g. by mothers of preterm infants). As long as there is frequent emptying of the breast, adequate milk output occurs despite the loss of the suckling-induced prolactin response.

Efficient *transfer* of milk from mother to baby is dependent on the milk ejection reflex and active 'sucking' by the baby. Both require that the baby is effectively fixed and positioned during a feed, ensuring an adequate mouthful of breast tissue to optimize reflex milk release and extraction.

### Routine breast-feeding management

Infants should be put to the breast in the delivery room. Frequent feeds (1–3 hourly) should be encouraged in the first few days, and later demand feeding (usually 5–7 feeds/day by 1 week). Infants and mothers should be in the same room at night. It is central to effective pain-free feeding that the baby takes an adequate volume of breast tissue (not simply the nipple) into the mouth, thus ensuring that the breast is not traumatized, and reducing the risk of sore nipples.

There should be *no restriction* of the duration or frequency of feeds, and babies should *not* be switched between breasts after an arbitrary time. Babies should feed from the first breast until they come off spontaneously. The second breast should then be offered, but whether or not it is taken, and for how long, should be dictated by hunger/satiety on the baby's part. A baby thus receives a balanced feed, in terms of the high-volume, low-fat *foremilk*, and low-volume, high-fat *hindmilk*. Adequate emptying of the breast is essential, as hindmilk is important in ensuring slower gastric emptying (thereby extending the inter-feed interval), maximizing intake of fat-soluble vitamins, and developing normal appetite control ('conditioned satiety').

If feeds are excessively long (> 30 min) or over-frequent (< 1-hourly), positioning may be incorrect. Suboptimal positioning is the commonest cause of failed or inadequate lactation, principally by compromising breast emptying. The essential steps for ensuring correct positioning are contained in a Royal College of 'Midwives' handbook entitled: *Successful Breast Feeding*. In the event of *breast feeding problems*, the advice of a skilled midwife should be sought. We also commend the benefits of a recognized local 'expert', with or without the input of local lay support groups (e.g. National Childbirth Trust breast-feeding counsellors).

## Special considerations

**Preterm infants** may feed competently from the breast as early as 30 weeks' gestation. Development of feeding skills may be impaired by the presence of, for example, gastric tubes or supplementary fluids given i.v. or enterally. An early trial of breast feeding is thus recommended. Even 'non-nutritive' sucking may improve the infant's progress and the establishment of breast milk supply.

**Electric pumps** are efficient at establishing breast milk flow, although the suckling-induced surge of prolactin wanes with repeated use. Treatment with *metaclopramide* will often offset any fall off in milk supply associated with prolonged pump use.

**Test weighing** is not a routine clinical procedure. When indicated, it should be conducted over a *24-hour period* and preferably in a familiar environment (i.e. at home). Simple mechanical scales are too inaccurate and an electronic balance must be used. 'Test weighing' over a single feed is not recommended.

**Ultrasound assessment of oral function** (using a submental sagittal view in real time or M-mode) may be useful in differentiating temporary problems from intractable neurological dysfunction.

## Clinical breast-feeding problems

### Oral anomalies which impair feeding

**Cleft lip and/or palate** This is one of the more obvious impairments to successful breast feeding, although babies with unilateral cleft lip are often successful. The cleft interferes with the negative pressure normally achieved in the mouth, impairing the teat-stripping action of the tongue. The early provision of a palatal prosthesis may allow successful feeding, although the presence of a plate will disturb the tactile stimulation necessary for the smooth translation of the peristaltic wave from the tongue to the pharynx, and may demand greater perseverance by the mother. One advantage is that earlier feeding will be possible after repair of the lesion.

**Sub-mucal cleft** A defect in the bony palate, but not involving the soft tissue, can interfere with feeding. Feeding is often very noisy, with a loud smacking sound generated as air enters the buccal cavity at the point when the soft tissue can no longer resist the high negative intra-oral pressure. Surgical repair may be necessary to prevent later speech or feeding problems.

**Pierre-Robin syndrome** The poor muscular development and retrognathia may be incompatible with early establishment of feeds, breast or artificial. Subsequent forward growth of the jaw may permit graduation from a spoon to the breast although, using special designs of bottle/teat, milk may be successfully squeezed into the oral cavity and artificial feeding established.

**Laryngomalacia** appears to impair the generation of normal negative intra-oral pressure, reducing feeding efficiency and milk intake, and occasionally contributing to failure to thrive.

**'Tongue-tie'** A severe tongue tie can prevent the normal forward thrust of the tongue to form a furrow around the nipple. This impairs the onset of the peristaltic stripping movement which forces milk from the lactiferous sinuses into the mouth. In the presence of breast-feeding difficulties surgical intervention is indicated.

**Nasal obstruction** Such obstruction (mucus, choanal atresia/stenosis, too close approximation of nares to the breast) will impair the normal 1:1 relationship of sucking to breathing. In the case of a positioning problem, rotate the baby to a better position, and do not press the breast away from the baby's mouth reducing the amount of breast tissue in the mouth.

**Oral thrush** This results in oral discomfort which, if untreated, can lead to an aversion to feeding. If there is itching, pain or discomfort to the mother she should be treated at the same time as the baby (see Chapter 17).

## Failure of lactation

**Retained placental fragments** These may secrete sufficient oestrogens to continue inhibition of prolactin.

**Primary failure of lactation** This is rare (< 2% of mothers), combining normal lactating prolactin levels (800–6000 mIU/L) with milk output below 150 mL/day at 1 month. Impaired end-organ responsiveness is suspected. Metaclopromide is ineffective, despite causing a further rise in prolactin.

## Insufficient lactation

**Breast milk insufficiency** This is found in about 5% of mothers, and is defined as milk output of 200–450 mL/day at 1 month. It may reflect the lower end of the normal range of output, but more frequently reflects suboptimal management. Careful assessment of technique is important, although supplementation with artificial formulae may be necessary.

**Impaired milk release** This may be due to impairment of the normal 'let-down reflex' and may be overcome by providing a relaxing, familiar environment and sensitive, skilled care. Occasionally it is due to reduced sucking efficiency by the baby (see above), and milk release can be encouraged by the use of an electric breast pump.

## Apparent lactation insufficiency

(Poor growth of an otherwise normal baby despite normal milk output of 500–800 mL/day.)

**Incorrect positioning** This is the commonest cause, the baby taking low-fat foremilk, resulting in volume or calorie depletion, and it is only usually correctable at an early stage before the infant becomes entrenched in a poor feeding habit.

**Inappropriate pattern of breast usage** Either exclusive single-breast feeding or rigid both breast policies may result in inefficient feeding, and may be overcome by the adoption of more flexible policies.

**Over-efficient maternal physiology** An over-vigorous ejection reflex, particularly in combination with either of the preceding two problems, may result in symptoms such as 'colic', overfeeding or symptoms of lactose malabsorption – flatus, 'wind' and loose frothy acid stools, possibly because of rapid gastric emptying and spillage of lactose into the colon.

## Maternal complications of breast feeding

**Engorgement** This is most common in the first week. Vascular engorgement, which resolves spontaneously, should be differentiated from milk engorgement, which is usually caused by restrictions on the baby's access to the breast. If the baby is unable to remove the milk, physical interventions are necessary (showers, manual expression, pump) to draw off milk and reduce areolar oedema.

**Mastitis/blocked duct** Infective and non-infective inflammation may present similarly. In the latter there is retrograde flow of milk under pressure from the lumen of the breast into the surrounding tissues, with local and general immune responses. Infective mastitis is usually associated with an infected lesion of the nipple and requires antibiotics. Breast feeds should be continued, even in the presence of infection, as cessation will exacerbate local swelling and may predispose to abscess formation, which usually requires surgical drainage. Breast feeding may still continue, unless sucking impinges on the abscess site.

## Breast milk contaminants

**Drugs** (see Chapter 28)

**Environmental pollutants** Fat-soluble contaminants may accumulate during the period of fat deposition in pregnancy and appear in high concentrations in the breast milk. No data on acceptable levels of pollutants exist and relative risks cannot be estimated.

**Viral infections** Vertical transmission of HIV may occur via breast milk. The risk is highest in situations where the mother contracts HIV postnatally, i.e. while breast feeding, and the infant has a high virus exposure. Where the mother is in a quiescent phase of the disease, viral transmission is low. For this reason, in countries where morbidity and mortality from infantile gastroenteritis are high, breast feeding is recommended, while in developed countries where the risk of gastroenteritis is low and safe formula milks are widely available, artificial feeding is recommended.

There is also evidence for vertical transmission of hepatitis C from mother to infant, but the risk attributable to breast feeding is unclear.

## ARTIFICIAL FEEDING

The unmodified milk of the cow, goat and ewe is unsuitable for feeding infants in the first months of life because the composition of these milks differs from that of human milk and may lead to an excessive renal solute load, late hypocalcaemia, and iron, folate or vitamin deficiencies, depending upon the milk used. Modern modified cow's milk formulae should be advised when mothers do not wish or are unable to breast feed. Table 13.1 shows the types and composition of the available modified formulae in the UK. Those with a casein:whey ratio resembling that of breast milk are most suitable. For each type, the various brands are similar so that the basis of preference is usually cost or local availability. However, there are differences, for example in lipid source, iron content, provision of long-chain polyunsaturated fatty acids, etc., and detailed information is always available from the manufacturers. There is no evidence to support the claim that the less modified formulae with a higher casein content are more 'satisfying' for the 'hungry and demanding baby'.

Offer a feed within 4 hours of birth and then feed on demand. The volumes recommended are given in Table 14.1.

*Infants at risk for hypoglycaemia* (see Chapter 16) should be fed early and more frequently, unless contraindicated by gastrointestinal or respiratory disease.

## Special formulae

Special formulae are used in the newborn period for the treatment of certain gastrointestinal and inherited metabolic disorders. These should only be prescribed with the advice and supervision of a paediatric dietician.

### Indications for use of special formulae

- *Specific gastrointestinal disorders*, e.g. for cow's milk protein intolerance a soya-based formula may be used, for disaccharidase deficiencies formulae with minimal lactose content are available, and for conditions with fat malabsorption formulae with predominantly medium-chain triglycerides (MCT) are available. After gastroenteritis, necrotizing enterocolitis or neonatal surgery, babies may be fed on a semi-elemental formula, e.g. 'Pregestemil', which is more easily absorbed.
- *Inherited metabolic disorders*, e.g. galactosaemia or phenylketonuria (see Chapter 16). Special formulae are available which compensate for the enzyme deficiency by reducing substrate intake, and ensure provision of essential nutrients.
- *Conditions with biochemical disturbances*, e.g. Di George syndrome, biliary atresia, renal failure, are usually managed with a combination of an appropriate special formula and careful dietary and nutritional monitoring.

## FEEDING PRETERM AND SICK INFANTS

Wherever possible preterm or sick infants should be enterally fed, as this is safer, cheaper, and nutritionally better than parenteral (intravenous) feeding.

### Preterm infants

The preterm infant requires 100–130 kcal/kg/day to grow at the rate achieved *in utero*. This requires 180–200 mL/kg/day of standard infant formula or expressed breast milk. Such high fluid intakes may be poorly tolerated and may predispose to the development of PDA (see Chapter 11) and NEC. Special formulae for preterm infants have a higher calorie content, permitting growth with lower volume intakes. Very preterm and low-birthweight infants (< 1250 g) will usually be started on intravenous feeding while enteral feeds are gradually increased.

It is important to avoid excess energy expenditure in preterm infants. Careful maintenance of a thermoneutral environment and measures to limit handling and excessive activity will minimize energy wastage.

*Human milk* from mothers of preterm infants has a higher sodium and protein concentration than the milk of mothers of fullterm infants, and is thus more suitable for preterm infants. Over the first few weeks the composition becomes more like that of term breast milk; it also varies widely between individuals. Supplementation with calories, protein, phosphate and sodium may be necessary. *Human milk fortifiers* are powder preparations which have been developed for this purpose. They contain the above nutrients, plus other minerals and vitamins, and aim to enhance growth and reduce the risk of osteopenia, while allowing the baby the benefits of breast milk (see Table 13.1). The dose of fortifier should be increased gradually as gastric emptying tends to slow, and vomiting may occur.

*Low-birthweight formulae* supply extra energy, protein and minerals to achieve intrauterine growth rates at intakes of 150–180 mL/kg/day (Table 13.1), and may be used in infants of < 1800 g. Note that these formulae have a variable sodium content, and further supplements may still be necessary to meet the needs of infants of < 1500 g. If extra fluid is needed (e.g. phototherapy) give water; do not increase the volume of low-birthweight formula. Hydration may be assessed by daily measurements of urine specific gravity (maintain SG at < 1.015), serum electrolytes and weight.

Only increase the volume of low-birthweight formulae above the volume recommended after full nutritional assessment, with biochemical screening, including – ideally – plasma amino-acid levels.

Low-birthweight formulae should only be used in hospital; it is usual practice to change to standard formula when the baby reaches 2000 g, or a few days before discharge.

Occasionally, babies with a very high calorie requirement (e.g. those with BPD, heart failure) will not gain weight adequately even on preterm formula. Calorie supplements containing carbohydrate with or without lipid may be used.

*Minimal enteral feeds* supplying 1–24 mL/kg/day have been shown to enhance both gut mucosal growth and overall gut function in very preterm infants. These 'non-nutritive' feeds are usually started in the first week of life in babies whose main nutritional support is provided by PN, and are then increased very gradually.

## FOOD ADDITIVES AND SUPPLEMENTS

### Vitamins

**Vitamin K** (see Chapter 4) The Department of Health recommends that infants at risk of nutritional deficiency should receive 5 drops/day of Children's Vitamin Drops (or a similar preparation) from 1 month to 2 years or until the mother's professional adviser believes that the infant is receiving an adequate vitamin intake in the diet. The compositions of suitable vitamin drops are as follows:

An infant who is being breast fed by a well-nourished mother should not need extra vitamins provided that an adequate mixed diet

| | Vitamin A | Vitamin C | Vitamin D |
|---|---|---|---|
| Children's Vitamin Drops (5 drops) | 214 mcg  (700 IU) | 21 mg | 7 mcg (280 IU) |
| Abidec* (Parke Davis 0.6 ml) | 1200 mcg (4000 IU) | 50 mg | 10 mcg (400 IU) |

* Also contains B vitamins.

is introduced between the fourth and sixth month of life. Those who are purely breast fed beyond 6 months should receive supplements as above. Formula-fed infants do not need extra vitamins. Proprietary baby foods are fortified with vitamins. Children's Vitamin Drops should be prescribed when the mixed diet is based on an inadequate family diet.

The following infants are particularly at risk of vitamin deficiencies.

**1** Low-birthweight infants (see below).
**2** Infants fed on unconventional diets.
- *unmodified cows', goats' or ewes' milk* should not be recommended for infants less than 6 months old because of their unsuitable composition, but if used vitamin supplements are needed. For those who are fed goats' or ewes' milk give Children's Vitamin Drops *plus* folate (100 mcg daily). If infants who are fed goats' milk have the milk boiled before use, vitamin $B_{12}$ will be needed, especially if they are weaned on to a diet low in the vitamin. In practice it is easier to give the total vitamin supplement as Ketovite tablets and liquid (Paines & Byrne, manufacturer).
- *Infants in traditional Asian households* or other ethnic groups known to be prone to vitamin D deficiency (e.g. *Rastafarians*) need vitamin supplementation with Children's Vitamin Drops during breast feeding and after the introduction of the family diet, and are recommended to continue up to the age of 5 years. If formula feeding is commenced, it should be encouraged until 12 months of age.
- *Infants of families on non-standard diets* may have nutritional requirements in addition to those provided in Children's Vitamin Drops. Mothers on *vegan, vegetarian* and *macrobiotic diets* should take additional vitamin $B_{12}$. Infants who are weaned on to these diets may be at risk of protein and calorie malnutrition.

Expert paediatric dietetic advice should be sought if in doubt.

## Fluoride

Fluoride supplementation is recommended where the drinking water contains less than 0.33 ppm, in order to reduce the incidence of dental caries. Fluoride drops are available to provide 0.25 mg daily in either two or five drops. A reduced dosage may be given for water supplies containing between 0.33 and 1.00 ppm fluoride. Information on the fluoride content of water in any area may be obtained from the Local Water Authority. Fluoride supplementation should be stopped when fluoride-containing toothpaste is used.

## Special requirements of the very preterm infant

**Vitamin D, calcium and phosphorus** Very preterm infants are at risk of metabolic bone disease or osteopenia resulting from failure to achieve intrauterine rates of phosphate and calcium accretion. We give *Vitamin D* supplements as Children's Vitamin Drops, 5 drops bd, i.e. twice the standard dose, which provides 560 IU daily. (Note that a double dose of Abidec is not recommended, as this will cause high vitamin A intake.)

*Calcium and phosphate* are not routinely supplemented for infants receiving artificial formulae, but phosphate supplementation ($K_2PO_4$, 2 mmol/kg/day) is necessary for very preterm children ($< 30$ weeks) receiving breast milk. Breast milk fortifiers provide phosphate which may be sufficient for babies receiving the maximum dose. Plasma calcium, phosphate and alkaline phosphatase should be monitored weekly. If serum phosphate falls below 1.8 mmol/L, phosphate supplements should be commenced. If signs of metabolic bone disease occur – hypocalcaemia, raised alkaline phosphatase, radiological signs of osteopenia or fractures – calcium supplements may also be required (2–4 mmol/kg/day). Vitamin D supplements of 400 IU/day are usually sufficient if adequate substrate is given, and there is no proven benefit of giving active vitamin D metabolites, such as 25-OHD, 1,25-OHD or 1-alpha-OHD, except in cases of cholestasis or metabolic disorders.

If both phosphate and calcium are being added to breast milk, the phosphate should be added first, and allowed to stand for at least 5 min before adding the calcium, in order to minimize co-precipitation.

**Vitamin E** The well-described vitamin E-deficient haemolytic anaemia is now rarely seen, as modern formulae contain the recommended vitamin E:polyunsaturated fatty acid ratio. Breast-fed babies appear to maintain adequate vitamin E levels. Randomized trials suggest that a single dose of vitamin E (25 mg/kg i.m.) may reduce the risk of severe degrees of IVH in babies below 33 weeks' gestation (see Chapter 12).

**Folic acid** Folic acid (50 mcg daily, orally) is given from 14 days until 6 weeks post-term to infants of < 33 weeks' gestation if they are being fed on breast milk or standard formula. Preterm formulae are supplemented with folic acid, so additional doses are not required while on this diet.

**Iron** There is controversy concerning how and when to provide iron supplementation. All infants experience a physiological fall in hae-moglobin concentration over the first 2–3 months of life. Preterm infants have low iron stores, and as their blood volume expands during rapid growth they require a dietary source of iron. Breast milk contains relatively little iron, but it is very well absorbed; most low-birthweight and standard formulae contain extra iron, but probably an insufficient amount to meet the needs of the smallest infants. However, extra iron may saturate the iron-binding capacity of lactoferrin, increasing the risk of gastroenteritis, as *E. coli* requires free iron in order to multiply. Iron absorption is related to age, growth rate and haemoglobin level, and is low during the first few weeks after birth.

The American Academy of Paediatrics Committee on Nutrition recommends 2 mg/kg/day iron supplementation to be started by at least 2 months of life. We currently supplement very preterm babies (< 33 weeks) with iron from 4 weeks until they are weaned (5–10 drops daily of Niferex, an iron-polysaccharide complex containing 0.6 mg elemental iron per drop, or 1 mL daily of Sytron, sodium ironedate, which contains 5.5 mg elemental iron/mL). If enteral feeding has been delayed and several blood transfusions have been given, treatment with iron is usually started later, at 6 to 8 weeks.

All babies who are being fed unmodified milks need iron supple-ments until thay are weaned. Term infants who are still fully breast fed at 6 months should have iron supplements.

## FEEDING TECHNIQUES

Infants of 34 weeks' gestation can usually co-ordinate sucking and swallowing, and should be offered breast or bottle feeds but, if unsuccessful, tube feeding may be necessary.

## Gastric feeding

Orogastric tubes are preferable to nasogastric tubes because they cause less airway obstruction. If taped over the mid-point of the lower lip, orogastric tubes are well tolerated.

Gastric feeding is usually intermittent (1 to 4-hourly) and the tube position checked (by testing aspirate for acidity) before each feed. Use a 5FG PVC tube, which should be changed every 2–3 days as PVC becomes stiff in use.

## Transpyloric (TP) feeding

This may be used in preference to i.v. feeding in infants who cannot tolerate gastric feeding (e.g. those with severe cardiac or respiratory disease). It is less physiological than gastric feeding, as digestion normally starts in the stomach with salivary amylase and lingual and gastric lipases, and should only be used if essential. Complications include displacement, obstruction, sepsis, ileus or NEC. If symptoms occur, stop feeds and X-ray the abdomen.

The tube (silicon rubber, *not* PVC) should be passed orally if tolerated, and may be fixed in place with a grooved dental plate or taped over the lower lip. Tube length equal to the distance from the baby's mouth to ankle is marked and passed with the baby lying on the right side. When the mark is at the level of the umbilicus, the tip is in the stomach (check aspirate for acidity). Slowly inject 1–2 mL of sterile water and advance the tube 1–2 cm every 5–10 min until the mark is at the mouth or nose. Slowly inject 1 mL of sterile water and gently aspirate on syringe. If there is resistance to aspiration the tip is probably in the duodenum or jejunum. Insert a gastric tube, inject a further 2–3 mL of sterile water into the transpyloric tube and aspirate the gastric tube. If nothing is obtained, the tube is almost certainly in the duodenum or jejunum, and the position may be checked by X-ray. The ideal position is in the second part of the duodenum – the jejunum is too far. Transpyloric feeds are given by continuous infusion, usually starting at 1–2 mL/hour and slowly increasing as tolerated. Aspirate the gastric tube 6-hourly.

## Cup feeding

This method is an alternative to tube feeding which is gaining in popularity. It provides oral stimulation, avoids nipple-teat confusion and reduces the need for passage of nasal or oral tubes. The baby is positioned in a sitting position and the cup tilted so that milk is at the lips – it is never poured into the baby's mouth. Sipping and sucking movements allow a small amount of milk to be swallowed; this method may be successful from 30 weeks onward.

## PARENTERAL NUTRITION (PN)

Parenteral (intravenous) feeding is an expensive and complex way of providing nutrition, and should be reserved for those situations in which enteral feeds are not practicable. It should only be undertaken by experienced medical and nursing staff and where adequate biochemical, bacteriological and pharmaceutical services are available. In preterm infants with low body nutrient stores, cautious use of intravenous nutrition can prevent catabolism, with its resultant negative nitrogen balance, until enteral feeds are established. Infants with serious gut disorders may require total parenteral nutrition for several weeks.

### Indications

Indications for parenteral nutrition include gastrointestinal surgery, extreme prematurity, necrotizing enterocolitis, severe illness such as septicaemia or cardiac failure – often with ileus, respiratory distress and severe intrauterine growth retardation.

### Nutrient supply

Nutritional requirements and fluid volumes are similar to those of enteral nutrition (see beginning of this chapter and Table 13.2).

*Calories* Are provided as glucose (0.4 calories/mL 10% dextrose) and as lipid emulsions (1.1 kcal/mL 10% intralipid, 2.0 kcal/mL 20% intralipid). Protein should be utilized for growth and not metabolized for energy (see below).

*Carbohydrate* Glucose is the main source. Sick newborn infants, particularly preterm, may be relatively intolerant, necessitating a gradual increase. Usually start with 10% dextrose and reduce the concentration if hyperglycaemic or increase if tolerated, to provide more calories. Dextrose concentrations of $>12.5\%$ should be given via a central line to avoid phlebitis.

*Protein* This is given as a synthetic crystalline amino acid solution. Special formulations are available for infants, although there is still

**Table 13.2** Guidelines for prescription of parenteral nutrition for newborn infants

| | Volume (mL/kg/day)* | Glucose (mg/kg/min)† | Amino acids (g/kg/day)‡ | Lipid (g/kg/day)§ | Na⁺ | K⁺ | Ca²⁺ (mmol/kg/day) | PO₄²⁻ (mmol/kg/day) |
|---|---|---|---|---|---|---|---|---|
| Day 1 | 80 | 4–6 | 0.5 | 0.5 | 2–5 | 1–3 | 0.5–1 | 0.5–1 |
| Day 2 | 100 | 4–6 | 1.0 | 1.0 | 2–5 | 1–3 | 0.5–1 | 0.5–1 |
| Day 3 | 120 | 6–8 | 1.5 | 1.5 | 2–5 | 1–3 | 0.5–2 | 0.5–2 |
| Day 4 | 140 | 6–8 | 2.0 | 2.0 | 2–5 | 1–3 | 0.5–2 | 0.5–2 |
| Day 5 | 160 | 8–10 | 2.5 | 2.5 | 2–5 | 1–3 | 0.5–2 | 0.5–2 |
| Day 6 | 160 | 8–12 | 2.5–3.0 | 3.0 | 2–5 | 1–3 | 0.5–2 | 0.5–2 |

*Total fluid volume may need to be adjusted depending on clinical status, electrolytes, phototherapy, etc.

†100 mL/kg/day of 10% dextrose provides 6.9 mg/kg/min (see Chapter 16).

‡'Vaminolact' (Pharmacia) contains 58 grams of protein/L, i.e. 0.58 g/10 mL.

§'Intralipid' (Pharmacia): 10%=0.1 g/mL; 20%=0.2 g/mL.

For preterm infants, especially if they are receiving some milk, we usually give a maximum of 2.5 g/kg/day of protein and 2.0 g/kg/day of lipid.

uncertainty about the ideal composition of such solutions – whether to mimic placental supply or breast milk composition. If no exogenous protein is provided, preterm infants will catabolize about 1 g/kg/day of body protein to meet their metabolic needs. Provision of 1–2 g/kg/day, with at least 60 kcal/kg/day of non-protein calories to provide for resting energy expenditure, will prevent this catabolism. Optimal protein requirements for growth are about 2 g/kg/day at term and 3–4 g/kg/day between 24 and 36 weeks.

**Fat** Given as an oil-in-water emulsion derived from egg phospholipid, soybean oil and glycerol. Fat provides a concentrated source of calories, but may be poorly tolerated by very small infants. Start at 0.5 g/kg/day (i.e. 5 mL/kg/day of 10% lipid emulsion), increasing to 2.0 g/kg/day for preterm infants and 3.0 g/kg/day for term infants. Soybean oil is rich in essential fatty acids (linoleic and alpha-linolenic acids), and 0.5–1.0 g/kg/day of 'intralipid' will provide adequate amounts. Blood triglyceride levels can be measured; keep levels below 150 mg/L. During periods of suspected and proven sepsis, thrombocytopenia (platelets $< 50 \times 10^9$/L), acidosis (pH $< 7.2$) and hyperbilirubinaemia (sufficient to warrant phototherapy), lipid infusion should be reduced to 0.5–1.0 g/kg/day or stopped for 24 hours until the baby is stable. Close monitoring is necessary in children with lung and liver disease.

**Minerals** The following are recommendations for term and preterm infants. Blood levels need to be closely monitored, particularly in the first week.

|  | Term | Preterm |  |
|---|---|---|---|
| Sodium | 2–3 | 3–5 | mmol/kg/day |
| Potassium | 1–2 | 1–2 | mmol/kg/day |
| Chloride | 1–2 | 2–3 | mmol/kg/day |
| Calcium | 1–2 | 2–4 | mmol/kg/day |
| Magnesium | 0.25 | 0.25 | mmol/kg/day |
| Phosphorus | 1–2 | 1–3 | mmol/kg/day |

NB It is often difficult to achieve the desired input of calcium and phosphate for preterm infants, because of solubility problems. This may improve with the availability of new organic phosphate solutions (sodium glycerophospate, glucose-1-phosphate).

**Trace elements** These are provided in a commercial mixture containing zinc, copper, manganese, selenium, fluorine and iodine. In prolonged total PN use levels may need to be measured, and other trace elements such as molybdenum and chromium may be required.

**Vitamins** A full range of vitamins must be provided in intravenous nutrition. Both water and fat-soluble vitamins are available in commercial paediatric preparations, but vitamin $B_{12}$ supplements are needed after about 1 month.

## Prescription and preparation

It has been shown that preterm infants will tolerate parenteral nutrition from day 1, and we aim to start within 24–48 hours in infants of < 1000 g birthweight in order to prevent catabolism. It is advisable to build up nutrient intake gradually, and a suggested regimen is shown in Table 13.2. In larger infants with some body nutrient stores, parenteral nutrition may be started later if enteral feeding is delayed. Clinical assessment of water requirement may make changes necessary (e.g. phototherapy, cardiac failure, use of muscle relaxants). When considering the sodium requirement, take account of sodium in arterial line infusate, flushes, and any measured losses.

Commercial products are available for the provision of parenteral nutrition. The most common method of delivery is to mix a single bag of water-soluble components – dextrose, amino acids, minerals, trace elements and water-soluble vitamins – and to give lipid emulsion, with fat-soluble vitamins, separately. The preparation must be carried out meticulously in a dedicated sterile area of pharmacy. The extent to which each baby's nutritional and metabolic needs can be individually met depends on local preference and staffing levels. A 24-hour supply is usually prepared.

## Administration

Parenteral nutrition may be administered via peripheral or central venous lines. Peripheral lines should be resited as quickly as possible to avoid hypoglycaemia. If given centrally, the caloric intake may be increased by the use of 15–20% glucose solutions (sclerosant to peripheral veins). Arterial lines are not suitable routes for i.v. nutrition.

PN may be infused via a standard infusion pump with a two-entry port burette. There should be a suitable bacterial filter in line before a Y-connector. The lipid emulsion is pumped into the other arm of this connector and thus into the baby. Both solutions should be protected from light.

Strict aseptic technique is necessary during preparation and administration. Ideally a separate i.v. line should be used purely for PN. With a peripheral line drugs may be given, if essential, so long as they are chemically compatible. They should be injected before the bacterial filter, and should be flushed through.

Glucose and amino acids are infused continuously. It used to be necessary to interrupt the lipid infusion for several hours, as lipid interferes with the measurement of serum sodium on laboratory analysers. With modern analytical equipment this is now rarely a problem, except in cases of extreme lipaemia (which will be obvious in the laboratory). Therefore lipid infusions can also be infused continuously over 24 hours. If in doubt, check with the local biochemist.

Lipid levels should be determined during and after at least 8 hours of lipid infusion.

## Cautions

- *Potassium* – extra care must be exercised during renal impairment, and potassium omitted or reduced if hyperkalaemic.
- *Hypocalcaemia* – occurs rarely as a result of excessive phosphate in the glucose-electrolyte mixture, and is corrected by reducing the phosphate concentration.
- *Never add bicarbonate* – as it will precipitate as $CaCO_3$.
- *Never add extra calcium to the glucose/amino acid mixture* – as it will precipitate out phosphate.
- *Polyunsaturated fatty acids* – are precursors of prostaglandins, and intravenous infusion may theoretically interfere with blood clotting, pulmonary artery vasodilatation, etc. Give with caution in sick infants.
- *Toxic levels of some amino acids* – may occur if high doses are given. If there is concern, urine amino acids should be measured.

## Complications

These can be classified into two main categories: infusion-related (usually problems with line) and infusate-related (usually metabolic).

### Infusion-related problems

***Sepsis*** This can be minimized by meticulous nursing and medical care of lines. Percutaneous long-lines should be inserted, and re-connections made, under full sterile conditions, and lines should be dedicated for PN.

***Malposition*** Check position with X-ray.

***Thrombosis*** With peripheral lines thrombophlebitis and skin ulceration may occur. Avoidance is by frequent inspection and resiting of lines. If PN 'tissues' under the skin, intradermal injection of saline may prevent further damage, and should be considered in conjunction with a plastic surgery opinion.

***Haemorrhage*** May occur shortly after insertion, or if the line is dislodged or disconnected.

### Infusate-related complications

***Hyperglycaemia*** Reduce the glucose concentration to 7.5% or even 5%. Consider sepsis. Occasionally low-dose insulin may be required.

***Hypoglycaemia*** Avoid by prompt resiting of i.v. lines. Increase glucose concentration if it persists. Consider sepsis or metabolic disorder.

***Hyperlipidaemia*** Can be identified by inspection or nephelometry of plasma or by measuring triglyceride and cholesterol levels. Stop lipid infusion for several hours and recommence at a lower rate.

***Cholestasis*** May occur after prolonged PN use and in relation to sepsis. It is not clear whether this is due to a toxic effect of one of the infusates (both amino acids and lipids have been implicated), or to the non-physiological effects of by-passing the GI tract, which produces many enzymes and hormones required for normal metabolism. Minimal enteral nutrition with 1 mL/kg every 2–4 hours (ideally breast milk) may help to prevent this.

## Monitoring

Clinical and laboratory monitoring is essential for all babies on parenteral nutrition.

### Clinical monitoring
This should include the following regular observations: daily weight; urine: volume, specific gravity, pH, glucose, protein and blood;

blood sugar, 4-hourly on first day, then 8 to 12-hourly or more frequently if unstable.

### Laboratory monitoring

- Full blood count, plasma urea, electrolytes, creatinine, bilirubin: daily first week, alternate days thereafter
- Plasma calcium, magnesium, phosphate and bilirubin: twice weekly until stable, then weekly.
- Lipid levels: weekly on infusions of more than 2 g/kg/day, twice weekly above 3 g/kg/day.
- Urine $Na^+$, urea, creatinine: daily if there is an excessive $Na^+$ requirement.
- Total and indirect bilirubin, albumin, alkaline phosphatase, transaminases: weekly.

## GASTROINTESTINAL PROBLEMS

### Gastro-oesophageal reflux (GOR)

Simple regurgitation of gastric contents is common in infancy. However, GOR may cause concern if it causes failure to thrive, aspiration pneumonia, apnoea or oesophagitis. It may also play a role in some cases of BPD. Predisposing factors include hiatus hernia, delayed gastric emptying and following repair of tracheo-oesophageal fistula.

#### Investigation

If available, *prolonged oesophageal pH monitoring* over 12–24 hours is the most accurate and sensitive method for the detection and quantification of GOR. If the pH is < 4.0 for more than 5% of the study time, this is an abnormal result, and a value over 15% indicates severe reflux. *Radiology* may be necessary to exclude hiatus hernia.

#### Management

Clinical reflux improves spontaneously with time, causing confusion over indications for treatment and assessment of its efficacy. The practice of sitting the baby at an angle of 60° is now considered more harmful than leaving the baby supine; the *anti-Trendelenberg position* (prone with head elevated) is the most effective postural treatment. Other interventions include the following.

*Small frequent feeds*

***Thickening agents*** e.g. Carobel or cornflour which make the baby more settled but do not improve GOR. Unsuitable for premature babies.

***Antacids*** e.g. Gaviscon.

***Cisapride*** Is a prokinetic agent which has been shown to reduce GOR significantly (and it may improve respiratory symptoms in babies with GOR and chronic respiratory symptoms).

***$H_2$ antagonists*** May be indicated in severe cases with oesophagitis.

***Omeprazole*** Proton pump inhibitor; may be helpful in severe reflux with oesophagitis.

***Surgical fundoplication*** May be necessary in very severe cases where medical treatment has failed.

## Necrotizing enterocolitis (NEC)

Although most common in very-low-birthweight babies, the frequency of NEC varies widely between centres. It is rare among babies who have not been fed. Recognized risk factors include:

- low birthweight;
- asphyxia;
- artificial feeds;
- intrauterine growth retardation;
- polycythaemia
- cardiac catheterization
- early feeding in association with the above.

### Aetiology

This is multifactorial (see Fig. 13.1). Developmental factors include immature bowel, abnormal motility and decreased host resistance. The pathogenesis remains unclear, but several important factors have been identified. Decreased vascular perfusion secondary to hypoxia or hypotension favours anaerobic bacterial overgrowth, and the combination of these factors leads to mucosal damage. Further exacerbation of mucosal injury may result from vasoactive agents (e.g. prostaglandins and cytokines) released by underperfused tissue and inflammatory cells. Subsequent invasion of damaged mucosa by

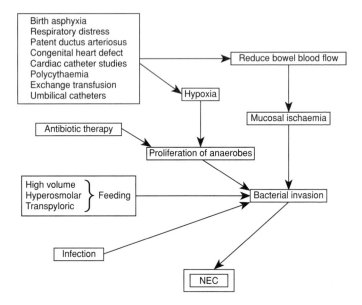

**Fig. 13.1** Causes of necrotizing enterocolitis in the newborn.

bacteria such as *Clostridia*, *Klebsiella* or *E. coli* results in severe tissue damage. The colon and ileum are the sites most frequently affected. Pathological changes include mucosal inflammation, necrosis, haemorrhage and pneumatosis.

### Clinical presentation

This is variable, and contributes to the difficulty of making an early diagnosis of NEC. The classical triad of abdominal distension, bile-stained aspirates and bloody mucousy stools may be accompanied in severe cases by temperature instability, inflammation of the abdominal wall, peritonitis, shock and apnoea. However, 30% of suspected cases have no blood in the stools, and most have a much milder illness.

***Radiological changes*** Are initially non-specific and include reduced bowel gas shadowing, free fluid and thickening of the bowel wall. Later findings include (diagnostic) air in the bowel wall (pneumatosis coli) or even in the portal tract. Free peritoneal gas indicates perforation.

*Laboratory findings* Include thrombocytopenia, coagulopathy, hyponatraemia, hypoproteinaemia and hyperbilirubinaemia.

**Management**

Because of the difficulty in diagnosis of early disease and the high mortality, a high index of clinical suspicion is necessary. Medical treatment consists of the following.

- Stop oral feeds (usually for 7–10 days) and apply continuous nasogastric drainage. Give parenteral nutrition.
- Full infection screen including stools for virology (usually negative), and begin treatment with antibiotics (use either penicillin or flucloxacillin with netilmicin and metronidazole).
- Optimize circulation – high losses of blood and colloid into the bowel are to be anticipated. Volume expansion is usually necessary, and ideally continuous monitoring of blood pressure and peripheral perfusion.
- Optimize oxygen delivery to the gut. Increase inspired oxygen or ventilate if necessary.
- Correct anaemia, coagulopathy, fluid and electrolyte imbalance.
- Isolate baby (risk of 'cluster' of cases).
- Repeat abdominal X-ray 12 to 24-hourly until pneumatosis is settling (watch for signs of perforation).
- Reintroduce feeds slowly after 7–10 days (breast milk or pregestimil are preferable to formula, as temporary lactose intolerance may occur).

*Surgical intervention* May be indicated if there is intestinal perforation, or peritonitis with deterioration despite medical treatment (see Chapter 9).

*Complications and prognosis* About 10% of cases will develop stricture and require surgery; short bowel syndrome may follow extensive resections. Mortality is highest in the very preterm. Gut function in most survivors appears normal in later infancy and childhood.

## Differential diagnosis of acute diarrhoea

- Congenital diarrhoeas – extremely rare.
- Gastroenteritis – viral and bacterial.
- Systemic infection – UTI, septicaemia, meningitis.
- Necrotizing enterocolitis.
- Metabolic disorders, e.g. adrenal insufficiency (see Chapter 16).
- Surgical conditions – Hirschsprung's disease (see Chapter 9).

- Other:
    lactose intolerance;
    immunodeficiency;
    prostaglandin therapy;
    opiate withdrawal;
    phototherapy.

## Gastroenteritis

Acute infectious disease presenting with watery diarrhoea and vomiting, which may occur in the newborn. The commonest pathogen is rotavirus, but other viruses, *E. coli*, *Salmonella*, *Campylobacter*, *Shigella* or *Yersinia* may be causative. Less common in breast-fed infants due to the presence of IgA, antiviral factors and iron-binding proteins (lactoferrin), which inhibit the growth of *E. coli*.

**Management** Stop formula feeds and isolate from other babies. Rehydrate with oral glucose electrolyte solution or i.v. fluids if severe; some breast feeding can continue. Slowly reintroduce enteral feeds when symptoms settle. Antidiarrhoeal drugs are not indicated.

## Lactose intolerance

**Secondary** May occur after gastroenteritis, NEC or gut surgery. Presents as diarrhoea with acid stools containing reducing substances. To avoid provoking symptoms it is wise to start feeding slowly with breast milk or hydrolysed cows' milk formula (pregestemil). Lactose containing milk may be reintroduced when the baby is thriving. Very small infants may have a gestation-dependent relative lactose intolerance on formula feeds.

**Primary** Very rare recessive disorder, presenting in the neonatal period with profuse watery diarrhoea. Sucrose and glucose are well tolerated.

## Congenital diarrhoea

Severe diarrhoea presenting at or soon after birth, leading to failure to thrive. The baby will need i.v. nutrition until a diagnosis is made and appropriate therapy instituted. It includes defects of intestinal transport ($Cl/HCO_3$ exchange; chloridorrhoea) and morphology (microvillous atrophy).

# BIBLIOGRAPHY

Bu'Lock, F., Woolridge, M.W. and Baum, J.D. (1990) Development of the co-ordination of sucking, swallowing and breathing: ultrasound study of term and preterm infants. *Dev. Med. Child Neurol.* **32**, 669–78.

Garza, C., Schanler, R.J., Butte, N.F. and Motil, K.J. (1987) Special properties of human milk. *Clin. Perinatol.* **14**, 11–32.

Gross, S.J., Geller, J. and Tomarelli, R.M. (1981) Composition of breast milk from mothers of preterm infants. *Pediatrics.* **68**, 490–93.

Henschel, D. and Juch, S. (1996) *Breastfeeding: a guide for midwives.* London: Books for Midwives Press.

National Breastfeeding Working Group (1995) *Breastfeeding: good practice guidance to the NHS.* National Breastfeeding Working Group. London: Department of Health.

Pereira, G.R. and Georgieff, M.K. (eds) (1995) *Clinics in perinatology: neonatal/perinatal nutrition.* Philadelphia, PA: W.B. Saunders Co.

Price, P., Kalhan, S., Fanaroff, A.A. *et al.* (1993) Nutrition and selected disorders of the gastrointestinal tract. In Klaus, M.H. and Fanaroff, A.A. (eds), *Care of the high-risk neonate*, 4th edn. Philadelphia, PA: W.B. Saunders Co., 130–88.

Ryan, S.W. (ed.) (1996) *Seminars in neonatology.* Vol. 1. *Enteral nutrition.* London: W.B. Saunders Co.

Tsang, R.C., Lucas, A., Uauy, R. and Zlotkin S. (eds) (1993) *Nutritional needs of the preterm infant: scientific basis and practical guidelines.* Baltimore, MD: Williams and Wilkins.

Woolridge, M.W. and Baum, J.D. (1988) The regulation of human milk flow. In Lindbald, B. S. (ed.) *Perinatal nutrition. Bristol-Myers Nutrition Symposium.* London: Academic Press, 243–57.

Woolridge, M.W. and Fisher, C. (1988) Colic, 'overfeeding', and symptoms of lactose malabsorption in the breast-fed baby: a possible artefact of feed management? *Lancet*, **II**, 382–4.

# Fluid and electrolyte therapy

The goal for the management of fluid and electrolyte therapy in newborn infants must be to achieve positive balance without overload. For the well infant this poses little problem and there is a reasonable margin for error. For the sick or very preterm infant the sensible management of fluid balance is crucial to improved outcome.

## WATER BALANCE

Throughout fetal life water comprises a decreasing proportion of body composition. At 30 weeks water comprises over 90% of body volume, 60% being in the extracellular compartment. By 40 weeks these proportions have fallen to 80% and 45%, respectively.

After birth, considerable changes in body water occur simultaneously, with changes in cardiac output, an increase in renal perfusion and a rapid rise in glomerular filtration rate (see Chapter 15). These combined events result in a diuresis, with proportionately greater loss of extracellular than intracellular water, and weight loss amounting to approximately 5% of birth weight. After preterm delivery the reduction in body water brings the body composition closer to that of the term infant. The normal diuresis may be delayed in sick or preterm infants, or if excessive fluids and sodium are administered, and may be a factor in delayed recovery from respiratory distress syndrome (RDS).

Preterm infants have immature renal function, and their mechanisms for sodium homeostasis are less efficient. In the very preterm this may lead to high baseline losses.

*Water balance* is controlled by renal plasma flow and the action of antidiuretic hormone (ADH) on the collecting duct. This posterior pituitary hormone is secreted in response to:

- a small rise in plasma osmolality (hypothalamic receptors);
- a fall in intravascular volume (left atrial stretch receptors);
- a fall in blood pressure (carotid sinus receptors).

In the very preterm infant, ADH action on the collecting duct is partially impaired. In the sick infant, ADH is secreted as a response to stress (oxygenation, intrathoracic pressure, IVH, brain injuries), and this may result in rapid swings in water excretion even with a normal GFR.

*Non-renal water loss* occurs via the respiratory tract (negligible if the infant is ventilated with humidified air) and, more problematically, via transepidermal evaporative loss. In the very preterm this may result in large losses, even up to 200 mL/kg for infants nursed naked under radiant heaters. For tiny babies, humidification of the environment or the use of barriers such as plastic wrappings or paraffin wax, may reduce this to tolerable levels. These methods also reduce concomitant heat loss (see Chapter 5). Humidification of 80–90% can be achieved in modern incubators with a reduction of transepidermal water loss of about 50% in babies of 24–27 weeks' gestation.

*Water therapy* must be planned with the help of *daily weights*, which are possible in all but the most unstable infants, and electrolytes. For the very preterm, *plasma sodium* may be the most reliable way of assessing loss in the child who is unable to be weighed, water intake being adjusted to maintain plasma sodium in the normal range. Sodium may need to be measured two or three times every 24 hours in the first few days. The measurement of urine output by collection is often very difficult and inaccurate, but it can be estimated by weighing the nappy shortly after voiding.

**Table 14.1** Suggested water, sodium and potassium intakes (these often need considerable modification from day to day depending on clinical course)

| Day Weight** | Water | | | | Sodium | | | | Potassium (all weights) |
|---|---|---|---|---|---|---|---|---|---|
| | <1 | −1.5 | −2.5 | >2.5 | <1 | −1.5 | −2.5 | >2.5 | |
| 1 | 100 | 80 | 60 | 60 | 0 | 0 | 0 | 0 | 0 |
| 2 | 120 | 100 | 90 | 90 | 5 | 4 | 3 | 1 | 0–2 |
| 3 | 150 | 130 | 120 | 110 | 5* | 4 | 3 | 1 | 2–3 |
| 4 | 180 | 150 | 150 | 130 | 5* | 4 | 3 | 1 | 2–3 |
| 5 | 180 | 180 | 170 | 150 | 5* | 4 | 3 | 2 | 2–3 |
| 6 | 180 | 180 | 170 | 150 | 5* | 4 | 3 | 2 | 2–3 |
| 7 | 180 | 180 | 170 | 150 | 5* | 4 | 3 | 2 | 2–3 |
| 8–13 | 180 | 180 | 170 | 150 | 5* | 4 | 3 | 2 | 2–3 |
| 14–20 | 160 | 160 | 150 | 150 | 4 | 3 | 2 | 1 | 2–3 |
| 21–27 | 160 | 160 | 150 | 150 | 3 | 2 | 2 | 1 | 2–3 |
| ≥28 | 160 | 150 | 150 | 150 | 2 | 2 | 2 | 1 | 2–3 |

These figures are for infants nursed in incubators or cots. Infants under radiant warmers may require higher volumes of water; those nursed in high humidity may require less.

Babies with RDS who have a delayed diuresis may require restricted fluid and sodium intake in the first few days.

*Sometimes higher requirements – check plasma sodium daily.

**Use birthweight or most recent weight whichever is greater.

*Normal water intake* in healthy breast-fed infants rises to about 150 mL/kg by the fifth postnatal day, forming the basis for the conventional 60, 90 and 120 mL/kg/day steps. This applies only to relatively mature infants. A suggested scheme for water, sodium and potassium intake is shown in Table 14.1. Any scheme must be tempered by close assessment of the state of hydration for each infant, urine output, insensible and observed losses, and plasma electrolytes. Note that water is an independent variable and the concentration of the various solutes (e.g. sodium, glucose) must be altered if the rate of water infusion is altered.

*Remember, when calculating intakes, that arterial flush solutions, and drugs contain extra sodium and water. Also, infusions of albumin (HAS or fresh frozen plasma) contain a considerable amount of sodium.*

*Always use the greater of birthweight or current weight, in calculations.*

## Management of oliguria and polyuria (see Chapter 15)

## SODIUM BALANCE

Sodium is normally excreted via the kidney, sweat and bowel losses being negligible. Term breast milk supplies less than 1 mmol/kg/day, implying that the kidney can conserve sodium and achieve positive balance and growth. Control is mediated via the renin-angiotensin-aldosterone system. This is equally active in the preterm, but tubular unresponsiveness leads to sodium wastage which is increased at lower gestation and in sick infants. This usually improves by 1–3 weeks. Normal requirements are usually 1–2 mmol/kg/day for term and 3–5 mmol/kg/day, or even more, for very preterm infants.

Monitor urinary electrolytes when there is a disturbance in electrolyte balance. Urinary sodium loss (fractional sodium excretion) may be calculated using the formula shown in Table 15.1. Normal is <1% in healthy term infants; sick preterm infants may have values up to 16% without implying renal failure.

Normative data for electrolyte concentrations are given in Chapter 29.

## HYPONATRAEMIA

**Definition** Plasma sodium < 130 mmol/L.

### Causes

**Water overload** May occur in first 24 hours due to excess administration of intravenous fluids to the mother, or later following excess administration to the infant. Occasionally it is secondary to ADH secretion which may occur following pneumothorax, IVH, brain injury or surgery.

**Acute renal failure** In oliguric phase before fluid restriction (dilutional) (see Chapter 16).

### Increased losses

**Excessive renal loss** In preterm infants is commonest, and is exacerbated during illness and by diuretic or aminophylline therapy.

*Inherited tubular disorders* Mimic poor preterm renal sodium handling, and infant should be given suitable replacements and referred to a specialist unit.

*Adrenal insufficiency* Associated with hyperkalaemia and dehydration, and will require replacement fluids, electrolytes and steroids (see Chapter 16).

*Excessive gastrointestinal sodium loss* During infection (gastroenteritis; see Chapter 13) or obstruction.

### Inadequate intake

*Late hyponatraemia* May occur during intravenous nutrition (with inadequate sodium concentration) or in preterm infants fed on breast milk or standard formula. Use of preterm formula or breast milk fortifier (see Chapter 13) provides a higher intake of sodium in the diet, reducing the need for early supplementation.

### Calculation of sodium deficit (mmol)

Sodium deficit $= (135 - $ plasma sodium$) \times 0.6 \times$ body weight (kg)

*Try to anticipate high losses*, such as those in preterm infants or gastrointestinal losses. If hyponatraemic, always slightly underestimate loss and replace *slowly* (e.g. $\frac{1}{3}$ deficit over 8 hours followed by $\frac{1}{3}$ over 16 hours and last $\frac{1}{3}$ over 24 hours). Add as 30% NaCl (5 mmol/mL) to bag or burette.

Emergency management of plasma sodium $< 120$ mmol/L with symptoms (irritability, apnoea, convulsions) should be started with a bolus of plasma or normal saline (15–20 mL/kg).

## HYPERNATRAEMIA

*Definition* Plasma sodium >145 mmol/L.

### Causes

#### Net loss of water

*Transepidermal water loss* in very preterm infants. Requires gentle volume expansion with 0.9% saline or plasma, followed by adjustment of water and electrolyte intake (see above). Anticipate higher fluid losses during phototherapy (Chapter 18), due to evaporative and stool losses.

**High rates of fluid loss** Occur during episodes of vomiting, diarrhoea or bowel obstruction.

**Glycosuria** Is a common cause of osmotic diuresis in the sick or very preterm.

It is important to rehydrate *slowly* and to start with isotonic solutions (plasma or 0.9% saline) to reduce the risk of inducing cerebral oedema.

### Excess sodium

Occurs if fluids and electrolytes are *mismanaged* or excess *bicarbonate* administered. Restrict sodium intake subsequently.

### Congenital hyperaldosteronism

Give diuretic (spironolactone) and refer to specialist unit.

## POTASSIUM BALANCE

Healthy term infants ingest about 1 mmol/kg/day, and most intravenous nutrition regimens supply about 2 mmol/kg/day, maintaining a positive potassium balance after 2–3 days.

## HYPOKALAEMIA

**Definition** Plasma potassium < 3 mmol/L.

## Causes

- Inadequate intake.
- Vomiting/diarrhoea.
- Alkalosis.
- Diuretics.
- Hyperaldosteronism.

## Management

Correct by increasing potassium input by 24-hour infusion or additions to milk; 1–3 mmol/kg/day is usually necessary.

Use strong potassium chloride (15%) or dipotassium hydrogen phosphate (17.42%), which contain 2 mmol/mL, diluted in a bag or burette.

## HYPERKALAEMIA

**Definition** Plasma potassium > 7 mmol/L.
ECG changes are a guide to toxicity: peaked *T*-waves; prolonged *PR* interval; absent *P*-waves; arrhythmias.

### Causes

- Artefactual due to sample haemolysis.
- Severe catabolism in sick infants.
- Acute renal failure.
- Hypoxia, shock, acidosis.
- Congenital adrenal hyperplasia (see Chapter 16).

### Management

ECG monitoring is needed.

1 Calcium gluconate (10%), i.v. 0.5–1 mL/kg, given over 2–4 min, cardioprotective for 30–60 min.
2 Correct acidosis (sodium bicarbonate 1–2 mmol/kg), effective for 1–2 hours.
3 Resonium A (sodium polystyrene sulphonate), 1 g/kg/day, orally or rectally.
4 Salbutamol, i.v. 4 mcg/kg by bolus injection (as effective as and safer than glucose/insulin infusion).
5 Glucose/insulin infusion (*dangerous*): give insulin 0.1 unit/kg with 4 mL/kg of 25% dextrose. Monitor blood sugar closely. Use in extreme circumstances, until dialysis is established.
6 Peritoneal dialysis (see Chapter 27).

**15**

# Renal disease in the newborn

## RENAL PHYSIOLOGY

During the last trimester the kidney undergoes rapid structural and functional development which continues after birth.

Renal blood flow, and thus glomerular filtration rate (GFR), is low at birth but increases rapidly during the first three postnatal days. Thereafter, GFR increases as a function of post-conceptional age (PCA) (i.e. gestational age plus postnatal age) rather than postnatal age, from 0.45 mL/min at 28 weeks' PCA to 5 mL/min at 42 weeks' PCA.

Plasma creatinine is used as a marker for GFR, as it is not practical to measure inulin or creatinine clearance routinely. At birth plasma creatinine reflects maternal levels, but it falls to infant levels by the second week. Creatinine levels are higher in the preterm infant and inversely related to gestational age (see Table 15.1). Isolated results should be interpreted with caution, as values vary with the type of assay used and interference by, for example, unconjugated bilirubin, ketones or drugs.

Creatinine excretion is reasonably constant (mean ± SD, $90 \pm 17 \, \mu$mol/kg/day), and urinary creatinine may be used to estimate urine volume and the sodium excretion rate (see Chapter 14). In contrast, urea generation rates may be very variable, and high in preterm infants as a result of catabolism. Urea excretion rates of up to 16 mmol/kg/day may be normal (contrast normal values of 1 mmol/kg/day in healthy term infants). A high blood urea in a sick infant does not therefore necessarily indicate dehydration or renal failure.

Renal tubular function is also immature. Urine-concentrating ability is limited by a reduced osmotic gradient between the cortex and the medulla, and also a reduced responsiveness to ADH. There is also a limited ability to excrete a water load. The term infant is able to conserve sodium efficiently. However, preterm infants have high sodium losses (see Table 15.1).

## Drugs

Because of both renal immaturity and potential toxicity, particularly from those drugs which alter renal blood flow, dosages of drugs with renal elimination must be adapted for use in the newborn (see Chapter 28). The following commonly used drugs should be used with caution.

- *Aminoglycosides* are excreted by glomerular filtration. Their half-life is related to PCA rather than postnatal age, and dosage schedules should be adjusted accordingly (see Chapter 28).
- *Frusemide* is excreted by glomerular filtration and secreted by a weak organic acid tubular mechanism. The effects are delayed

**Table 15.1** Normal values for neonatal renal parameters

| | Term infants | | | Preterm infants (<37 weeks' gestation) | | |
|---|---|---|---|---|---|---|
| | Gestation (weeks) | Value | Postnatal age | Gestation (weeks) | Value | Postnatal age |
| Fractional sodium excretion (FeNa)* | | 1% | 2 | >33 | 1% | 2–14 |
| | | | | <33 | 3–5% | 2–14 |
| Maximal attainable urine osmolality | | 800 mOsm/kg | <14 | | 500–700 mOsm/kg | <14 |
| GFR (creatinine clearance) | 38 | 2.5 mL/min | >3 | 28 | 0.45 mL/min | >3 |
| | 40 | 3.5 mL/min | >3 | 30 | 0.7 mL/min | >3 |
| | 42 | 5.0 mL/min | >3 | 32 | 0.9 mL/min | >3 |
| | | | | 34 | 1.3 mL/min | >3 |
| | | | | 36 | 1.8 mL/min | >3 |
| Plasma creatinine (±2 sd) | | 50±36 μmol/L | 7 | 28 | 84±32 μmol/L | 7 |
| | | 38±20 μmol/L | 14 | | 72±32 μmol/L | 14 |
| | | | | 29–32 | 83±41 μmol/L | 7 |
| | | | | | 69±32 μmol/L | 14 |
| | | | | 33–36 | 68±44 μmol/L | 7 |
| | | | | | 55±36 μmol/L | 14 |

*FeNa = $\dfrac{\text{urine Na}}{\text{urine creatinine}} \times \dfrac{\text{plasma creatinine}}{\text{plasma Na}} \times 100$.

and prolonged. The magnitude of response varies widely, particularly in sick infants who may have a low GFR.

- *Indomethacin*, a prostaglandin synthetase inhibitor, alters renal haemodynamics and may produce a fall in GFR, fractional excretion of sodium and free water clearance without any change in systemic blood pressure. The effects are usually transient and recover on stopping the drug.
- *Tolazoline* is an alpha-adrenergic blocking agent with a non-adrenergic vascular relaxant effect. It causes an increase in renal vascular resistance and a consequent fall in renal perfusion. The use of tolazoline in the presence of hypoxaemia, if systemic arterial blood pressure is not maintained, may lead to acute renal failure. It is therefore important to maintain adequate blood pressure during its administration (see Chapter 10).
- *Aminophylline* may have a diuretic and natriuretic effect when given as a rapid infusion, by temporarily increasing GFR, but maintenance doses probably do not have important effects.

## CIINICAL FEATURES OF RENAL DISEASE

### Family history

Some renal diseases are inherited in a Mendelian fashion either alone, e.g. polycystic kidney disease (autosomal dominant and recessive), nephrogenic diabetes insipidus (X-linked), congenital nephrotic syndrome (autosomal recessive), or as part of a syndrome, e.g. Alport's (X-linked), Towne's (autosomal dominant), Meckel's (autosomal recessive). Autosomal recessive renal abnormalities, particularly tubular defects, are also seen in association with several metabolic disorders, e.g. tyrosinosis, fructose intolerance, galactosaemia and cystinosis. Vesico-ureteric reflux is common and also genetically determined, probably as an autosomal dominant with reduced penetrance.

### Perinatal history

Oligohydramnios suggests renal agenesis, dysplasia or hypoplasia, or bilaterally obstructed urinary tracts (e.g. posterior urethral valves). It may be associated with deformation of the infant, together with lung hypoplasia, i.e. Potter's syndrome (see Chapter 7).

Less than 4% of liveborn children with a single umbilical artery have significant associated genito-urinary abnormalities.

A placenta weighing more than 25% of the infant's weight is suggestive of congenital nephrotic syndrome. There may be oligohydramnios, and the infants are often small for dates, preterm and have fetal distress. Prenatally, diagnosis may be suggested by a raised alpha-fetoprotein (see Chapter 1).

## Antenatal ultrasound

Congenital abnormalities of the genito-urinary tract can be detected as early as 12–15 weeks' gestation; 90% of fetal kidneys can be identified by 17–20 weeks and 95% by 22 weeks. Overall, urinary tract abnormalities are reported in 0.1–0.9% of pregnancies, the variation being related to the timing of the antenatal scan.

Accuracy, even in the most experienced hands, is limited and misinterpretation is common. For example, in the presence of renal agenesis the misshapen adrenal may be mistaken for a kidney. Moreover, the distinction between multicystic kidney and pelviureteric junction obstruction may be difficult, and dilated calyces may mimic renal cysts. In addition, the normal increased echogenicity of the fetal kidney, and physiological dilatation of the collecting system, are commonly open to misinterpretation. Thus, although antenatal ultrasound may pick up lesions that would be detectable clinically only in a minority of cases, the technique cannot always define the diagnosis accurately.

## Postnatal evaluation

The first investigation should be repeat ultrasonography, which should be done when the baby is 4 to 5 days old, as scans performed on day 1 can be misleadingly 'normal', and only if the abnormality is confirmed is further investigation indicated. The presence of suspected severe bilateral obstruction (e.g. posterior urethral valves or severe pelvi-ureteric junction obstruction) requires prompt management and is the only lesion for which early further postnatal investigation is indicated. Elective investigation of other abnormalities, especially where radiology is dependent on renal function (IVP, renal isotope scans) to define the lesion further, is better postponed for a few weeks. The presence of vesico-ureteric reflux or obstruction predisposes to urinary tract infection and therefore, in the presence of a dilated urinary tract, prophylactic antibiotics (e.g. trimethoprim, 2 mg/kg/day) are commenced until the diagnosis and

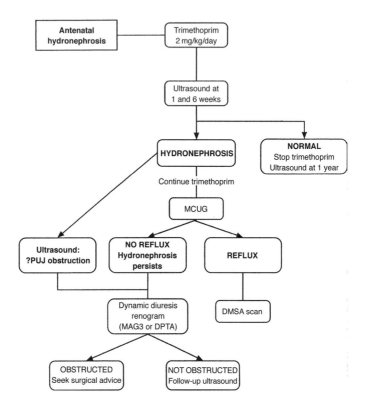

**Fig. 15.1** Suggested scheme for postnatal investigation and management of a baby with hydronephrosis diagnosed antenatally.

subsequent management plan is clear. A suggested scheme of investigation is shown in Fig. 15.1.

## Abdominal masses

More than two-thirds of abdominal masses detected in the newborn period arise in the genito-urinary system. Causes are listed in Table 15.2. Ultrasound is the primary investigation, and subsequent management is dependent on the findings (see Fig. 15.2).

An enlarged bladder in a male is commonly due to posterior urethral valves; ultrasound is followed by a micturating cystourethrogram (MCUG). Bladder drainage (urethral or suprapubic)

**Table 15.2** Causes of renal enlargement

| Unilateral | Bilateral |
|---|---|
| • Multicystic kidney | • Polycystic kidneys |
| • Solitary cyst | • Cystic dysplasia |
| • Hypertrophied single kidney | • Acute renal injury (hypoxia, ischaemia) |
| | • Twin-to-twin transfusion (recipient) |

**Unilateral or bilateral**

• Obstructive uropathy
  • Pelvi-ureteric junction obstruction
  • Vesico-ureteric junction obstruction
  • Bladder outflow obstruction
• Renal vein thrombosis
• Mesoblastic nephroma/Wilm's tumour

**Miscellaneous**

• Horseshoe kidney
• Pelvic kidney

should be discussed with the surgeon or specialist centre. Relief of the obstruction may lead to a marked post-obstructive diuresis, and natriuresis, which will require careful monitoring and fluid replacement.

## Bladder and genital abnormalities

*Bladder exstrophy and epispadias* Requires urgent referral for specialist advice. The bladder mucosa should be protected by applying gauze dressings soaked in saline.

*Hypospadias* The site of the meatus, severity of chordee, and any accompanying abnormalities, e.g. meatal stenosis, inguinal hernia or cryptorchidism, should be identified. If hypospadias is perineal or is part of an ambiguous genitalia presentation, careful investigation is required (see Chapter 16). Infants with coronal and distal shaft hypospadias require surgical review in out-patient clinics. Perineal and penoscrotal hypospadias is an indication for renal investigation which should be conducted in conjunction with the surgical team. Infants with hypospadias should not be circumcised, as the prepuce may be needed for the repair of the defect.

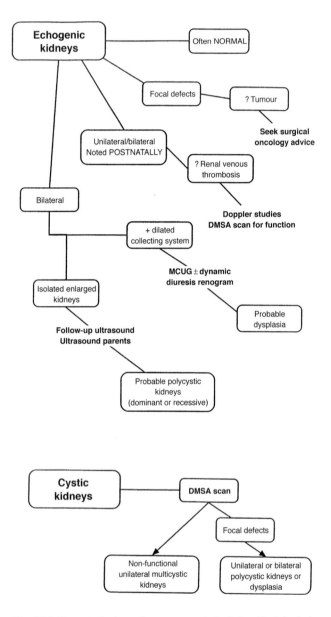

**Fig. 15.2** Suggested scheme for management of a baby with abdominal masses shown on ultrasound to be either echogenic or cystic kidneys.

*Cryptorchidism* Unilateral cryptorchidism is present in 2–3% of term male infants. Follow-up (usually by the family doctor) is required so that if descent has not occurred by the age of 1 year the child can be referred with a view to orchidopexy being performed before the age of 2 years. Bilateral cryptorchidism with hypospadias requires urgent investigation (see Chapter 16).

## Oliguria

To remain in solute balance, the minimum rate of urine production depends on the dietary solute load and renal concentrating ability. In infants this is in the range 0.5–1.0 ml/kg/hour. Oliguria may present antenatally (as oligohydramnios) or postnatally. It may be due to obstruction, poor renal perfusion, intrinsic renal failure, or increased antidiuretic hormone (see Chapter 14). Obstruction should be excluded by clinical or ultrasonographic examination, and the other conditions differentiated on plasma and urinary biochemistry (see p. 271).

## Polyuria

Polyuria may be seen in the recovery phase of acute renal failure, following relief of urinary obstruction, with certain drugs (e.g. diuretics and aminoglycosides) and in nephrogenic diabetes insipidus. A postnatal weight loss of more than 10% in an otherwise healthy infant whose urine is hypo-osmolar may be the first sign of nephrogenic diabetes insipidus. Rehydrate and ask for advice before embarking on a water deprivation test which may be dangerous.

## Haematuria

Gross haematuria is rare, although up to 10% of newborns may have microscopic haematuria ($> 10$ RBC/µL). Distinguish between haematuria, discoloration of urine by pigment (haemoglobin, urate) and contamination of urine by vaginal blood. Causes of haematuria include:

- birth trauma;
- systemic embolism (e.g. from umbilical artery catheter);
- cortical and medullary necrosis;
- acute renal failure;
- hydronephrosis;
- mesoblastic nephroma/Wilm's tumour;
- infection;

- following hypoxic, ischaemic or infective episode;
- drugs;
- Alport's syndrome;
- a bleeding disorder may rarely present with haematuria.

Investigation should include microscopy and urine culture, blood count, clotting studies, renal function tests and renal ultrasound. Consider referral for specialist advice.

## Renal venous thrombosis

Around 75% of renal venous thromboses occur in the first month of life. Presenting features include macro/microscopic haematuria, oliguria, renal failure and palpably enlarging kidneys. Proteinuria is minimal and nephrotic syndrome is rare. Anaemia and thrombocytopenia are common.

Haemoconcentration, hyperviscosity and hyperosmolarity predispose to renal venous thrombosis, and important risk factors include perinatal asphyxia, especially in infants with congenital renal anomalies, infants of diabetic mothers, hypernatraemic dehydration and infusion of hypertonic solutions (e.g. radiological contrast media).

Ultrasound reveals an enlarged kidney with a normal appearance or increased echogenicity. Doppler studies may confirm absent flow in the renal veins, although visualization may be difficult, in which case the diagnosis can be made with certainty only by venography (contraindicated in the sick infant).

Management is conservative. Anticoagulants and fibrinolytics have not been shown to be of value. Radionuclotide scans (DMSA) may be useful to document the function of the unaffected kidney or to predict recovery of the affected kidney. Long-term sequelae include renal atrophy and hypertension.

## Leukocyturia

Normally there are less than 25 (male) or 50 (female) WBC/µL. Pyuria is often associated with urinary tract infections but is not pathognomic, and an increased white cell excretion rate may be seen in any patient with a fever.

## Proteinuria

Protein excretion varies with gestational and postnatal age. Transient proteinuria is common in the first few days of life, and dipsticks frequently give false positive results with alkaline urine. Pathological causes include:

- infection;
- renal venous thrombosis;
- congenital infection (syphilis, toxoplasmosis, CMV);
- drugs (mercury);
- idiopathic familial congenital nephrotic syndrome.

Investigation should include renal function tests, urine protein excretion as protein/creatinine ratio, plasma proteins, congenital infection screen and renal ultrasound. Consider referral for specialist advice.

## Oedema

Renal causes include excessive water and salt administration, acute renal failure, obstructive uropathy and congenital nephrotic syndrome. Differentiation from non-renal causes such as anaemia, cardiac failure, tissue injury (anoxia, hypothermia, ischaemia) and hypoproteinaemia (non-renal) is usually evident clinically.

Investigation should include dipstick urinalysis for blood and protein, renal function tests and plasma proteins.

## Acidosis

The commonest causes of metabolic acidosis in the newborn will be shock and sepsis, with or without renal failure, and will be associated with an increased anion gap. The presence of metabolic acidosis with a normal anion gap suggests a renal tubular acidosis (RTA). During the first few postnatal days most infants will have a urine pH of around 6, although the capacity to alter pH in response to bicarbonate is present. The excretion of an inappropriately alkaline urine in the presence of acidosis may occur in various RTA syndromes, but also with severe respiratory distress syndrome (RDS).

### Hyponatraemia and hypernatraemia

See Chapter 14.

### Hypertension

The upper limits for systolic and diastolic BP in term infants are 100 mm Hg and 75 mm Hg respectively (see Figs 29.1 and 29.2). Use a cuff width at least two-thirds of the upper arm length, and record

**Table 15.3** Causes and management of hypertension

| Mechanism | Causes | Management |
|---|---|---|
| Renin mediated | Coarctation of aorta | See Chapter 11 |
| | Renovascular | Vasodilator and beta-blockade |
| | Obstructive uropathy Cystic kidneys | |
| Salt and water retention | Excess administration | Fluid restriction, diuretic |
| | Renal failure | Dialysis |
| | Adrenal disorders | See Chapter 16 |
| Catecholamine drive | Stress (pain, cold), hypovolaemia, drugs, e.g. dopamine | Correct underlying cause |
| Raised intracranial pressure | Cerebral oedema; IVH | See Chapter 12 |

BP only when the infant is at rest. BP that is persistently $> 110$ systolic and/or $> 80$ diastolic requires treatment regardless of the presence of symptoms, although such symptoms (e.g. vomiting, irritability, fits) may occur at lower levels. Of the renal causes of hypertension over 90% will be renovascular, the commonest of which is renal artery thrombosis following umbilical artery catheterization.

Treatment of hypertension depends on the cause (see Table 15.3). Hydralazine, 0.5–1 mg/kg i.v., can be given to control BP acutely. Mild hypertension may respond to diuretics. More severe hypertension may require the use of beta-blockers, which must be used with caution because of the risk of cardiac failure. The long-term effects of beta-blockade on the endocrine system are unknown. Captopril (100–300 mcg/kg/dose 8-hourly) may be useful in severe hypertension unresponsive to other agents, but renal function should be carefully monitored.

## Urinary tract infection

A urinary tract infection should be considered in any infant who is unwell, jaundiced, vomiting, febrile or failing to thrive.

Diagnosis is confirmed by finding $> 100\,000$ organisms on culture from at least two clean catch specimens, or preferably by obtaining any growth from a suprapubic aspiration sample. No growth from a bag urine will rule out a urinary tract infection, but a bag urine cannot be relied upon to make a positive diagnosis because of the high incidence of contamination. The baby should be examined for evidence of renal disease, and blood culture, lumbar puncture, and renal function checked prior to commencing therapy.

### Management

Before sensitivity results are available an aminoglycoside and ampicillin are usually effective (common organisms are *E. coli*, *Proteus*, *Pseudomonas* and *Streptococcus faecalis*). When sensitivities are known, change to the most appropriate and least toxic antibiotic.

Many neonatal urinary tract infections are haematogenous in origin, but all cases should have radiological investigation of the urinary tract to exclude abnormality. A renal ultrasound examination should be performed at the time of diagnosis, followed by an elective MCUG, which may be performed later. All babies should be kept on prophylactic antibiotics until vesico-ureteric reflux has been excluded. A DMSA scan several weeks after the infection will identify any scarring.

## ACUTE RENAL FAILURE

Acute renal failure is characterized by a sudden fall in glomerular filtration rate (GFR) which leads to disturbances in water and electrolyte balance and acid-base homeostasis, and to the accumulation of nitrogenous products. Oliguria is usually the first sign of acute renal failure, although a 'normal' urine output does not exclude the diagnosis and, because of the practical difficulties in measuring a baby's urine output, oliguria may escape observation. Furthermore, hypercatabolism, which is common in sick infants, leads to uraemia and hyperkalaemia due to protein breakdown, despite a normal GFR. Plasma creatinine is a reliable indicator of GFR. Although a single value is of limited usefulness (see Chapter 29), a rise of $> 20$ $\mu$mol/24 hours does suggest a fall in GFR.

Acute renal failure may be secondary to circulatory insufficiency without structural damage (pre-renal), parenchymal damage (intrinsic renal failure), or due to urinary tract obstruction (post-renal) (Table 15.4).

### Symptoms and signs of renal failure

- *Symptoms of renal failure*, e.g. poor feeding, vomiting, seizures, bleeding, cardiac arrhythmias.
- *Signs*, e.g. fluid overload (hypertension, oedema, excess weight gain, hepatomegaly, tachypnoea), fluid depletion (poor peripheral perfusion, hypotension), renal abnormality (palpable kidney, bladder).

### Investigation

This should include:

- weight;
- blood pressure;
- infection screen;
- renal ultrasound.

**Table 15.4** Causes of acute renal failure

---

**Pre-renal**

Hypovolaemic
   Blood loss
   Plasma loss
   Insensible loss (e.g. phototherapy in VLBW infants)
   Gastrointestinal loss (diarrhoea, vomiting)
   Polyuria
   Inadequate intake (e.g. fluid restriction after birth asphyxia)

Normovolaemia
   Hypoxia
   Septicaemia
   Hypotensive drugs (e.g. tolazoline)

**Intrinsic renal failure**

Uncorrected pre-renal failure
Acute tubular necrosis
Acute medullary necrosis
Acute cortical necrosis
Renal vessel thrombosis
Nephrotoxinas (e.g. gentamicin)
Congenital renal abnormality

**Post-renal**

Posterior urethral valves
Vesico-ureteric obstruction
Pelvi-ureteric junction obstruction
Neurogenic bladder

---

**Urine**
- dipstick;
- microscopy (look for casts);
- urea and electrolytes;
- creatinine;
- osmolality.

**Blood**
- electrolytes;
- urea and creatinine;
- acid-base status;
- glucose;
- calcium, magnesium;
- albumin;
- blood count (film and platelets);
- clotting studies.

It is important to differentiate between the three main causes of renal failure, as their treatments differ.

*Obstruction* is usually easily confirmed or excluded on renal ultrasound examination.

*Differentiation between pre-renal and intrinsic renal failure* is often more difficult, and may be further complicated by the fact that the former may lead to the latter.

Indices which differentiate between pre-renal and intrinsic renal failure (see Table 15.5) are often less helpful than in the older child because a low-protein diet and a high urinary sodium excretion affect both osmolality and those indices which rely on urinary sodium. All indices are less reliable in preterm infants, and a high fractional excretion of sodium (FeNa) in particular does not necessarily indicate renal failure.

If doubt exists about the extent of the pre-renal component, an intravenous isotonic fluid challenge may help (see below – use with caution because of risk of fluid overload).

**Table 15.5** Indices to differentiate between pre-renal and intrinsic renal failure

|  | Pre-renal | Renal |
|---|---|---|
| Urine/plasma urea | >10 | <10 |
| Urine/plasma osmolarity | >2 | <1 |
| FeNa* | <1% term<br><5% preterm | >3% |

*See Table 15.1.

## MANAGEMENT OF RENAL FAILURE

**Pre-renal** Restore circulating volume with colloid or isotonic saline, 10–20 mL/kg i.v. quickly over 30–60 min. With hypotension (see Fig. 29.1) in the absence of fluid depletion give an infusion of an inotrope, e.g. dopamine 5–10 mcg/kg/min.

**Post-renal** Relieve obstruction surgically or by suprapubic or urethral catheter as appropriate.

**Intrinsic renal failure** Restore circulating volume if indicated.

Replace all fluid losses (urine and gastrointestinal tract) together with insensible losses (see Chapter 14). One-third of insensible loss is respiratory (negligible if the infant is ventilated). The volume of drug infusions may exceed the infant's losses, and the highest safe infusion concentrations should be used (check with pharmacy).

Electrolyte losses should be calculated and replaced (measure urine electrolytes and estimate gastrointestinal losses according to site). Conservative measures to lower plasma potassium (see Chapter 14) should be used only temporarily until the cause of the renal failure is corrected or dialysis instituted.

Severe acidosis (pH < 7.2) requires correction.

Monitor blood glucose: hypoglycaemia is a common complication during fluid restriction. In contrast, during polyuric renal failure (as seen after relief of urinary obstruction) the replacement of large urine volumes with glucose solutions may lead to hyperglycaemia, especially if the infusion rate is higher than normal utilization rate (5–8 mg glucose/kg/min).

Regular clinical (input/output charts, weight, blood pressure, peripheral/core temperature gradient) and biochemical assessments are required. Caloric needs can rarely be met in an oliguric or anuric infant despite infusions of 10–15% glucose and this may be an indication for dialysis.

### Dialysis

Dialysis is seldom required but urgent indications include:

- severe fluid overload ± pulmonary oedema;
- severe metabolic acidosis (pH < 7.2 with $PaCO_2$ < 40 mm Hg);
- severe hyperkalaemia (K ≥ 8.0 mmol/L despite conservative measures).

If there is an immediate prospect of renal recovery, dialysis should be commenced prior to the development of fluid and electrolyte imbalance and allow administration of adequate calories and supportive drugs (see p. 427 for practical procedure for dialysis).

## BIBLIOGRAPHY

Birch, D.M., Griffiths, M.D., Malone, P.S. and Attwell, J.D. (1992) Fetal vesicoureteric reflux: outcome following conservative postnatal management. *J. Urol.* **148**, 1743–5.

Coulthard, M.G. and Sharpe, J. (1995) Haemodialysis and ultrafiltration in babies under 1000g. *Arch. Dis. Child.* **73**, F162–F165.

Coulthard, M.G. and Vernon, B. (1995) Managing acute renal failure in very low birthweight infants. *Arch. Dis. Child.* **73**, F187–F192.

Donaldson, M.D.C., Spurgeon, P., Haycock, G.B. and Chantler, C. (1983) Peritoneal dialysis in infants. *B.M.J.* **286**, 759–60.

Holliday, M.A., Barratt, T.M. and Avner, E.D. (1993) *Paediatric nephrology*, 3rd edn. Baltimore, MD: Williams & Wilkins.

Koff, S.A. and Campbell, K. (1992) Non-operative management of unilateral neonatal hydronephrosis. *J. Urol.* **148**, 525–31.

Leiberman, K.V. (1987) Continuous arteriovenous haemofiltration in children. *Pediatr. Nephrol.* **1**, 330–38.

Thomas, D.F.M. and Gordon, A.C. (1989) Management of prenatally diagnosed uropathies. *Arch. Dis. Child.* **64**, 58–63.

# Metabolic and endocrine problems

## GLUCOSE

### Hypoglycaemia

*Hypoglycaemia and alternative fuels* In normally grown, healthy term babies, a fall in blood glucose concentration is usual immediately after birth; blood glucose levels rise spontaneously thereafter and should not normally need to be measured. After delivery, relatively high blood lactate concentrations help to fuel the neonatal brain. Subsequently, ketone concentrations rise, providing further alternative fuels and thus minimizing the baby's glucose requirement while maternal lactation is established. Because of this ability to utilize alternative substrates, the term baby is probably not at risk of hypoglycaemia-associated neuronal injury over the first few days, whereas preterm babies and those with growth impairment do not produce ketones and are at risk.

**Definition of hypoglycaemia** Blood glucose < 2.6 mmol/L. However, there is no agreed definition for hypoglycaemia in the newborn, nor are there grounds for considering that SGA babies or preterm infants, both of whom produce less alternative fuels, have a lower risk of neurological damage from hypoglycaemia than older children. Maintaining the blood glucose concentration above 2.5 mmol/L may prevent long-term developmental deficits in preterm babies. Furthermore, glucose levels below this value appear to produce measurable neurophysiological dysfunction in infants and term babies.

**At risk population** Hypoglycaemia (after the first 2 to 3 hours) is a biochemical *symptom*, and usually means that the baby has failed to make adequate perinatal metabolic adaptation. Babies at risk of such maladaptation should be identified early and managed prospectively:

**At risk babies:**
- small-for-dates infant;
- preterm;
- starvation (including delayed resiting of infusions);
- cold stress;
- hypoxia;
- infection;
- polycythaemia;
- maternal β-blockers/glucose infusion;
- maternal diabetes.

---

**Conditions associated with hypoglycaemia:**
- decreased adrenal or pituitary function;
- inborn errors of metabolism (e.g. galactosaemia);
- hyperinsulinism:
  - infant of a diabetic mother;
  - Beckwith-Wiedemann syndrome;
  - severe haemolytic disease;
  - nesidioblastosis/islet cell adenoma.

---

Cerebral fuel deficiency in term babies may be manifested as a reduction in the level of consciousness and/or seizures. Jitteriness is not a useful discriminating symptom. As the level of consciousness drops, the cry changes, movements decrease, feeding becomes poor, and there are long respiratory pauses or apnoea.

*Blood glucose measurement* is indicated:

- if the baby is at risk (above situations present or suspected);
- in the investigation of coma or convulsions;
- during neonatal intensive care;
- occasionally in relatively small babies who are slow to establish feeds.

Blood glucose measurements should be made using quality-assured, laboratory-grade equipment, by staff trained in its use. The use of test-strip readings in babies is no longer recommended (*Safety Notice 9616*, Medical Devices Agency, 1996), but until laboratory grade equipment is widely available these will continue to be the first-line investigation in many units.

### Prevention of hypoglycaemia (in at-risk children)

Use the algorithm (Fig. 16.1).

- Beware of the baby who appears wasted and in whom this may represent growth retardation in a baby who was destined to be large. These children may be at the same risk of hypoglycaemia as one who is small-for-dates; if in doubt, measure the mid-arm:head circumference ratio (Table 16.1).
- Feed early and frequently (at least 8 feeds per day).
- Aim for a total intake of at least 90 mL/kg/day from day 1.
- It is only necessary to measure blood glucose once, before the second feed, if the baby shows no subsequent signs of cerebral fuel deficiency.
- Consider continuous nasogastric milk feeds if the baby is intolerant of volume (often necessary to maintain intake).

Failure to tolerate enteral feeding, together with an inability to maintain a blood glucose concentration of > 2.5 mmol/L, constitute grounds for intravenous therapy. Babies of < 3rd centile for birth-weight are at particularly high risk of hypoglycaemia (and hypothermia), and should be monitored carefully.

***During intensive care*** Clinical detection of hypoglycaemia is almost impossible in the sick or preterm baby and in babies prone to seizures for some reason other than hypoglycaemia (e.g. encephalopathy). In these situations routine measurements of blood glucose are the only option. When clinically stable, glucose should be measured at least once each day, but more frequently in the child who is sick or unstable.

### Management of hypoglycaemia

Coma and convulsions (see p. 199):

- insert an i.v. cannula;
- draw blood to measure glucose and other investigations;

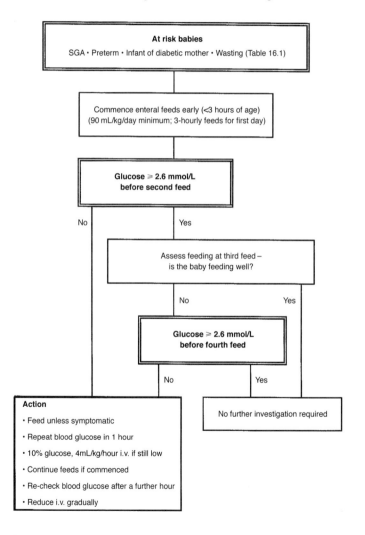

**At risk babies**
SGA · Preterm · Infant of diabetic mother · Wasting (Table 16.1)

Commence enteral feeds early (<3 hours of age)
(90 mL/kg/day minimum; 3-hourly feeds for first day)

**Glucose ≥ 2.6 mmol/L
before second feed**

No      Yes

Assess feeding at third feed –
is the baby feeding well?

No      Yes

**Glucose ≥ 2.6 mmol/L
before fourth feed**

No      Yes

**Action**

- Feed unless symptomatic
- Repeat blood glucose in 1 hour
- 10% glucose, 4mL/kg/hour i.v. if still low
- Continue feeds if commenced
- Re-check blood glucose after a further hour
- Reduce i.v. gradually

No further investigation required

**Fig. 16.1** Algorithm for management of hypoglycaemia.

**Table 16.1** Consider a baby to be wasted if the ratio of mid-arm circumference to head circumference (MAC:HC, both measured in cm) is less than the values shown in the table

| Gestation (weeks) | MAC:HC |
| --- | --- |
| 36 | 0.26 |
| 37 | 0.28 |
| 38 | 0.28 |
| 39 | 0.28 |
| 40 | 0.29 |
| 41 | 0.29 |
| 42 | 0.30 |

- if symptoms persist, give a bolus of 2 mL/kg 10% glucose and observe the response;

*NB If there is a delay in establishing i.v. access;*

- take capillary sample for blood glucose;
- give glucose concentrate gel (e.g. Hypostop 0.5 mL/kg) orally;
- continue to establish i.v. access.

*NB Never use boluses of 25% or 50% glucose: they are unnecessary and can be dangerous.*

A term baby with reduced conscious level and a low blood glucose (< 2.6 mmol/L) has fuel deficiency. The choice of management is as follow:

- give some milk (as a tube feed if the suck is poor);
- give glucagon (100 mcg/kg i.m.; useful for infants of diabetic mothers who have low glucagon levels at birth);
- give intravenous 10% glucose, 2 mL/kg;
- follow with suitable change in energy intake (see below).

These options have not been subject to controlled evaluations. Discuss the options with the baby's mother concerning which to try first, but one option *must* be taken. Always repeat blood glucose measurement 1 hour after action has been taken, to ensure that the concentration has risen.

If the baby is already receiving an intravenous 10% glucose infusion, consider:

- increasing the infusion concentration to 12.5%–20% (depending on the response);

- increasing the rate of fluid administration if the clinical situation allows this;
- using a percutaneous silastic 'long' line if the glucose concentration is > 12.5%;
- calculating the glucose infusion rate (Fig. 16.2).

If not on continuous i.v. infusion:

- always follow a bolus of glucose by a continuous infusion of 10% glucose at 6–7 mg/kg/min (4 mL/kg/hour);
- continue or increase enteral milk feeds, if the enteral route is appropriate.

Do not discontinue milk feeds if a baby becomes hypoglycaemic because:

- milk contains nearly twice the energy of 10% glucose;
- milk promotes ketone body production;
- if the mother intends to breast feed it is important for her to see her own milk being given to her baby;
- enteral feeding, especially with breast milk, promotes metabolic adaptation.

*Special investigations* are required if:

- glucose infusion rates to prevent hypoglycaemia are persistently > 12 mg/kg/min (Fig. 16.2), in a well-grown or large-for-gestational-age baby (small-for-gestational-age babies quite often need high glucose infusion rates for several days);
- there is evidence of hypothalamic dysfunction such as unstable temperature;
- profound hypoglycaemia occurs unexpectedly in a well-grown term baby;
- hypoglycaemia is associated with other abnormalities (exomphalos, coloboma);
- there is a family history of sudden infant death, Reye's syndrome, severe developmental delay, poorly defined neuropathy or myopathy, or other evidence suggestive of an inborn error of metabolism.

Babies with a high glucose requirement behave as if they are 'hyperinsulinaemic', although their circulating insulin levels may not be different to those of other healthy babies of the same gestation.

In children, circulating insulin concentrations are usually undetectable (< 1 mU/L) when blood glucose concentration is < 4.5 mmol/L, but in the newborn infant it is *normal* to have

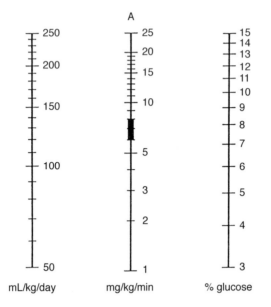

**Fig. 16.2** Glucose rate calculator. Use a straight-edge to determine the glucose infusion rate (column A) in mg/kg/min. The normal glucose requirement in the newborn infant is 6–8 mg/kg/min. If this is insufficient to maintain adequate blood levels, there is evidence of increased utilization, e.g. due to cold stress or hyperinsulinism. (From Klaus, M.H. and Fanaroff, A.A. (eds) (1979) *Care of the high-risk neonate.* London: W.B. Saunders Co.)

circulating insulin concentrations up to 10 mU/L even when the blood glucose concentration is 3 mmol/L or less.

In large babies with high glucose requirements take blood for simultaneous insulin and glucose measurement (usually arrange for 2 mL plasma to be frozen in case endocrine assays prove to be needed).

Depending on the other clinical features of the baby, consider:

- collecting urine for acyl carnitines and organic acids (freeze it at weekends), for inborn errors of metabolism such as beta-oxidation defects;
- arranging cranial ultrasound examination (for septo-optic dysplasia);
- arranging abdominal ultrasound examination (for insulinoma);

- doing a glucagon test (to exclude glycogen storage disease by demonstrating that glucose can be mobilized from the liver). Give glucagon, 30 mcg/kg, and measure blood glucose at 0, 15 and 30 min. A rise of 3 to 4 mmol/L in blood glucose is normal;
- investigating for pituitary dysfunction or other inborn errors of metabolism.

### Managing hyperinsulinism

If you suspect or have confirmed genuine hyperinsulinism:

- insert a central line to secure an uninterrupted glucose infusion, particularly if giving 15% or 20% glucose;
- if the glucose requirement is very high, e.g. 20 mg/kg/min, give somatostatin (as octreotide, 1 mcg/kg subcutaneously every 4 hours), to which glucagon can be added if necessary;
- if the glucose requirement is less dramatic, but normoglycaemia cannot be maintained even with calorie-fortified milk feeds, start diazoxide 5 mg/kg, and chlorothiazide 10 mg/kg, both 12-hourly;
- failure to contain the situation medically may necessitate 95% pancreatectomy – consult a centre skilled in the management of these conditions early on.

## Hyperglycaemia

Very-low-birthweight infants do not always reduce their hepatic glucose output, or increase their peripheral uptake, when circulating glucose concentrations rise, particularly when they are stressed by lung disease or infection. A rise in blood glucose concentrations may herald clinical deterioration, but is non-specific. Transient diabetes mellitus is a very rare complication in infants who are usually also small for dates.

**Definition** Renal immaturity protects against osmotic diuresis until the urinary glucose concentration is enough to register ++ on dipstick. In practice, blood glucose concentrations up to 10 mmol/L are of no clinical significance. Levels in double figures, particularly if glycosuria is ++ or more on dipstick testing, always require careful monitoring and may need action if blood concentrations are sustained or rising, or if associated with a diuresis (diagnose by weighing the baby serially or measuring fluid balance).

### Management

- Reduce the glucose infusion rate by reducing the infused glucose concentration to 5%, but maintain the total infused volume.

- If unsuccessful, replace the glucose completely with normal or 0.5N saline for 1 or 2 hours.
- Insulin infusion is hazardous, but may be necessary if the baby must continue to receive parenteral nutrition or is fully milk fed. Give soluble insulin by infusion, with a starting dose of 0.05 units/kg/hour.
- Glucose concentrations must be monitored closely, avoiding abrupt changes in energy supply.

## CALCIUM AND MAGNESIUM

Circulating calcium concentrations normally fall from birth until 48 hours of age, and then stabilize and rise. Illness may exacerbate this normal pattern. Cardiac function does not seem to be impaired by these physiologically low levels, and increasing the serum calcium concentration by infusing calcium does not improve it.

### Hypocalcaemia (see also p. 235)

**Definition** Total calcium concentrations may appear low because of low concentrations of albumin. The ionized calcium concentration is more relevant, and is routinely measured on some of the newer blood gas analyzers. Hence apparent 'hypocalcaemia' should not be taken at face value. Symptoms of hypocalcaemia only occur when the total calcium concentration is less than 1.5 mmol/L.

*Measurement* of calcium should be made:

- in any infant with convulsions or tetanus (together with glucose, magnesium, sodium and phosphate);
- in encephalopathy;
- in renal failure;
- when Di George syndrome is suspected;
- in any disorder of maternal calcium metabolism;
- in babies fed on unmodified cow's milk (due to high phosphate load).

Serum calcium concentrations in the first 72 hours are difficult to interpret, and measurements are of limited value. Early nutritional support with milk or parenteral feeding (see Chapter 13) rapidly restores circulating calcium concentrations to the normal range.

The daily requirement is between 1 and 2 mmol/kg/24 hours (10% calcium gluconate contains 0.225 mmol $Ca^{2+}$ in 1 mL and 10%

calcium lactate contains 0.32 mmol $Ca^{2+}$ in 1 mL). Observe i.v. sites carefully as extravasation may cause severe tissue injury. Adding calcium to bicarbonate or phosphate solutions may cause precipitation.

*Hypomagnesaemia* may accompany hypocalcaemia. Measure magnesium in:

- convulsions (together with calcium, glucose, sodium and phosphate);
- refractory hypocalcaemia.
- If calcium infusion fails to maintain normocalcaemia, give 50% magnesium sulphate (0.2 mL/kg intramuscularly).
- Consider intramuscular magnesium sulphate if the serum magnesium level is < 0.7 mmol/L.
- Rarely, oral maintenance therapy is required (magnesium sulphate, 0.2 mL/kg/day).
- Larger doses may be necessary in malabsorptive states.

## Hypercalcaemia (> 2.8 mmol/L)

- Infusing calcium unaccompanied by phosphate sustains normocalcaemia in the short term, but can easily lead to 'overshoot' hypercalcaemia after a day or two. Stop infusion or give additional phosphate.
- Hypercalcaemia may be an unintended side-effect of treatment with vitamin D or alphacalcidol (stop medication).

## INBORN ERRORS OF METABOLISM

Inborn errors may present with:

- encephalopathy;
- isolated seizures;
- unexplained acidosis;
- hypoglycaemia;
- liver disease (prolonged, conjugated jaundice);
- very non-specifically lethargy, poor feeding and weight loss.

   Be alert for an inborn error if:

- there is a high rate of consanguineous marriage in the local population;

- there is a family history of unexplained neonatal or infant deaths;
- there is a family history of unexplained neuropathy or myopathy;
- there are persistent, unexplained symptoms.

Initial investigations should include:

- full infection screen;
- renal and liver profiles;
- blood glucose;
- blood ammonia;
- blood gases;
- urine for microbiology, electrolytes and creatinine, glucose and other reducing substances, and ketones.

Specific tests should always be performed in close liaison with the laboratory, and in consultation with a paediatrician or chemical pathologist with special expertise in the diagnosis and management of these conditions.

Focus additional specific investigations as follows.

### Acidosis

- blood for lactate, ketones, amino acids, carnitine.
- urine for amino acids and organic acids, including orotic acid.

### Hypoglycaemia

Collect samples, whenever possible, at the time of hypoglycaemia. Investigate as for hypoglycaemia (see p. 280), but if an inborn error seems likely:

- blood for lactate, ketones, alanine and glycerol, amino acid profile, carnitine, and red blood cell galactose-1-phosphate uridyl transferase assay;
- urine for organic acids.

### Acute liver disease

- Blood for amino acids, carnitine, red blood cell galactose-1-phosphate uridyl transferase assay, alpha$_1$-antitrypsin.
- Urine for reducing substances, amino acids, organic acids.

### Neurological signs, or encephalopathy

- Blood as for metabolic acidosis, + uric acid + very-long-chain fatty acids.
- Urine as for metabolic acidosis, + sulphite.

- CSF for microscopy, culture, protein, glucose, lactate and amino acids.

### Immediate management

- Give general supportive care (intensive care if necessary), maintaining tissue perfusion and attempting to control acidaemia.
- Reduce the load on metabolic pathways: stop milk feeds or parenteral nutrition and maintain the baby on a glucose infusion giving at least 8 mg/kg/min (Fig. 16.2).
- Give L-carnitine, 100 mg/kg/day (as four oral doses or continuous i.v. infusion) to help conjugate toxic metabolites.
- Treat hyperammonaemia if more than 150 μmol/L: sodium benzoate or sodium phenylbutyrate, 250 mg/kg loading dose over 90 min followed by 250 mg/kg/day.
- Consider dialysis or haemofiltration if the urine output is poor or hyperammonaemia cannot otherwise be controlled.
- Avoid high-dose multivitamins in the absence of a specific diagnosis.

If the baby dies, it is still extremely important to try to make a diagnosis, particularly with regard to advice concerning future pregnancies. Specimens must be taken as soon after death as possible, with parental assent, and remember to discuss the importance of an autopsy, *since the diagnosis may be not be an inborn error at all.*

- *Blood* (can be taken from the heart): at least 10 mL. Arrange for immediate separation of the plasma and ask for it to be frozen at − 20°C in 2-mL aliquots. Make sure the cellular fraction is stored at + 4°C for tests requiring intact red and white cells (may be stored for up to 2 days).
- *Urine*: 20 mL should be frozen at − 20°C in 5-mL aliquots.
- *Liver*: needle biopsy, freeze immediately in liquid nitrogen or dry ice.
- *Skin*: full-thickness skin biopsy for fibroblasts. *For skin biopsy,* use aseptic conditions. Clean the skin with chlorhexidine in spirit and clean off with an alcohol swab. Take at least 1 mm$^2$ of skin. Place in culture medium or, if this is not available, in normal saline. Store at + 4°C, getting the specimen to an appropriate laboratory as quickly as possible.

### Screening for metabolic disease

Phenylketonuria (birth prevalence 1 in 6000) and hypothyroidism (1 in 3000 – see below) are routinely sought by neonatal screening. A heel-prick spot of blood is collected on filter paper or in a capillary tube at 5–10 days of age, depending on locality. This procedure may need to be repeated if the child has not been on milk feeds for 48 hours before testing. A variety of techniques are used to detect excess phenylalanine. The original Guthrie test uses a bacteriological assay (so antibiotics in the baby's circulation can potentially interfere and yield a false negative result). Modern techniques usually rely on chromatography.

More recent generic technologies (e.g. tandem mass spectrometry) can potentially detect any aminoacidopathy and many other inborn errors of intermediary metabolism on a single blood spot.

## AMBIGUOUS GENITALIA

This includes:

- bilateral cryptorchidism;
- perineal hypospadias;
- frankly ambiguous genitalia.

Do not ask the parents to choose the gender, and *never guess*. If you are in any doubt as to the sex of the baby, say so straight away. Explain to the parents that it will take time, investigation and discussion before gender can be confirmed, and that an expert in these conditions will be contacted immediately to help them. Reassure the parents that the baby will be either a boy or girl, not 'in between'.

Review the history with the parents, with particular reference to:

- drugs taken during pregnancy;
- family history (ambiguous genitalia; infertile aunts);
- neonatal or infant deaths (congenital adrenal hyperplasia).

Make a careful examination for:

- any other dysmorphic features;
- size of phallus;
- position of urethral orifice;
- gonads, anywhere from the inguinal ring downwards;
- blood pressure.

### Investigation

The danger to the baby is the possibility of congenital adrenal hyperplasia (CAH) with substantial salt loss and hypoglycaemia. While expert help is on the way, organize:

- chromosomes;
- appropriate blood and urine samples for CAH (see below).

## CONGENITAL ADRENAL HYPERPLASIA (CAH: 21 HYDROXYLASE DEFICIENCY)

CAH may present in the neonatal period as ambiguous genitalia, sometimes accompanied by pigmentation of the nipples and/or the scrotum. These infants may develop a high serum potassium before the classical finding of hyponatraemia with paradoxically high urinary sodium. About 75% are strong 'salt losers' and may present with dehydration and collapse during the second or third postnatal week.

*Diagnosis* of 21-hydroxylase deficiency is based on the plasma concentration of 17-hydroxyprogesterone (17-OHP), normally < 30 nmol/L in blood taken more than 24 hours after birth to avoid the presence of placental 17-OHP. In untreated CAH, values are usually > 200 nmol/L. Save samples of plasma and 10 mL of urine, as these may prove diagnostically important if the diagnosis is *not* 21-hydroxylase deficiency.

Because of the unpredictable degree of salt loss, initially daily measurements of the following are needed:

- plasma electrolytes and creatinine;
- urine electrolytes and creatinine;
- blood pressure;
- weight.

The fractional excretion of sodium can then be calculated (see Table 15.1).

Immediate management is by replacement therapy. By the time salt loss is diagnosed, the baby will be in considerable negative sodium and water balance, so the priorities are as follows.

- Infuse 0.9% saline, 20 mL/kg rapidly if the baby is collapsed, then at 150 ml/kg/day (in 5–10% glucose if the baby is not being fed): only 24–48 hours of treatment may be needed.

- Give hydrocortisone: this can be started as an infusion (1 mg/hour for 24 hours) if the baby is collapsed, and then continued orally.
- Give 9-alpha-fludrocortisone, 100 mcg daily orally.

The out-patient follow-up and long-term management of babies with CAH requires the specialist services of a paediatric endocrinologist supported by paediatric surgeons, and is beyond the scope of this book.

## THYROID DISORDERS

### Congenital hypothyroidism

Few babies 'present' with symptoms consistent with congenital hypothyroidism, which is one of the main justifications for the screening programme. Some of the features described are:

- prolonged gestation;
- temperature instability;
- poor tone;
- large tongue;
- delayed passage of meconium;
- poor feeding;
- lethargy.

#### Causes
Most cases are due to failure of normal thyroid gland development:

- aplasia;
- hypoplasia;
- ectopy.

Rarely, hypothyroidism with an enlarged thyroid, or goitre, may be caused by:

- maternal drugs (antithyroid drugs or iodine) (note that most babies are unaffected);
- dyshormonogenesis.

#### Diagnosis
Most cases are picked up through the neonatal screening programme (local practices vary):

- the birth prevalence is about 1 in 3000;

- a blood spot is collected on filter paper at 5–10 days at the same time and on the same paper as the test for phenylketonuria;
- the concentration of thyroxine or thyroid-stimulating hormone (TSH) is measured.

### Investigation

If hypothyroidism is suspected clinically, full thyroid function tests, including free thyroxine ($T_4$), tri-iodothyronine ($T_3$) and TSH assays, should be performed. These results are available so quickly that performing an X-ray of the knee to look for absent epiphyses in a term infant is no longer justifiable.

The normal range for $T_4$ is 90–195 nmol/L in infants over 1 week old, and for TSH is < 5 mU/L. Small, sick preterm infants may show biochemical evidence of transient hypothyroxinaemia, but this is not the same as congenital hypothyroidism, and is probably analogous to the 'sick euthyroid' situation seen in adults.

**Treatment** This is with thyroxine 10 mcg/kg given daily, starting immediately after definitive diagnosis. Aim to maintain $T_4$ values in the upper part of the normal range. TSH values should eventually return to normal, but do not always suppress in the first few weeks. Subsequently, monitor the dosage by maintaining a normal TSH level. The dose relative to body weight gradually decreases with age.

## Neonatal hyperthyroidism

This may occur in infants born to mothers with active or non-active Graves' disease. It is due to transplacental passage of a thyroid-stimulating IgG immunoglobulin. The infants may be protected initially by maternal antithyroid drugs, but can show signs of thyrotoxicosis at birth. Usually presentation is at 7–10 days with signs of thyrotoxicosis such as sweating, tachycardia, jitteriness, exophthalmos, lid lag, vomiting and diarrhoea, which may progress to heart failure and hyperthermia.

### Investigation

In mothers with Graves' disease, take cord blood for thyroid-stimulating immunoglobulin because high titres increase the likelihood of neonatal problems. In any baby with suspected thyrotoxicosis take blood for free $T_4$, $T_3$ and TSH.

### Management

This is usually symptomatic. The problem is self-limiting and therapy is rarely needed beyond 2 months.

The mainstay of treatment is:

- propranolol (up to 0.5 mg/kg every 6 hours);
- propylthiouracil (5–10 mg/kg/24 hours given in three equal doses).
  Alternatively, consider:
- Lugol's iodine (5% iodine and 10% potassium iodide), 0.1 mL orally 8-hourly;
- sodium ipodate, 500 mg every third day, orally.

## HYPOPITUITARISM

This is normally congenital, and is usually associated with other midline defects:

- septo-optic dysplasia;
- rarely, with cleft lip and palate.

**Presentation** May be with temperature instability, hypoglycaemia, micropenis, and other symptoms of specific endocrine deficiency.

**Investigations** These should include:

- cerebral ultrasound scan;
- possibly CT or MRI imaging;
- random blood for growth hormone, cortisol, TSH, $T_4$ and $T_3$;
- Synacthen test.

These and further tests should always be undertaken in collaboration with a paediatric endocrinologist, since growth hormone replacement and possibly testosterone therapy will become an issue.

**Immediate management** This comprises:

- correcting blood glucose as for hypoglycaemia;
- giving hydrocortisone (starting dose 12 mg/m$^2$/day);
- starting thyroxine as for hypothyroidism.

## BIBLIOGRAPHY

Aynsley-Green, A. and Soltész, G. (1985) *Hypoglycaemia in infancy and childhood. Current Reviews in Paediatrics. Vol. 1.* London: Churchill Livingstone.

Brook, C. (1995) *Clinical paediatric endocrinology.* London: Blackwell Science.

Holton, J.B. (1994) *The inherited metabolic diseases*, 2nd edn. Edinburgh: Churchill Livingstone.

Medical Devices Agency (1996) *Safety Notice 9616.* London: Medical Devices Agency.

Ward Platt, M.P. and Hawdon, J.M. (1993) Hypoglycaemia in the neonate. In Gregory, J.W. and Aynsley-Green, A. (eds), *Hypoglycaemia. Ballière's clinical endocrinology and metabolism. Vol. 7.* London: Ballière, 669–82.

The UK Directory of Laboratories Diagnosing Inborn Errors of Metabolism can be found on the Internet at http://www.ncl.ac.uk/~nchwww/SSIEM/bimdg.html.

# Perinatal infections

Congenital infections
Other maternal infections during pregnancy
Neonatal infections
Superficial infections
Systemic infections
Investigation of infant suspected of infection
Virus infections of the newborn
Fungal infections

The newborn infant is particularly susceptible to infection because of reduced defence mechanisms, and is rapidly colonized by whatever organisms are in the environment. Humoral immunity is mainly by transplacental IgG, and IgA levels are low. Neutrophils have decreased chemotaxis, phagocytosis and bactericidal activity. Complement is reduced and B- and T- cell function is impaired. Consequently, even weak pathogens may cause serious infection.

## CONGENITAL INFECTIONS

Primary infection of the mother during pregnancy with cytomegalovirus, rubella, toxoplasma, treponema, herpes or parvovirus can cause fetal disease. Often this is asymptomatic, but in a minority of cases it can be severe with long-term sequelae.

### Cytomegalovirus

The commonest congenital infection, occurring in 1–2% of all births. Ninety per cent are asymptomatic, but multisystem disease may occur in 10% of cases. Fetal damage is more severe if maternal infection occurs in early pregnancy.

### Clinical signs

- Small for dates.
- Microcephaly with cerebral calcification.
- Jaundice.
- Thrombocytopenia.
- Hepatosplenomegaly.
- Anaemia.
- Chorioretinitis.

Long-term sequelae of sensorineural deafness and mental retardation occur in 15% of cases.

***Diagnosis*** By CMV-specific IgM; virus isolation from urine.

## Rubella

Now uncommon (2 in 100 000 births), due to immunization.

### Clinical signs

- Microcephaly.
- Cataracts.
- Retinal pigmentation.
- Congenital heart defect.
- Mental retardation.

## Toxoplasmosis

Most infants are asymptomatic but if untreated have a high risk of long-term handicap. Treatment of the infected mother in pregnancy improves the outcome.

### Clinical signs

- Hydrocephalus or microcephaly.
- Cerebral calcification.
- Chorioretinitis.
- Microphthalmia.

***Diagnosis*** By *Toxoplasma*-specific IgM.

***Treatment*** With pyrimethamine and sulphadiazine.

## Treponemia

Uncommon, but increasing in incidence. Routine screening ante-natally is universal, but many cases of congenital syphilis have no antenatal care.

### Clinical signs

- May not appear until several months after birth.
- Hepatosplenomegaly.
- Jaundice.
- Lymphadenopathy.
- Thrombocytopenia.
- Anaemia.
- Rash.
- Osteochondritis.
- Periostitis.

**Diagnosis** By specific antitreponemal IgM and reactive CSF VDRL in all cases at risk.

**Treatment** With i.m. penicillin for 10 days.

## Herpes simplex

HSV-2 is the usual cause of genital herpes and hence of neonatal infection, but HSV-1 can also cause neonatal infection. It is usually acquired intrapartum. There is a 50% risk of neonatal infection following vaginal delivery in a mother with primary active HSV lesion, but only a 3% risk with recurrent genital lesions. The risk is claimed to be lower if delivery is by Caesarean section.

### Clinical signs

- May be delayed for up to 2 weeks after delivery.
- Localized skin vesicles are the commonest sign and progress to generalized disease in 70% of cases if untreated.
- May be localized pneumonitis or encephalitis.
- Generalized disease involves liver, adrenals, lungs and brain, with jaundice, hepatosplenomegaly, thrombocytopenia and DIC.
- Often fulminant and fatal.

**Diagnosis** High index of suspicion as early treatment is essential. HSV immunofluorescence of vesicle fluid, viral culture from vesicles, nasopharynx, CSF.

**Treatment** With Acyclovir i.v.
*Prophylaxis* (part exposure) – if the mother has an active, recurrent genital lesion, send cultures from the infant's conjunctiva and nasopharynx at 24–48 hours. If these are positive start treatment with Acyclovir.

## Parvovirus (B19)

Infection occurs in up to 3% of pregnancies, usually with no adverse effect on the fetus, but in up to 2% of infected cases there may be fetal hydrops due to anaemia and cardiac failure. Infection may cause stillbirth or recover spontaneously.

## OTHER MATERNAL INFECTIONS DURING PREGNANCY

### Human immunodeficiency virus

Perinatal transmission is the major route of infection with HIV in children, with a transmission rate of about 20%. Two-thirds of cases are infected during delivery and the remainder are infected either *in utero* or within a few months of birth.

Treatment of the mother with Zidovudine orally during pregnancy and i.v. during labour, and oral treatment of the baby for 6 weeks after birth, reduces the perinatal transmission by about 60%. Caesarean section may have some protective value.

Certain groups of women are at greater risk of HIV infection:

- intravenous drug abusers;
- natives, residents or visitors of Central Africa or Haiti;
- sexual partners of HIV-positive or high-risk individuals;
- prostitutes;

Testing for HIV in pregnancy should be offered to all women in these groups after counselling. High-risk women who refuse screening for HIV should be managed as if proven positive.

The risk of infection to staff or other patients is very low, provided that appropriate precautions are taken in handling blood, lochia and other body fluids from sero-positive women (e.g. use gloves and impermeable protective gowns, disposable bedding, etc.).

The baby should be bathed in the delivery room. Breast feeding increases the risk of infection by at least 10%. The neonate is usually asymptomatic, and signs of HIV infection may not occur until 3–6 months of age.

Diagnosis in the neonatal period is difficult. Maternal IgG is present in the baby even if not infected; uninfected infants become seronegative at about 9–15 months. The baby's status may be uncertain during this time, but the risk of pneumocystitis infection in infected babies starts at about 3 months, so all babies of HIV-positive mothers should start on Co-trimoxazole prophylaxis at 1 month of age.

BCG vaccination should not be given to infants born to HIV-positive mothers.

## Varicella zoster

Fetal infection rarely causes limb defects, microcephaly and ocular abnormalities.

Maternal rash within 5 days before delivery or an infant rash 5 days after delivery may be associated with severe neonatal illness. Zoster immunoglobulin may reduce the severity of the illness.

Consider treatment with Acyclovir.

## Hepatitis B

Cross-infection precautions for hepatitis B must be taken during the delivery for the following groups of patients, whose infants should be given immunization after birth:

- intravenous drug abusers;
- patients who have been resident in psychiatric institutions;
- patients with chronic active hepatitis, cirrhosis or polyarteritis nodosa;
- patients who have had acute hepatitis within the past 6 weeks;
- consort of a man who has been in prison in the past year;
- all natives of the Far East (Chinese, Phillipino, Vietnamese, etc.), Africans and Caribbean people born and raised in their country of origin;
- sexual partner of any of the above;
- mothers known to be hepatitis B surface antigen positive. If these mothers are e-antigen positive and e-antibody negative, the children are at especially high risk. If the e-antibody is positive and e-antigen is negative, the risk is low. The risk to infants of mothers with neither e-antigen nor e-antibody is intermediate.

**Hepatitis B immunization** Infants of mothers in all of the above 8 groups should be given hepatitis B vaccine, 0.5 mL i.m. shortly after birth and again at 1 and 6 months. Infants of mothers who are e-antigen positive and e-antibody negative should also be given human anti-hepatitis B immunoglobulin, 200 international units by deep i.m. injection (NB *not i.v.*) as soon as possible after birth, and not later than 48 hours. The first dose of hepatitis B vaccine should be given at a different site at the same time or within a few days.

Follow-up arrangements should be made to assess the serological evidence of immunity in all of these infants at the age of 1 year and at yearly intervals until the age of 5 years.

## Tuberculosis

- *Mothers with active or open tuberculosis.* Immunize infant with isoniazid-resistant BCG within a few days of birth and start isoniazid on day 1. Continue isoniazid until the mother is sputum-negative for TB and the infant has a positive skin tuberculin test. The mother and baby should be kept separated until the mother has been on antituberculous treatment for 2 weeks (i.e., start treatment *before* delivery if possible).
- *Mothers with healed or inactive tuberculosis.* Chest X-ray and sputum cultures during pregnancy, as reactivation may occur. If there is no evidence of reactivation, give the infant BCG within the first week after birth (and arrange follow-up after 4–6 weeks to ensure successful immunization).

NB Masks are of *no* value in preventing infection of the baby if the mother has active TB, and are unnecessary if she has not. Breast feeding is contraindicated only with active or open tuberculosis.

*BCG immunization* of the newborn is normally recommended where the infant:

- is known to be a contact of a case of active respiratory TB;
- belongs to an immigrant community characterized by a high incidence of TB;
- will reside in or travel to any area where the risk of TB is judged to be high.

For these infants, BCG should be given soon after birth and testing for sensitivity is unnecessary. There are two different immunization techniques:

- BCG vaccine, 0.05 mL strictly intradermally (not subcutaneously) at the insertion of the deltoid muscle near the middle of the left upper arm. Injection at a high site may lead to keloid formation; or
- percutaneous BCG immunization by multiple puncture technique. This is a much easier technique using a multiple

puncture gun and special percutaneous BCG vaccine. Use the same site on the left arm. With this technique there is usually no local reaction.

When BCG is given to infants there is no need to delay the primary immunizations, but no further immunizations should be given for at least 3 months in the arm used for BCG because of the risk of regional lymphadenitis.

## NEONATAL INFECTIONS

*Early-onset* infections presenting within 48 hours of birth have probably been acquired *in utero* or during birth. An increased risk is associated with:

- prolonged rupture of membranes (> 24 hours);
- prolonged labour;
- multiple obstetric procedures;
- preterm labour;
- fetal distress;
- maternal pyrexia/infection, especially urinary or enteral;
- foul-smelling liquor.

The commonest organisms are those in the normal vaginal flora, in particular Group B streptococcus, and less frequently *E. coli, Haempohilus influenzae*, gonococcus, *Listeria*, herpes and *Candida*. *Late-onset* infections presenting after the age of 48–72 hours have probably been acquired postnatally and may be associated with:

- preterm delivery;
- meconium aspiration;
- males > females;
- malformations, e.g. spina bifida, urogenital anomalies, gastrointestinal malformations;
- infusions, especially with long lines and parenteral nutrition;
- umbilical catheters; peripheral arterial lines;
- endotracheal tubes;
- cross-infection from staff, parents and other patients.

The commonest organisms are: *Staphylococcus albus and Staphylococcus aureus, E. coli, Pseudomonas*, streptococci, *Candida* and, less commonly, *Proteus* and *Klebsiella*.

## Management of suspected intrapartum infection

Any infant born after any of the above factors should be regarded as potentially infected and must have broad-spectrum antibiotic cover.

Children with PROM > 24 hours and *no* symptoms should be observed (4-hourly TPR) for at least 24 hours. In this situation, an infection screen and antibiotic therapy should be started if any symptoms develop.

Babies of < 36 weeks' gestation who develop RDS after an elective delivery with no infection risk should have a blood culture, but do not require antibiotics unless there are indicators of infection, such as low platelets, high or low white cell count, or abnormal chest X-ray appearances.

Where one twin is treated with antibiotics within 72 hours of birth, the other twin must be screened and started on antibiotics as a matter of urgency.

All symptomatic infants must have an infection screen and start antibiotics.

In all cases, if cultures are negative after 48 hours then antibiotics can be stopped. If the mother has been given antibiotics before delivery these may suppress neonatal cultures and the baby should be treated for 5 days even if the cultures are negative.

## SUPERFICIAL INFECTIONS

### Ophthalmia neonatorum (see Chapter 20)

### Skin infections

Usually due to *Staphylococcus aureus*, and may present as scattered pustules or blisters, particularly in axillae and groins, paronychia, breast abscess, or rarely as toxic epidermal necrolysis. Routine use of 0.33% hexachlorophane powder will reduce the risk of staphylococcal infection. Isolated spots may be treated with topical Fucidin ointment, but more widespread infection needs systemic flucloxacillin.

### Umbilicus

The umbilicus should be cleaned daily with chlorhexidine. The catheterized umbilicus should be treated daily with povidone-iodine.

If the abdominal wall around the umbilicus becomes inflamed, do a blood culture and start systemic antibiotics.

## SYSTEMIC INFECTIONS

The clinical signs of sepsis in the newborn are non-specific and overlap with the signs and symptoms of many other disorders, particularly respiratory, cardiac and haematological ones. The work-up of any ill infant must include a sepsis screen.

### Signs suggestive of infection

*Non-specific change in condition*: poor colour; lethargy; poor feeding; temperature instability; hypothermia; fever. The following signs are also suggestive of infection:

- vomiting;
- loose stools;
- distended abdomen; splenomegaly;
- jaundice;
- purpura; bleeding;
- irritability; convulsions;
- cyanotic or apnoeic attacks;
- grunting; tachypnoea;
- tachycardia;
- hypotension;
- disordered glucose metabolism } hypoglycaemia; hyperglycaemia and glycosuria.

## INVESTIGATION OF INFANT SUSPECTED OF INFECTION (SEPSIS SCREEN)

| Sample | Investigation | Abnormal findings |
|---|---|---|
| Skin lesions, nose, throat and umbilical swabs | Gram stain | Pus cells and bacteria seen |
| | Virology/electron microscopy | Growth |
| | Culture | |
| Stools | Culture and virology | Pathogens isolated |

| Urine, clean catch or suprapubic aspiration (not bag sample) | Microscopy | Bacteria and white cells seen |
| | Culture | Growth |
| Blood | Culture (aerobic and unaerobic) | Growth |
| | Haemoglobin (Hb) | Low |
| | Platelets | <80 000/dL |
| | Total WBC | <4000 or >20 000/dL |
| | Differential WBC | Neutrophils <2000 or >15 000/dL |
| | Film | Shift to left. Toxic granulation Burr cells |
| CSF | Microscopy | White cells >30/mm$^3$ and >50% polymorph organisms seen |
| | Culture/virology | Growth |
| | Protein | Raised >1.5 g/L |
| | Sugar | Low compared to blood level |

## Other investigations

- Chest X-ray, even in the absence of respiratory symptoms.
- Abdominal X-ray, if any signs are suggestive of NEC.
- Blood: glucose, urea, electrolytes, pH and gases CRP.
- Urine: sugar, protein and blood.

### Infection screens

Neonates who are being screened for 'infection risk' within the first 24 hours do not require a lumbar puncture unless meningitis is seriously considered. The 'screen' thus effectively means a blood culture, full blood count, peripheral swabs (from infected sites only) and X-rays as appropriate, but there should be a low threshold for performing a lumbar puncture – see section on meningitis.

After the first 24 hours, all children who are placed on broad-spectrum antibiotics must have a lumbar puncture. This may be delayed by a *few hours* if a child is particularly unstable, but should not be left without discussion with a consultant. Lumbar puncture in children who are unstable should be performed by an experienced doctor and not a junior doctor in the first weeks of his or her new post.

After 7 days all children should have a urine sample taken *before* commencing antibiotics. If it is urgent to start antibiotics, then an SPA should be performed under ultrasound guidance.

**Target** Within 1 hour of a decision to perform a screen and start antibiotics, the screen, including LP, should be completed and the antibiotics given.

## General management of the septic infant

1 General support as described in Chapter 5.
2 Respiratory support for apnoea, abnormal blood $PaO_2$, and $PaCO_2$ (see Chapter 10).
3 Correct hypotension with fresh frozen plasma, 10 mL/kg; this may also correct defective opsonization.
4 Transfuse if anaemic (Hb < 12 g/dL).
5 Correct fluid, electrolyte and glucose imbalance (see Chapter 14).
6 In cases of severe toxic shock an exchange transfusion may be beneficial.
7 Antibiotics must be started at once before bacteriological diagnosis, and must therefore be broad spectrum. However, the age at onset of symptoms will help in choosing a suitable antibiotic regimen:

  - *Onset within 48 hours of birth* – use penicillin + aminoglycoside;
  - *Onset after 48 hours of birth* – use flucloxacillin + aminoglycoside.

### Course length
Antibiotics should be stopped at 48 hours post-screen unless positive cultures are reported. The decision to continue antibiotic therapy beyond this point in the face of negative cultures is a consultant decision.

- *Staphylococcus epidermidis*: 5-day course.
- Gram-negative or other Gram-positive other: 7–10 day course.
- Meningitis: 14-day course.

This regimen should be modified according to the illness being treated (see below) and subsequent isolation of organisms and sensitivities (see Tables 17.1 and 17.2).

**Septicaemia** Probable organism depends on route of infection and age of onset (see p. 298). Treat as described above.

**Table 17.1** Common organisms causing neonatal infection and recommended antibiotics

| Organism | Recommended antibiotics (for parenteral use) (see Chapter 28) |
| --- | --- |
| Group B streptococcus | Penicillin<br>Ampicillin |
| *Staphylococcus aureus* | Flucloxacillin<br>Cefuroxime, fusidic acid<br>Teicoplanin |
| *Staphylococcus epidermidis* | Netilmicin<br>Flucloxacillin<br>Cefuroxime<br>Vancomycin<br>Teicoplanin |
| *E. coli*<br>*Klebsiella*<br>*Proteus* | Netilmicin<br>Cefuroxime<br>Cefotaxime |
| *Pseudomonas* | Netilmicin+<br>   azlocillin<br>Ceftazidime |
| *Haemophilus* | Ampicillin<br>Cefuroxime, cefotaxime |
| *Listeria* | Ampicillin<br>Netilmicin |
| *Chlamydia* | Erythromycin |
| *Candida* (systemic infections only) | Amphotericin +5 flucytosine, fluconazole |

Wherever possible, monitor blood levels of antibiotics and adjust dosage accordingly.

**Pneumonia** May be congenital due to ascending or intrapartum infection, especially streptococcal. Postnatal infection is related to aspiration syndromes, endotracheal intubation and hypostatic. Treat as described above.

**Group B streptococcal (GBS) disease** *Early onset*: acquired from vaginal flora, usually in preterm infants, with prolonged rupture of membranes, but may be normal term delivery. Early respiratory symptoms occur, which mimic RDS and may progress to apnoea and

**Table 17.2** Neonatal infections and their treatment

| Disorder | Recommended antibiotics* |
|---|---|
| Septicaemia | |
|   (<48 hours old) | Penicillin+netilmicin |
|   (>48 hours old) | Flucloxacillin+netilmicin |
| Second-line therapy for failure of above | Cefotaxime (cefuroxime) |
| Meningitis† | Cefotaxime |
| Pneumonia | As for septicaemia |
| Urinary infection | Ampicillin+netilmicin |
| NEC | Penicillin+netilmicin+metronidazole |
| Osteomyelitis‡ (*Staphylococcus aureus*) | Flucloxacillin+fusic acid |

*All confirmed infections should be treated for 5 days at least.
†Continue treatment for 14 days after the first negative CSF culture.
‡Continue treatment for 4–6 weeks.

severe shock. GBS are found in gastric aspirate. The baby may have septicaemia and meningitis as well as pneumonia. There is a high mortality rate. Treat with high-dose penicillin and full intensive care support (see Chapter 10).

*Late onset* (1–2 weeks old): probably a nosocomial infection. Typically, meningitis presents in previously well term infant, often due to type III GBS. There is a low mortality rate. Treat with high-dose penicillin for 14 days.

Mothers who have had a previously infected baby are at significant risk in subsequent pregnancies and should be given ampicillin i.v. in labour.

**Neonatal meningitis** There may be no physical signs of meningitis in the neonate, and all babies with suspected sepsis, fits or apnoeic attacks must have their CSF examined. Normal values are given in Table 29.3. In cases of a bloody tap the 'normal' ratio of WBC to RBC is taken as 1:1000. The baby will usually have septicaemia as well, and general environmental and respiratory support may be needed. The most suitable antibiotics are cefotaxime, or penicillin for streptococcal infection. Aminoglycosides have poor CSF penetration and are not suitable for treatment of meningitis; intrathecal administration by the lumbar route is of no value, although intraventricular aminoglycosides may be useful in treating ventriculitis.

CSF examination should be repeated daily for 2–3 days to ensure effective therapy and antibiotic therapy continued for 2 weeks from the date the CSF becomes sterile.

**Urinary tract infection** Usually presents insidiously with poor feeding, vomiting and jaundice, but may be acute. Always culture the urine of every sick infant by SPA (see Chapter 15 for management of urinary tract infection).

**Necrotizing enterocolitis** (see Chapter 13).

**Gastroenteritis** Uncommon in the newborn in the UK, but epidemics of rotavirus in SCBUs have been reported. Sporadic cases of *Salmonella, Shigella, Campylobacter* and pathogenic *E. coli* enteritis do occur, usually acquired from the mother during delivery. Isolate. Stop feeds and give i.v. fluids if dehydrated. Antibiotics are not necessary.

**Osteomyelitis** Insidious onset, usually not moving a limb, which is inflamed, oedematous and tender to touch. Do blood culture, and get orthopaedic advice on aspiration of fluid from infected bone or joint for culture. The commonest organism in the neonate is *Staphylococcus aureus*. X-ray changes may not appear for 2–4 weeks. Treat with flucloxacillin and fusidic acid for 6 weeks.

**Listeriosis** Infection with *Listeria monocytogenes* acquired transplacentally or intrapartum produces a clinical illness similar to Group B streptococcus. There is commonly a history of maternal pyrexia within a few days before delivery, and the amniotic fluid may have a green discoloration. Mothers may acquire the organism from 'cook-chill' foods, paté, soft cheeses, milk, etc. *Listeria* will grow at low temperatures (6–10°C) on such foods.

*Early onset* Pneumonia: X-ray looks like aspiration pneumonitis but may mimic RDS or miliary pneumonia. Transient salmon-coloured papular rash on trunk. Disseminated disease (granulomatosis) may occur and is commonly fatal unless treatment is started within 1 or 2 hours of birth.

*Delayed onset* of meningitis at 2–3 weeks old. Peripheral white count usually shows increase in polymorphs and monocytes.

**Treatment** (early and delayed onset): i.v. ampicillin, 200 mg/kg/day, (or high-dose penicillin) + i.v. netilmicin (or gentamicin).

**Chlamydial infections** infection with *Chlamydia trachomatis* acquired intrapartum from the vagina usually presents as ophthalmia at the end of the first week, unresponsive to usual therapy. There may be late onset (1–3 months) of pneumonia and sometimes otitis media. Chest X-ray shows diffuse interstitial infiltration.

*Diagnosis* is by chlamydial culture of eye swabs and specific IgM.

*Treatment* Ophthalmia is treated with topical tetracycline and oral erythromycin for 2 weeks. Pneumonia is treated with oral erythromycin for 3 weeks.

**Ureaplasma urealyticum** is commonly found in the liquor of mothers in premature labour, and is associated with chorioamnionitis. Colonization occurs in up to 60% of their babies.

*U. urealyticum* is thought to be a common cause of congenital pneumonia, particularly in very-low-birthweight babies, and to be associated with the development of chronic lung disease of the neonate.

Pneumonia should be treated with erythromycin i.v. As yet, there are no data to suggest that antibiotic prophylaxis is of value in preventing the development of chronic lung disease.

## VIRUS INFECTIONS OF THE NEWBORN

Clinical features are indistinguishable from bacterial sepsis. Investigation and management are similar, and until viral diagnosis is confirmed and bacterial cultures are negative, antibiotics are usually given. Appropriate samples (throat swabs, CSF, urine, stools, blood) should be sent for specific virology.

### Viral meningitis

Usually caused by enterovirus. There are clinical signs of infection, but not severe.

*CSF*: normal sugar, raised cell count – polymorphs in first day of illness becoming predominantly lymphocytes. Remember to send separate samples of CSF for bacterial and viral cultures.

There is no specific treatment. Isolate.

### Myocarditis

Usually caused by Coxsackie types B1–5, but may also be caused by congenital infection agents, and be one feature of generalized viral illness (+ meningitis). Presents with pyrexia and signs of cardiac failure, cyanosis and poor cardiac output. Hepatosplenomegaly. Large heart on X-ray. ECG shows low-voltage **QRS**, prolonged **QT**, and flat **T**-waves. Ventricular ectopics and arrhythmias. Differential diagnosis of septicaemia, diabetic cardiomyopathy (see Chapter 11), cardiomyopathy, endocardial fibro-elastosis (see Chapter 11). Give environmental and respiratory support as indicated, digoxin and diuretics. Obtain cardiological advice. There is significant mortality.

## ECHO virus infection

A severe illness with collapse, disseminated intravascular coagulation and adrenal, CNS and gastrointestinal haemorrhage. May also cause meningitis, pneumonia, hepatitis and diarrhoea.

## FUNGAL INFECTIONS

### Oral thrush

White spots on the tongue and buccal mucosa; may be associated with poor feeding, especially if there is also an oesophagitis. Treat with oral nystatin or miconazole. Maternal vaginal thrush predisposes to this infection.

### Perianal thrush

Red rash over napkin area, with scattered satellite lesions, which is commonly associated with oral thrush. Very common. Keep area as dry as possible; nurse exposed (in warm room); avoid waterproof napkin cover or pants. Treat with oral and topical nystatin or miconazole.

### Systemic candidiasis

There is a high risk of candidiasis in association with antibiotic therapy, parenteral nutrition (particularly via a central line) and preterm delivery. It usually presents as oral/perianal thrush becoming systemic with candidal septicaemia, meningitis and renal infection. Babies at risk should have regular cultures of blood and SPA urine for *Candida*, and should be given prophylactic nystatin.

**Presentation and diagnosis** *Clinical signs* of sepsis failing to respond to antibiotics, and becoming chronic. Recurrent apnoea. Do blood culture (arterial and venous), SPA urine and CSF for *Candida*, taking care to avoid skin contamination of samples.

**Treatment** Liposomal amphotericin is significantly less toxic than plain amphotericin and should be used in preference, especially where there is concern about nephrotoxicity.

*Dose*: Liposomal amphotericin, 1 mg/kg/day infused i.v. over 15 min. This dose may be increased if necessary to 3 mg/kg/day.

Combine with oral 5-flucytosine, 50 mg/kg 6-hourly. Continue therapy for 4–6 weeks. Monitor renal function carefully. Check candidal cultures weekly. Alternatively, may be treated with fluconazole, 3 mg/kg i.v. every 72 hours in neonates less than 2 weeks old, and every 48 hours in neonates over 2 weeks old.

## BIBLIOGRAPHY

Isaacs, D. (ed.) (1996) *Seminars in neonatology. Vol. 1, No. 2. Fetal and neonatal infections.* London: W.B. Saunders.

Isaacs, D. and Moxon, E.R. (1991) *Neonatal infections.* Oxford: Butterworth-Heinemann.

# Neonatal jaundice

Bilirubin, produced from the breakdown of haemoglobin, myoglobin, cytochromes and other haem-containing compounds, mainly in the spleen, liver and bone marrow, is fat-soluble and toxic in high concentrations, particularly to the CNS. Conjugated bilirubin (mainly water-soluble diglucuronide) is less toxic. In fetal life, unconjugated bilirubin is excreted via the placenta, but from birth it is excreted in the bile, after conjugation. Unconjugated bilirubin is transported to the liver bound to albumin. An acceptor protein, ligandin, transports bilirubin into the liver cells where conjugation to bilirubin diglucuronide occurs. Water-soluble conjugated bilirubin is then secreted into the bile and excreted via the bowel. Some of the bilirubin reaching the gut is deconjugated by bacterial glucuronidase activity, reabsorbed and returned to the liver (enterohepatic circulation).

## PHYSIOLOGICAL JAUNDICE

The change-over from fetal to neonatal bilirubin metabolism results in a rise in circulating bilirubin levels in normal infants, with a peak on the third or fourth day, falling over the next 4–5 days to a mean of less than 30 μmol/L at 10 days of age.

Bilirubin levels above 150 µmol/L in the first 24 hours after birth, or above 350 µmol/l at any time in normal-term infants are not physiological, and warrant investigation. Approximately 6% of term infants develop significant neonatal jaundice (> 300 mmol/l).

## PATHOLOGICAL JAUNDICE

Pathological processes may affect the metabolism of bilirubin at any stage of the pathway, from production to excretion (Table 18.1).

**Albumin binding** Unconjugated bilirubin is carried in plasma bound to albumin. If dissociated from albumin, bilirubin can readily diffuse into cells of the CNS, causing damage by uncoupling oxidative phosphorylation, increasing glycolysis and decreasing protein synthesis. Bilirubin can be displaced from albumin by certain drugs (e.g. sulphonamides, salicylates), by plasma non-esterified fatty acids (NEFA) (which increase with fasting, cold stress and sepsis), or by acidosis. The bilirubin-binding capacity of albumin varies widely (70–140 µmol bilirubin per gram of albumin), according to clinical circumstances. Techniques developed to identify 'free' or unbound bilirubin, or to quantify serum bilirubin binding, have not proved useful.

**Bilirubin encephalopathy (kernicterus)** The term kernicterus refers to the yellow staining of the basal ganglia and hippocampus found at autopsy in infants dying with bilirubin toxicity.

The clinical picture of bilirubin encephalopathy may not develop for several hours after toxic levels of bilirubin have occurred. During the prodromal syndrome (poor feeding, temperature instability, irritability, decreased reflexes, 'cycling' movements of the arms and lethargy) prompt treatment by exchange transfusion may prevent sequelae. Progression within a few hours may include generalized stiffening, with extension and tight fisting of the arms, crossed extension of the legs, opisthotonos, and a high pitched cry, and there may be 'sun setting' of the eyes from paralysis of extra-ocular muscles, and seizures. Gastric or pulmonary haemorrhage may be a terminal event. In survivors, extensor spasms may give way to generalized hypotonia, poor feeding and developmental delay. Long-term consequences vary and may include spastic or choreo-athetoid cerebral palsy, paralysis of upward gaze, severe mental impairment, dental enamel dysplasia and high-tone hearing loss.

The pattern of bilirubin encephalopathy may be different in very preterm infants, who may only show fisting, increased tone and possibly apnoea in the acute phase.

Bilirubin encephalopathy is rarely seen in term infants without underlying haemolysis (e.g. rhesus disease; glucose-6-phosphate dehydrogenase deficiency) or at bilirubin levels below 500 μmol/L, but

**Table 18.1** Pathophysiology of neonatal jaundice

**Unconjugated hyperbilirubinaemia**

*Acute intravascular haemolysis* (may present in first 48 hours after birth)
  Haemolytic disease (Rhesus, ABO, other)
  Red cell abnormalities (glucose-6-phosphate dehydrogenase deficiency, spherocytosis)
  Intrauterine infections (CMV, toxoplasma, herpes , other)
  Bacterial sepsis

*High red cell mass* (polycythaemia)

*Sequestered blood*
  Swallowed (fetal or maternal)
  Bruising (cephalhaematoma, breech delivery)
  Intraventricular haemorrhage

*Decreased conjugation*
  Crigler-Najjar syndrome (glucuronyl transferase deficiency)
  Sepsis

*Increased enterohepatic circulation*
  Breast milk jaundice
  Delayed passage of meconium (meconium plug, late feeding, hypothyroidism)
  Bowel obstruction (below ampulla of Vater: atresia, stenosis, meconium ileus, Hirschsprung's disease)

**Conjugated hyperbilirubinaemia**

*Impaired hepatocellular function/excretion of conjugated bilirubin*
  Intrauterine infections (hepatitic presentation)
  Metabolic disorders (galactosaemia, tyrosinosis, alpha-1-antitrypsin deficiency, other)
  Rare familial conditions (Dubin-Johnson or Rotor syndrome)
  Prolonged intravenous nutrition
  Inspissated bile syndrome (follows severe Rhesus disease)

*Obstruction to bile flow*
  Biliary atresia
  Choledochal cyst
  Common bile duct obstruction by band

in preterm or low-birthweight infants, particularly in the presence of acidosis, RDS, sepsis or perinatal asphyxia, it may occur at much lower levels. These babies also tend to have lower albumin levels.

## THE JAUNDICED BABY

Jaundice is usually first noticeable in the face and neck; as the level rises it gradually becomes more apparent over the trunk, the limbs and finally on the palms and soles. In dark skinned infants jaundice may be difficult to detect, but it is usually apparent on the sclera, on the skin of the nose when blanched or, if more severe, on the palms or soles.

### When to investigate jaundice

- Jaundice in the first 24–36 hours (suggests haemolysis).
- Marked jaundice at any age (see Fig. 18.1).
- Jaundice persisting beyond 14 days (term) or 21 days (preterm).

### History

Important points in the history are the mother's (and father's) blood groups; past obstetric history (particularly if any previous children were jaundiced); ethnic origin of parents; maternal drugs; gestation; mode of delivery; known isoimmune antibody status.

### Examination

The presence of bruising, cephalohaematomata, or plethora may suggest increased red cell destruction. Hepatosplenomegaly suggests infection or haemolysis, and pallor of the mucous membranes supports the latter. Delayed passage of meconium may suggest functional bowel obstruction (e.g. meconium ileus, Hirschsprung's disease) or hypothyroidism.

### Investigation (< 7 days)

If bilirubin is in or above zone 4 in Fig. 18.1, check:

- blood groups (infant and mother);
- Coomb's test (on cord blood or infant's blood);
- full blood count, blood film and PCV;
- urine for reducing substances (test for galactosaemia – see Chapter 16);

and if baby is unwell:

- a full infection screen (see Chapter 17).

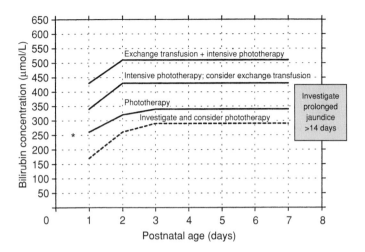

**Fig. 18.1** Guidelines for the management of jaundice in healthy term infants (adapted from American Academy of Pediatrics (1994) Practice parameter: management of hyperbilirubinaemia in the healthy term newborn. *Pediatrics* **94**, 558–65). * Jaundice appearing before 24 hours – investigate, treat with phototherapy and consider exchange transfusion if rate of rise is > 10 µmol/L/ hour.

If bilirubin is close to the 'exchange' line in Fig. 18.1:

- serum albumin and acid-base status (low pH or albumin increase risk of kernicterus at a given bilirubin level);
- direct (i.e. conjugated) bilirubin (if > 10% total bilirubin is conjugated this suggests hepatocellular damage or biliary obstruction – use the *unconjugated* bilirubin level as a guide to the need for exchange transfusion).

### Management

In any child whose bilirubin levels appear to be rising rapidly and may require intervention, repeat bilirubin estimations should be made every 4–6 hours until it is clear that the rate of rise is unlikely to require attention.

***Early neonatal jaundice*** Jaundice in the first 24–36 hours should be urgently assessed. If there is evidence of isoimmune haemolytic disease (e.g. positive Coomb's test), then exchange transfusion is likely to be necessary and should be performed if the bilirubin goes into zone one in Fig. 18.1, especially if the rate of rise is greater than 10 μmol/L/hour (see p. 413). In haemolytic disease there is an impression that earlier exchange transfusion may reduce later jaundice.

**Healthy term babies** Guidelines for management of the otherwise well term infant are summarized in Fig. 18.1. This graph is a *rough guide* only, and policy will vary from unit to unit. Recently there has been concern that jaundice in this population is overtreated (e.g. Dodd, 1993). For term infants there is no evidence that the use of phototherapy for lower levels of jaundice than those shown in Fig. 18.1 will decrease the need for exchange transfusion, although it may decrease the duration of jaundice.

**Preterm or sick babies** Phototherapy and exchange transfusion should be used at lower levels, e.g. for a well infant of 30 weeks' gestation the 'exchange transfusion' line would approximate to the 'phototherapy' line for a term infant (Fig. 18.1). The indication for phototherapy in such an infant would be correspondingly lower. Again practice varies widely, but a commonly adopted 'rule-of-thumb' is to use the formula *(gestational age (weeks)* × 10) to indicate a conservative exchange level, in μmol/L, and to subtract 100 to indicate a level over which to consider phototherapy if the child is more than 48 hours old. Early-onset jaundice is managed as for a term infant.

**Treatment** The mainstay of treatment is phototherapy, which is used to lower bilirubin levels and thus to avoid an exchange transfusion, which carries greater risk. Recent work has suggested that tin-mesporphyrin (a haem oxygenase inhibitor) may reduce bilirubin production and decrease the need for other intervention.

**Phototherapy** Unconjugated bilirubin when exposed to light is iso-merized to a more water-soluble form ('photobilirubin') which can then be excreted in the bile without conjugation. Blue light (wave-length 400–500 nm) is most effective, but is unpleasant for parents and staff, so white or mixed blue/white lights are commonly used. Efficiency of phototherapy is improved by increasing the area of exposed skin, removing plastic covers, and decreasing the distance from the light to the baby. The intensity and efficacy of phototherapy may be increased by using two phototherapy units or a high intensity lamp. Stopping phototherapy for up to 3 hours in 4 does not significantly decrease effectiveness, and facilitates feeding, changing and visiting. The main adverse effect of phototherapy is increased fluid loss, particularly in the stools, so extra fluids (about 1 mL/kg/hour extra) are needed. This may be given as extra feeds. There is no evidence that supplemental water fed to term babies affects the progress of the condition. Although there is no good evidence that phototherapy damages the eyes, it is a reasonable precaution to cover the infant's eyes whilst he or she is under the light. These covers should be removed when the infant is receiving nursing care. Phototherapy reduces skin bilirubin, so the colour of exposed skin is not a good indicator of serum bilirubin, rendering transcutaneous bilirubin meters unreliable.

Phototherapy should not be used for infants with high conjugated bilirubin levels, as it is unnecessary and may lead to an unpleasant bronzed appearance of the skin.

***Exchange transfusion*** Rough guidelines on when exchange transfusion is needed in term infants are given in Fig. 18.1. Practical details are provided in Chapter 27.

If the infant has *severe haemolytic disease* (with hypoproteinaemia, oedema, cardiac failure, severe anaemia or frank hydrops fetalis), exchange transfusion may lead to major potentially fatal fluid shifts (see Chapter 27). For such infants the first exchange transfusion has the aim of correcting anaemia and raising serum albumin levels, rather than removing bilirubin. This exchange should therefore be of only 30–60 mL/kg.

An exchange transfusion of 160 mL/kg (i.e. twice the infant's blood volume) will remove approximately 80% of the infant's red cells, and reduce the serum bilirubin by about 50%. Check the bilirubin level 4–6 hours after the exchange, as there is commonly a rapid 'rebound', with a much slower rise thereafter.

## Prolonged neonatal jaundice

Jaundice persisting beyond 14 days in a term baby (21 days in preterm) is usually considered to be pathologically prolonged (Fig. 18.1). The most important investigation is the measurement of *conjugated bilirubin* which dictates further investigation and management.

### Unconjugated hyperbilirubinaemia (>90% unconjugated)
Investigations should include:

- thyroid function tests (TSH, $T_3$, $T_4$);
- urine – microscopy and culture – reducing substances;
- blood count and film.

If these investigations are normal and the child breast fed, the jaundice is usually benign ('breast milk jaundice') and is probably due to the presence of α-glucuronidase in the milk. This results in deconjugation of bilirubin in the bowel and an increased enterohepatic circulation. It is of no clinical significance; breast feeding should *not* be interrupted (unless exchange transfusion is being considered), and the mother should be strongly reassured.

Prolonged unconjugated jaundice is common in very preterm infants, in whom delayed feeding may lead to both decreased bile flow and gut motility, resulting in increased reabsorption of deconjugated bilirubin. It is also common in the presence of polycythaemia.

### Conjugated hyperbilirubinaemia (> 20% conjugated)

Prolonged conjugated jaundice may occur with resolving haemolytic disease, hepatic damage from infection (CMV, toxoplasma, other), metabolic disease or obstruction to bile flow (Table 18.1). It may also occur after a prolonged period of intravenous nutrition, often where there has been associated sepsis; most of these infants make a full recovery. Investigations should exclude the common causes (as listed in Table 18.1):

- serum for antibodies to CMV, toxoplasma, rubella and other viruses as appropriate;
- plasma amino acids;
- serum for α-1-antitrypsin phenotype;
- three freshly voided urines for viral culture;
- urine for  reducing sugars
          amino acids
          organic acids.

***Further investigation*** Once the common causes have been excluded, difficulty may be encountered in distinguishing *biliary outflow obstruction* from *neonatal hepatitis*. These probably represent opposite ends of a single disease spectrum, arising from damage by an unknown agent to the hepatobiliary system at different stages, from the middle trimester of pregnancy (biliary atresia) to several weeks after birth (neonatal hepatitis). Both conditions are characterized by conjugated hyperbilirubinaemia, which may date from the first week or sometimes not be noticed until 2–4 weeks (onset after 4 weeks makes biliary atresia unlikely). In both conditions there is commonly enlargement of the liver, disordered coagulation, and elevated transaminase levels. Infants with biliary atresia are often remarkably well despite having severe jaundice, and usually have very pale stools. Ninety per cent of infants with biliary atresia have extrahepatic atresia, with absence or hypoplasia of the hepatic duct, cystic duct, common bile duct or any combination of these. The importance of distinguishing biliary atresia from neonatal hepatitis is that surgery for the former (biliary drainage by a Kasai portoenterostomy) is most successful if carried out within the first 6 weeks. Beyond that age irreversible liver damage progressively occurs, making drainage unlikely to succeed. Several investigations have been used to try to distinguish between biliary atresia and hepatitis, including serum alphafetoprotein (elevated in hepatitis, but usually normal in atresia) and a radionucleotide excretion scan (usually HIDA), but none is entirely satisfactory. If significant doubt remains, liver biopsy is indicated; if this is equivocal, then a laparotomy with an operative cholangiogram may be necessary.

Even with early diagnosis and surgery, successful long-term biliary drainage is achieved in only 20–30% of infants with biliary atresia. Liver transplantation is required in a further 30%, and 80% of children transplanted for biliary atresia become long-term survivors with a good prognosis. One-third of infants will die of liver failure in infancy. In contrast, most infants with neonatal hepatitis make a complete recovery, but may have complications from bleeding, sepsis, or malabsorption of vitamins A, D and K, and should be given suitable vitamin supplements (see Chapter 13).

## ISOIMMUNE HAEMOLYTIC DISEASE

### Aetiology
The rhesus antigen system consists of five distinct antigen types: 'C', 'D' and 'E' are dominant and 'c' and 'e' are recessive traits. About 85% of Caucasians have 'D' antigen, termed 'rhesus positive'. Other non-rhesus antigens may cause haemolytic disease, notably Kell and Duffy (Fy).

Leakage of fetal red cells across the placenta into the maternal circulation may lead to the formation by the mother of IgG antibodies directed against fetal antigens which she does not possess herself. Most commonly such antibodies are produced by rhesus-negative women (i.e. 'dd' genotype) and directed against rhesus-positive fetal cells (i.e. 'Dd' or 'DD' genotype). These IgG antibodies cross into the fetus and may cause destruction of circulating red cells. Severe cases are usually associated with anti-D, -c, -e and -Kell and occasionally anti-Fy antibodies. Rhesus haemolytic disease is more common if both mother and fetus are of the same ABO blood group.

IgG antibodies are not usually produced on first exposure to an antigen, but require initial sensitization, with an amplified response on second or subsequent exposure. Thus significant rhesus haemolytic disease is uncommon in first pregnancy, and increases in incidence and severity with increasing parity. Sensitization may occur from mismatched blood transfusion, or from fetomaternal bleeding at abortion. Small fetomaternal leaks may occur spontaneously or after amniocentesis or external cephalic version, and may account for the occasional cases of rhesus haemolytic disease in first pregnancies. Most spontaneous leaks occur in the last trimester, and prophylactic anti-D given to the mother at 28 and 34 weeks' gestation significantly reduces the incidence of subsequent rhesus disease.

The earlier the antibody crosses into the fetus, the more severe the disease. Haemolysis starting in the second trimester may cause severe anaemia with hepatosplenomegaly, liver damage, and hypoproteinaemia, cardiac failure and generalized oedema with ascites (hydrops fetalis; see Chapter 1). In severe cases there is a conjugated hyperbilirubinaemia.

When haemolysis starts nearer to term, the infant is born less severely anaemic but often develops severe neonatal jaundice.

### Prevention of rhesus haemolytic disease

Since 1969 the incidence of rhesus haemolytic disease has fallen dramatically as a result of the prevention of sensitization in rhesus-negative women. All non-sensitized rhesus-negative women should be given human rhesus hyperimmune gamma globulin (100–200 mcg i.m.) within 60 hours after any procedure which might result in sensitization (e.g. birth of a rhesus-positive infant, amniocentesis, termination of pregnancy). The gamma globulin binds to fetal cells and expedites their removal from the maternal circulation.

### Antenatal management

Routine screening of all rhesus-negative pregnant women for the presence of rhesus antibodies allows the identification of most affected fetuses. Where the partner is heterozygous, fetal genotype can be determined from amniotic fluid for the D, Kell and Fy antigens. Past history, levels and rate of rise of antibody, amniotic fluid $\Delta OD_{450}$ and chemiluminescence (to determine the avidity of the antibody) are the best predictors of disease severity short of direct fetal sampling. Ultrasound surveillance for signs of hydrops is also important in monitoring affected pregnancies.

The best management of an affected pregnancy remains controversial. However, it should always be in conjunction with a tertiary referral centre where cordocentesis, measurement of haematocrit and blood group, and direct fetal transfusion can be performed if necessary. The relative merits and demerits of each technique in the third trimester have not been established, and it is still unclear whether it is best to proceed to early delivery in the light of excellent neonatal survival from 30 weeks' gestation, or to continue with cordocentesis and transfusion, with their attendant risks, until spontaneous labour ensues.

### Management of the infant with rhesus haemolytic disease (see Fig. 18.2)

Continued low-grade haemolysis in infants who do not need exchange transfusion may rarely lead to late anaemia (after 2–3 weeks) which may necessitate a top-up transfusion. Early supplementation with iron and folic acid may reduce the severity of this anaemia.

Children who have received repeated intrauterine transfusions are born with significant marrow suppression and may not become jaundiced after birth. Red blood cell production may not commence for several weeks after birth, and close monitoring of haemoglobin and reticulocyte levels is necessary, as are frequent transfusions.

### Jaundice from ABO incompatibility

Infants of blood group A (or more rarely B) born to mothers of blood group O may develop early jaundice from haemolysis caused by transplacental passage of maternal antibodies directed against the A (or B) antigen. The severity of haemolysis does not correlate well with the level of maternal circulating anti-A or anti-B antibody. Although approximately 25% of pregnancies are potentially affected (mother O, fetus A or B), only 1 in 45 of these infants is affected. The incidence and severity are the same in firstborn or subsequent children.

Most infants with ABO incompatibility show only mild or moderate early jaundice, but in some the bilirubin may rise to levels requiring exchange transfusion. Hepatosplenomegaly is not a feature of ABO incompatibility, and late anaemia (see above) is rarely a problem.

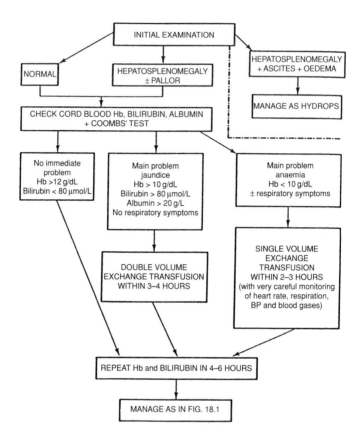

**Fig. 18.2** Management of the infant with suspected rhesus haemolytic disease (e.g. previous affected sibling or rising Rh antibody titres during this pregnancy).

## BIBLIOGRAPHY

American Academy of Pediatries (1994) Practice parameter: management of hyperbilirubinaemia in the healthy term newborn. *Pediatrics* **94**, 558–65.

Dodd, K. (1993) Neonatal jaundice – a lighter touch. *Arch. Dis. Child.* **68**, 529–32.

Newman, T.B. and Maisels, M.J. (1992). Evaluation and treatment of jaundice in the term newborn: a kinder, gentler approach. *Pediatrics* **89**, 809–18 (see also commentaries after the paper).

Otte, J.B., De Ville de Goyet, J., Reding, R. *et al.* (1994) Sequential treatment of biliary atresia with Kasai portoenterostomy and liver transplantation: a review. *Hepatology* **20**, 41S–48S.

Ozolek, J.A., Watchko, J.F. and Mimouni, F. (1994) Prevelance and lack of significance of blood group incompatibility in mothers with blood type A or B. *J. Pediatr.* **125**, 87–91.

Weiner, C.P. (1994) Fetal hemolytic disease. In James, D.K., Steer, P.J., Weiner, C.P. and Gonik, B. (eds), *High risk pregnancy: management options.* London: W.B. Saunders, 783–802.

Yao, T.C. and Stevenson, D.K. (1995) Advances in the diagnosis and treatment of neonatal hyperbilirubinaemia. *Clin. Perinatol.* **22**, 741–58.

# 19

# Haematological problems

Normal values
Bleeding and clotting disorders
Anaemia
Polycythaemia

## NORMAL VALUES (see Chapter 29)

### Haemoglobin and haematocrit

- Haemoglobin (Hb) and haematocrit (Hct) values are increased by delayed cord clamping (particularly if the placenta is above the level of the baby).
- Hb and Hct both rise after birth (by 2–3 g/dL and 3–6%, respectively), to peak at 3–12 hours of age.
- Capillary values for Hb and Hct are consistently higher than venous (or arterial) values:
  at 28 weeks' gestation: mean capillary Hb = 1.2 × venous Hb;
  at 40 weeks' gestation: mean capillary Hb = 1.1 × venous Hb.

### White cell count

- Increase in immature (band) neutrophils suggests infection.
- Increase or (more important) decrease in total neutrophil count also suggests infection.

## Platelets

- Normal platelet count does not change significantly with gestation:

    $275 \pm 60 \times 10^3/\text{mm}^3$ at 30 weeks' gestation;

    $310 \pm 70 \times 10^3/\text{mm}^3$ at 40 weeks' gestation (mean $\pm$ SD).
- A platelet count of $< 100 \times 10^3/\text{mm}^3$ is abnormal at any gestation, and values of $100\text{--}150 \times 10^3/\text{mm}^3$ warrant further investigation.
- Platelet counts commonly fall with neonatal sepsis.
- The platelet count rises to $3\text{--}400 \times 10^3/\text{mm}^3$ by 3–4 weeks in term and preterm infants.

# BLEEDING AND CLOTTING DISORDERS

## Assessment of the bleeding infant

### History

Family history; maternal illness (e.g. idiopathic thrombocytopenic purpura, systemic lupus erythematosus); previously affected siblings; isoimmunization; infections during pregnancy; maternal drugs (e.g. aspirin, indomethacin, phenytoin, phenobarbitone, thiazides); labour and delivery.

### Examination

- Site of bleeding? Petechiae? Hepatosplenomegaly?
- Is the infant sick?

### Investigations

Platelet count; prothrombin time (PT); partial thromboplastin time (PTT); blood film (to look for fragmented red cells) $\pm$ thrombin time (TT); fibrin degradation products (FDP).

*Apt's test* on vomited blood (to determine whether it is fetal or maternal). To 5 mL of water in a test-tube add 3 drops of vomited blood and 1 mL of sodium hydroxide. Adult Hb turns brown within 1–2 min. Fetal Hb stays pink. Always use controls of known Hb F and Hb A.

## Differential diagnosis of bleeding in the newborn
(see Tables 19.1 and 19.2)

**Table 19.1** A summary of the results of laboratory screening tests in the differential diagnosis of the bleeding infant*

| Platelets | Laboratory studies | | Likely diagnosis |
|---|---|---|---|
| | PT | PTT | |
| **'Sick' infants** | | | |
| Decreased | Increased | Increased | DIC |
| Decreased | Normal | Normal | Platelet consumption (infection, necrotizing enterocolitis, renal vein thrombosis) |
| Normal | Increased | Increased | Liver disease |
| Normal | Normal | Normal | Compromised vascular integrity (associated with hypoxia, prematurity, acidosis, hyperosmolality) |
| **'Healthy' infants** | | | |
| Decreased | Normal | Normal | Immune (auto or allo) thrombocytopenia; occult infection or thrombosis; bone marrow hypoplasia (rare) |
| Normal | Increased | Increased | Haemorrhagic disease of newborn (vitamin K deficiency) |
| Normal | Normal | Increased | Hereditary clotting factor deficiencies |
| Normal | Normal | Normal | Bleeding due to local factors (trauma, anatomical abnormalities); qualitative platelet abnormalities (rare); Factor XIII deficiency (rare) |

*From Glader and Buchanan (1976) *Pediatrics* **58**, 548.

**Table 19.2** Screening tests of blood coagulation in term and preterm infants

|  | Preterm | Term newborn | > 1–2 months |
|---|---|---|---|
| Platelet count ($\times 10^3/mm^3$) | 150–400 | 150–400 | 150–400 |
| Platelets on peripheral smear* | 10–20 | 10–20 | 10–20 |
| Prothrombin time (PT) (sec)† | 14–22 | 13–20 | 12–14 |
| Partial thromboplastin time (PTT) (sec)† | 35–55 | 30–45 | 25–35 |
| Thrombin time (TT) (sec)† | 11–17 | 10–16 | 10–12 |
| Fibrinogen (mg/dL) | 150–300 | 150–300 | 150–300 |

* Platelets per oil immersion field, including one or two small clumps.
† Normal values may vary from one laboratory to another; PT and PTT may remain prolonged in infants of < 1500 g despite vitamin $K_1$ having been given.
Modified from Glader and Buchanan (1976) *Pediatrics* **58**, 548 and Gross and Stuart (1977) *Clin. Perinatol.* **4** 259.

# Disseminated intravascular coagulation (DIC)

DIC results from widespread activation of the clotting mechanism in sick infants, leading to secondary thrombocytopenia and clotting disorder (depletion of factors II, V and VIII and fibrinogen).

## Causes

- Infection (e.g. bacterial, congenital infections, NEC).
- Hypothermia.
- Asphyxia.
- Acidosis.
- Hypoxia.
- Hypotension.
- Severe rhesus disease.

## Diagnosis

- Bleeding from puncture sites ± petechiae ± thromboses (e.g. gangrenous necrosis of skin).
- ↓ Platelets; ↑ PT and PTT; ↑ TT.
- ↑ FDP in blood and urine.
- Blood film may show fragmented red cells.

## Management

- Treat underlying condition (e.g. sepsis, hypoxia).
- Replace clotting factors by transfusion with fresh frozen plasma, 10–15 mL/kg.

- Give 1 mg vitamin K$_1$ i.v.
- In severely ill infants or those with persisting bleeding/clotting disorder, exchange transfusion (with fresh blood) may be life-saving (see Chapter 27).

## Haemorrhagic disease of the newborn

Vitamin K stores at birth are very small and rapidly depleted. Breast milk contains very little vitamin K, and breast-fed infants may develop bleeding from depletion of factors II, VII, IX and X. Phenobarbitone and phenytoin given during pregnancy interfere with vitamin K metabolism, and may cause extreme depletion of factors II, VII, IX and X in the fetus, with bleeding at birth.

### Diagnosis

Bleeding from umbilical cord, melaena, haematemesis, bleeding into the skin or from puncture sites – usually between 24 and 72 hours after birth (occasionally up to 2–3 weeks in breast-fed infants). ↑ PT and PTT; platelets, TT and FDP normal.

### Prevention (see Chapter 4)

All babies should be given vitamin K on the day of birth. Normal infants should receive 500 mcg (0.25 mL Konakion) orally. Breast-fed infants should have second and third oral doses at 1 week and 4–6 weeks respectively.

High-risk babies should be given 100 mcg (0.05 mL Konakion) i.m./i.v.

### Management of the bleeding infant

*(1) If significant haemorrhage has occurred and the infant is shocked:*
(BP < 35 mm Hg; pH < 7.25. *NB* Hb may not fall for 2–3 hours).

- The baby may have cold peripheries with poor capillary perfusion and a capillary return of > 2 sec. Blood pressure may not fall until potentially life-threatening blood loss has occurred.
- Transfuse rapidly over 5–15 min with 15–20 mL/kg uncross-matched O-negative blood. If the infant is still shocked, give a further 15–20 mL/kg over 15–20 min.
- Monitor blood pressure and central venous pressure closely.
- Aim to achieve BP > 40 mm Hg (in term infant) and CVP < 8 cm H$_2$O.
- If necessary give further transfusion, cross-matched against the mother's blood (10–30 mL/kg over 2–3 hours, accompanied by 1–2 mg/kg frusemide i.v.).

### (2) If the infant is not shocked:

- Give vitamin K$_1$, 1 mg i.v.
- Transfuse with cross-matched packed cells to raise Hb to 10–12 g/dL (over 2–3 hours, with 2 mg/kg frusemide i.v.).
- NB 10 mL/kg of packed cells will raise Hb by 2–3 g/dL or the Hct by about 10%.

## Hereditary bleeding disorders

These may present with bleeding from puncture sites or incisions (e.g. circumcision).

- *Haemophilia*: X-linked, factor VIII deficiency;
- *Christmas disease*: X-linked, factor IX deficiency.
- *von Willebrand's disease*: factor VIII deficiency and platelet defect, autosomal dominant.

**Diagnosis** Family history; specific factor assay.

## Thrombocytopenia (see Chapter 1)

Thrombocytopenia usually presents with petechiae, bruising and cephalhaematoma. Rarely, major haemorrhage (e.g. intracranial, intrahepatic) may occur as a result of birth injury.

**Diagnosis** See Fig. 19.1.

## Autoimmune thrombocytopenia (ITP)

Mothers with SLE or ITP may have circulatory IgG antiplatelet antibodies which cross to the fetus and cause fetal/neonatal thrombocytopenia in 50% of cases. Neonatal ITP has a wide spectrum ranging from transient to up to 3 months' duration, and from minor to severe bleeding. Prediction of neonatal ITP before delivery can be assessed by:

- maternal platelet count; 70% risk if her count is < 100 000;
- maternal HPA-antibody; 92% risk if levels are elevated;
- maternal splenectomy; high risk. The mother's platelet count may be normal but still have many antibodies crossing to the baby;
- cordocentesis to measure fetal platelet count;
- fetal scalp blood sample for platelet count in labour. This is not recommended because of the danger of severe fetal bleeding.

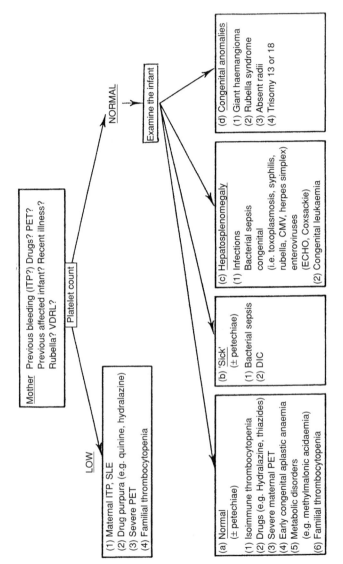

**Fig. 19.1** The diagnosis of haematological problems in the newborn.

There is little evidence that delivery by Caesarean section is of benefit in reducing the risk of fetal bleeding, but it is advisable to treat the mother with steroids or immunoglobulin for 5 days before delivery.

## Alloimmune thrombocytopenia

Analogous to rhesus disease. The mother produces IgG antibodies to HPA-1a antigen on the infant's platelets, leading to severe fetal and neonatal thrombocytopenia. The recurrence rate in subsequent pregnancies is 75%.

### Management

The baby's platelet count may be normal at birth and not fall for 2 days, so do a platelet count at birth and 12-hourly for 72 hours, and thereafter according to level.

Avoid i.m. injections.

There is an increased risk of bleeding in preterm babies with platelets < 50 000 and in term infants with platelets < 20 000. Transfused donor platelets may be used in ITP but will be rapidly destroyed in alloimmune thrombocytopenia; i.v. immunoglobulin will increase the platelet count more quickly than steroids.

- If the platelet count is < 10 000 or there is evidence of
  continuing bleeding, give 1 unit (20 mL/kg) of donor platelets to babies with maternal ITP. In alloimmune thrombocytopenia you must use either HLA-matched platelets or washed and irradiated maternal platelets.
    Start a course of i.v. immunoglobulin (e.g. Sandoglobulin)
    1 mg/kg/day for two consecutive days.
- If the platelet count is 10–20 000, treat with immunoglobulin as above.
- If the platelet count is 20–50 000, with petechiae or purpura,
  treat with prednisolone 2 mg/kg/day until the condition resolves.

Treatment with steroids or repeated courses of immunoglobulin may be needed for several weeks.

## ANAEMIA

## Definition

Haemoglobin level < 12 g/dL in the first week, or < 10 g/dL after the first week.

### Early anaemia

The cause is commonly apparent from the history.

**Causes**

*Haemorrhage*

- Fetomaternal (NB Kleihauer test)
- Twin-to-twin
- Placental (at or before delivery)
  - placenta praevia
  - vasa praevia
  - placental abruption
  - incision of placenta at Caesarean section
- Fetoplacental (after delivery)

Neonatal (e.g. intracranial, intrahepatic, gastrointestinal, pulmonary, sub-aponeurotic, from umbilical cord, from venous or arterial cannula).

*Haemolysis*

- Rhesus isoimmunization
- Haemoglobinopathies (e.g. alpha-thalassaemia).
- Congenital infections.
- Bacterial infections.

**Investigations**

- Full blood count, film and reticulocyte count.
- Serum bilirubin (direct and total).
- Blood group and Coomb's test.
- Kleihauer test on the mother's blood.
- (Clotting studies and platelet count).
- (Congenital infection screen).
- (Hb electrophoresis).

**Management**

As for haemorrhagic disease (p. 326).

### Late anaemia (i.e. > 7 days of age)

**Causes**

*Haemorrhage*

- Small perinatal haemorrhage.
- Excessive blood sampling.

- Haemorrhagic disease.
- Intraventricular haemorrhage.
- Chronic gastrointestinal blood loss.

*Haemolysis*

- Rhesus, ABO incompatibility.
- Sepsis (+ DIC).
- Haemoglobinopathies.
- Red cell defects (e.g. spherocytosis).
- Vitamin E deficiency.

*Decreased red cell production*

- Anaemia of prematurity.
- Infection (bacterial or viral).
- Folic acid deficiency.
- Drugs.
- Congenital marrow aplasia) ⎫ very rare.
- Congenital leukaemia) ⎭

### Investigation

- Full blood count, film and reticulocyte count.
- Serum bilirubin (direct and total).
- Blood group and Coomb's test.
- Urine microscopy and culture.
- Check stools for occult blood.
- Blood culture.

### Management

- Treat underlying cause. Give iron and folate supplements (see Chapter 13).
- Transfuse with packed cells (see p. 326) if Hb < 8 g/dL or if symptomatic.

## POLYCYTHAEMIA

## Definition

Haematocrit values from automated blood cell counters are calculated and may be inaccurate. It is better to measure haematocrit directly on a capillary-tube sample.

Venous haematocrit (packed cell volume) > 65% in a newborn infant (capillary haematocrit is commonly 3–5% higher). Blood viscosity rises linearly with Hct up to 65%, but exponentially above that, particularly in vessels with low flow velocity (i.e. veins and capillaries).

## Causes

### (1) Increased intra-uterine erythropoiesis

Placental insufficiency
 (SGA infants)
Post-term infants
Maternal pre-eclamptic toxaemia
Maternal drugs (e.g. propranolol)
Maternal smoking

Maternal diabetes
Maternal heart disease
Neonatal thyrotoxicosis
Trisomy 13, 18 or 21
Beckwiths' syndrome
Congenital adrenal
 hyperplasia

### (2) Secondary to red cell transfusion

Placental transfusion
 (delayed cord clamping)

Maternofetal transfusion
Twin-to-twin transfusion

### (3) Capillary permeability and plasma loss

Cold stress
Hypoxia

Preterm infants
Hypovolaemia

**Clinical features** Commonly plethoric but asymptomatic. However, may show:

Lethargy
Irritability
Hypoglycaemia
Vomiting
Hepatomegaly
Thrombocytopenia
Cardiac failure
NEC
Renal venous thrombosis

Hypotonia
Poor feeding
Cyanosis
Acidosis
Jaundice
Respiratory distress
Convulsions
Peripheral gangrene

### Investigations

- Full blood count, platelet count, venous and capillary haematocrit.
- Blood sugar.
- Serum calcium and bilirubin.

*If cardiorespiratory symptoms*:

- chest X-ray (may show cardiomegaly ± prominent vasculature ± pleural fluid);
- ECG (see Chapter 11).

**Management**

Several studies have shown a significant incidence of long-term neurological sequelae, but the precise level of Hct which warrants treatment is controversial.

*If symptomatic* (e.g. cardiorespiratory or neurological signs of symptoms:

- dilution exchange transfusion with 20–30 mL/kg HAS, 4.5%, over 20–30 min (see Chapter 27).

  *If asymptomatic*:

- repeat venous Hct 6- to 12-hourly until < 65%;
- monitor blood sugar carefully;
- ensure adequate fluid intake (monitor urine specific gravity);
- dilution exchange as above if venous Hct > 75% or infant becomes symptomatic.

## BIBLIOGRAPHY

Hann, I. M., Gibson, B.E.S. and Letsky, E.A. (eds) (1991) *Fetal and neonatal haematology.* London: Ballière Tindall.

McClelland, B. (ed.) (1996) *Handbook of transfusion medicine,* 2nd edn. London: HMSO.

# 20

# Ophthalmic disorders

## EXAMINATION OF THE NEWBORN EYE

Examination of the eyes of newborn infants forms part of the routine examination (see Chapter 4). Unless correctable abnormalities which interfere with the development of vision are detected early, permanent changes develop in the higher visual pathways which preclude good acuity later, even if the original condition is subsequently treated.

Most neonatal eye conditions are recognizable by simple inspection and testing for a red reflex, with pupillary dilatation and fundal examination with the direct ophthalmoscope if indicated. For detailed examination of the peripheral retina, indirect ophthalmoscopy with an aspheric condensing lens is necessary.

A family history is very helpful in the detection of inherited eye disorders. Routine examination should include assessment of visual function by observation of fixation and horizontal following of a face, large coloured object, or light. Any definite constant squint is abnormal. The examination should be conducted systematically, starting from the lids and progressing posteriorly to fundus and orbit.

Pupillary dilatation is achieved where necessary with one drop of homatropine (1%), to which one drop of phenylephrine (2.5%) can be added for additional effect. The dose may be repeated after 20 min if necessary.

## Indications for direct ophthalmoscopy

- Positive family history.
- Congenital infection.
- Other external ocular abnormalities.

## Indications for indirect ophthalmoscopy (usually by an ophthalmologist)

- Retinopathy of prematurity suspected.
- Any fundal abnormality detected.
- Inability to see the fundus.

Parents of children with any significant ocular condition should be counselled by an ophthalmologist and a paediatrician after definition of the lesion.

## SQUINT

An occasional deviation of the visual axis up to the age of 6 months may not be abnormal. A definite diagnosis of squint requires the cover test to be performed accurately.

A *constant squint* is abnormal at any age and requires investigation by an ophthalmologist. Such a squint may cause amblyopia which must be corrected as soon as possible to prevent permanent visual impairment. Fundal examination is mandatory to exclude serious pathology such as retinoblastoma.

## CONJUNCTIVITIS AND OPHTHALMIA NEONATORUM

The signs of conjunctivitis are purulent discharge, conjunctival injection and lid oedema. The cornea should be bright and clear. If bacterial infection is acquired from the maternal genital tract, the signs are present from the first or second day ('ophthalmia neonatorum') and usually bilateral. If due to failure of the nasolacrimal duct to open, signs are usually delayed for 1 week, and although usually bilateral initially, may be unilateral.

Conjunctivitis may be the result of early bacterial infection (gonococcus, now rare), perinatal infection with *Chlamydia trachomatis* (inclusion conjunctivitis presents after 3 days), later infection with environmental organisms, or occasionally chemical irritation from, for example, meconium. After discussion with the laboratory, conjunctival swabs should be taken for direct microscopy of a smear preparation (gonococcus – first 72 hours), and for a direct immunofluorescent test (*Chlamydia*), in addition to routine bacteriological swabs. Chlamydia should be sought even in the presence of gonococcal infection as the two may co-exist.

Suspected gonococcal ophthalmia requires urgent treatment before the bacteriological results are available, to avoid possible corneal perforation. Resistance to penicillin is not infrequent, and the recommended treatment is a single i.m. injection of cefotaxime (100 mg/kg).

Chlamydial conjunctivitis is treated with chlortetracycline ointment 4 times a day for 1 month, combined with a full 2-week course of oral erythromycin once the infecting agent is confirmed. A full course of erythromycin is important for the prevention of later pneumonitis.

Infection by other bacteria is usually covered by the administration of 0.5% neomycin eye ointment/drops, which has the advantage that subsequent cultures for *Chlamydia* are possible, unlike the situation after treatment with chloramphenicol.

### Nasolacrimal duct obstruction

Conjunctivitis is due to non-pathogenic organisms pooling in the conjunctival sac, and should be treated conservatively with cleaning of the lids, use of antibiotic drops if there is much discharge, and instructions to the parents regarding massage of the lacrimal sac to attempt to open the lower end of the nasolacrimal duct. Only if this has been ineffective by the age of 1 year should probing of the nasolacrimal ducts be carried out under general anaesthetic.

# RETINOPATHY OF PREMATURITY

### Aetiology

ROP develops during recovery of the immature retina from ischaemia, which may be as a result of hyperoxia. ROP particularly affects infants of < 28 weeks' gestation, and is rare after 32 weeks' gestation. No 'safe' upper limit for $PaO_2$ has been identified, and there is much confusion as to the true aetiology. It is recommended that $FiO_2$ is adjusted to maintain $PaO_2$ between 50 and 80 mm Hg (6.5–10.4 kPa) during the early neonatal course. Instability of perfusion and oxygenation may be important factors contributing to the progression of ROP, and care should be aimed at minimizing swings in these variables.

### Pathophysiology

Retinal vascularization begins at the optic disc from 14 weeks' gestation, progressing outwards to reach the peripheral retina (ora serrata) at term. The growth of retinal vessels is inhibited if ischaemia occurs during this phase. Subsequently, the unvascularized ischaemic peripheral retina may release a vasoproliferative factor (similar to that postulated for proliferative diabetic retinopathy), to stimulate the growth of new vessels from the peripheral edge of the vascularized retina (the demarcation line). These vessels grow forward into the vitreous cavity, stimulate the growth of glial tissue, exert vitreoretinal traction, and thereby cause visual loss from vitreous haemorrhage, retinal distortion and detachment.

### Detection

All infants of < 31 weeks' gestation or < 1501 g birthweight should be examined by an ophthalmologist using an indirect ophthalmoscope. Infants born at < 26 weeks' gestation should be screened first at 6–7 weeks postnatal age and then 2-weekly until 36 weeks' gestation. Infants of 26 weeks or more gestation should be screened at 6–7 weeks of age and again at 36 weeks' gestation. If signs of ROP have not developed by 36 weeks', no further examinations are necessary.

### Grading

- Stage 1 – flat demarcation line between pink normally vascularized posterior retina and white unvascularized ischaemic peripheral anterior retina.
- Stage 2 – demarcation line raised into vitreous cavity.

- Stage 3 – new vessels elevated into vitreous cavity from raised demarcation line, with or without vitreous haemorrhage.
- Stage 4 – traction retinal detachment.

'*Plus*' is added to each grading if there are dilated retinal vessels in the normal posterior retina, and implies progressive disease.

### Treatment
Stages 1 and 2 usually resolve spontaneously without sequelae. For Stage 3 ROP, laser or cryotherapy to the ischaemic peripheral retina has been shown to be effective in many cases in halting the progress of the disease if performed early. For very preterm children treatment of stage 2 'plus' disease with laser may be beneficial.

### Prevention
Careful monitoring of $PaO_2$, with the avoidance of high and low levels, is recommended. Despite many studies, vitamin E administration has *not* been shown to have a beneficial effect.

## DISORDERS OF THE EXTERNAL EYE

## Lids

*Coloboma* Gap in lid margin, usually upper and nasal; may lead to exposure keratitis and require surgical repair; associated with Goldenhaar's syndrome.

*Cryptophthalmos* Unilateral or bilateral absence of a palpebral fissure and formed globe; no treatment.

*Blepharophimosis* Partially or completely fused lids, normal in very preterm infants (< 26 weeks) in whom they open spontaneously; occasionally requires surgery.

*Ptosis* Usually unilateral, may be associated with superior rectus muscle weakness, with Horner's syndrome, or may be mechanical due to a lid tumour; congenital ptosis does not normally require further investigation for a systemic cause. It may require surgery later to avoid amblyopia, or for cosmetic reasons.

*Port-wine stain* As part of Sturge-Weber syndrome may be associated with congenital glaucoma.

## Tumours

**Dermoid cyst** Sometimes has orbital component, usually outer part of upper lid; may need excision on cosmetic grounds later.

**Capillary haemangioma** Increases in size in first year, spontaneous involution over up to 5 years in most cases. May cause ptosis and subsequent amblyopia, but is otherwise best left untreated.

## Orbit

**Proptosis** Due to traumatic haemorrhage, orbital tumours (hae-mangioma and lymphangioma are the commonest in the first year), and with shallow orbits, as in craniostenosis and Crouzon's disease (craniofacial dysostosis).

## Cornea

**Corneal opacities** *In all cases where there is significant corneal opacity, an ophthalmologist should be involved early in an attempt to avoid gross amblyopia.*

**Birth trauma and congenital glaucoma** May cause splits in Descemet's membrane which allows fluid to enter the cornea, causing opacification.

**Sclerocornea** A developmental abnormality that causes partial or complete opacification. Opacities may be associated with the *anterior chamber cleavage syndrome* where there is incomplete formation of the structures bordering the anterior chamber – cornea, drainage angle, iris and lens.

**Dermoid tumours of the cornea** Can occupy a variable extent of the cornea from the limbus. Their surface is irregular, unlike sclerocornea.

**Corneal ulceration** A rare cause of opacification. The most likely agent is the gonococcus or pseudomonas. Swabs and ulcer scrapings should be taken for culture and sensitivity as soon as possible. A broad-spectrum antibiotic (such as ciprofloxacin) should be given topically, before sensitivities are available.

**Metabolic causes** These are very unusual at birth, perhaps because the absent enzyme crosses the placenta from the maternal circulation. Mucolipidosis Type IV does, however, cause opacification at birth.

# INTERNAL EYE DISORDERS

## Iris

*Aniridia* Frequently autosomal dominant with significant later ocular problems. In sporadic cases it is sometimes associated with a chromosomal deletion and a high risk of later Wilms' tumour.

*Coloboma* May be autosomal dominant. It is due to failure of closure of the fetal fissure. Always inferior or infero-nasal, it may be associated with a choroidal coloboma, frequently bilateral, the extent of which determines the visual prognosis. No treatment.

*Corectopia* An eccentric pupil. It may be autosomal dominant, and is sometimes associated with glaucoma or subluxation of the lens. Otherwise it carries a good visual prognosis.

*Anisocoria* Unequal pupils. It may be a simple local abnormality with no systemic associations, or it may be part of congenital Horner's syndrome, or part of a third cranial nerve palsy. In most circumstances, intensive systemic investigation is not required and the visual prognosis is good.

*Albinism* Generalized albinism (autosomal recessive) and ocular albinism (X-linked) cause lack of melanin pigment in the retinal pigment epithelium and choroid, resulting in macula hypoplasia, poor acuity and nystagmus. It is caused by defects in tyrosine metabolism.

## Pupil

### Leucocoria
An abnormal white reflex from the pupil and a serious prognostic sign. The causes, listed below, are dealt with in the relevant sections:

- retinoblastoma;
- cataract;
- coloboma of the choroid;
- persistent hyperplastic primary vitreous;
- retinopathy of prematurity;
- infection – toxoplasma, cytomegalovirus, herpes simplex;
- Norrie's disease and incontinentia pigmenti (Bloch-Sulzberger syndrome).

## Lens

### Cataract

Many syndromes include cataract as an occasional feature, reflecting the fact that cataract represents the final common path of many varied insults to the fetal and neonatal lens:

Causes include the following:

- isolated autosomal dominant and no other abnormality, rarely autosomal recessive or X-linked;
- intrauterine infection, usually rubella;
- metabolic disorders:
    galactosaemia,
    hypoglycaemia;
- chromosomal disorders –
    trisomy 13, 18, 21,
    Turner's syndrome;
- associated with other ocular abnormalities –
    microphthalmos,
    persistent hyperplastic primary vitreous;
- systemic syndromes (see Jones, 1997).

After general examination, investigations include chromosome analysis, intrauterine infection screen (toxoplasma, rubella, cytomegalovirus, herpes simplex), and urine chromatography for amino-aciduria.

Bilateral and unilateral congenital cataracts sufficient to obscure the fundus view should be treated at the earliest opportunity.

## Vitreous

***Persistent hyperplastic primary vitreous*** Persistence of the fetal hyaloid vascular system that extends from the optic disc to the posterior lens surface, causing opacity on and behind the posterior lens capsule. Immediate referral is advised.

## Retina

**Retinopathy of prematurity** (see separate section above).

### Retinoblastoma

***Pathophysiology*** A malignant tumour of embryonic retinal tissue, appearing as a white mass arising from any part of the retina, posterior or peripheral, occasionally present at birth but usually presenting before 5 years. Those that present in the neonatal period are important in that they are often autosomal dominant and may be bilateral or multicentric. The remainder are spontaneous mutations, normally present later and are unilateral (because the mutation is somatic) and not usually inherited.

**Presentation** After routine examination in the presence of a relevant family history, or the appearance of a white mass in the pupil (one cause of leukocoria), or squint due to visual loss – an important reason for early fundal examination of any child found to have a constant squint.

**Management** Urgent ophthalmological referral is necessary if retino-blastoma is suspected. Children of affected parents and siblings of affected children must be followed up frequently by an ophthalmo-logical department from birth.

### Retinal haemorrhage
Usually due to birth trauma or asphyxia. Dome-shaped (under the internal limiting membrane) or flame-shaped (in the nerve fibre layer). They disappear spontaneously, normally without visual sequelae.

## Choroid

**Albinism** (see under iris)

**Choroidal coloboma** (see under iris)

### Congenital toxoplasmosis
Fundal appearance of choroido-retinitis is that of a white lesion due to destruction of the pigment epithelium and underlying choroid, usually with surrounding pigment proliferation. It is normally in-active at the time of birth, but may cause blindness in the affected eye if the macula region is affected.

## ABNORMALITIES OF GLOBE SIZE

## Congenital glaucoma (buphthalmos)

Unilateral or bilateral, usually sporadic, sometimes autosomal re-cessive. May be associated with *systemic abnormalities* (Jones, 1997).

**Signs** These include:

• corneal opacity;

- watering eye;
- enlargement of globe;
- photophobia;
- eye rubbing.

**Treatment** Requires urgent referral for glaucoma surgery, usually goniotomy, to prevent permanent visual loss and unsightly enlargement of the globe.

## Microphthalmos

This is associated with:

- other ocular abnormalities;
- intrauterine infections;
- many syndromes (Jones, 1997).

## BIBLIOGRAPHY

Committee for the Classification of Retinopathy of Prematurity (1984) An International Classification of Retinopathy of Prematurity. *Arch. Ophthalmol.* **102**; 1130–4.

Jones, K.L. (1997) *Smith's recognisable patterns of human malformation*, 5th edn. Philadelphia, PA: W. B. Saunders.

Lepage, P., Bogaerts, J., Kestelyn, P., and Meheus A, (1988) Single dose cefotaxime intramuscularly cures gonococcal ophthalmia neonatorum. *Br. J. Ophthalmol.* **72**; 518–20

Lucey, J.F. and Dangman, B. (1984) A re-examination of the role of oxygen in retrolental fibroplasia. *Pediatrics* **73**; 82–96.

Marlow, N. (1997) Clinical care and the prevention of retinopathy of prematurity. *Clin. Risk* **3**; 37–41.

Royal College of Ophthalmologists and British Association of Perinatal Medicine (1995) *Retinopathy of Prematurity: Guidelines for Screening And Treatment – Report of a Joint Working Party.* London: Royal College of Opthalmologists and British Association of Perinatal Medicine.

# 21

# Neonatal skin disorders

Common harmless eruptions
Vesiculobullous eruptions
Pustular disorders
Erythrodermas
Eruptions in the napkin area
Dermatitis
Treatment of neonatal skin disorders

The appearance of the skin at birth is one of the features used to assess gestational age (see Chapter 22). The epidermis and dermis of the full-term baby are similar in structure and function to those of the adult. In the preterm baby the epidermis is more permeable and the dermis is thinner with immature vasculature, reflected in the readiness with which generalized hyperaemia, cutis marmorata (marbling) and harlequin colour change occur. Many congenital disorders and acquired diseases are recognized through skin changes.

**Table 21.1**

| Condition | Clinical features | Distribution | Pathology |
|---|---|---|---|
| **Common harmless eruptions** | | | |
| Sebaceous gland hyperplasia | Yellow pinpoint papules | Face, areolae, genitalia | Maternal androgen |
| Milia | Firm white papules | Face, especially nose | Follicular keratin cysts |
| Miliaria | Crops of tiny vesicles and/or papules with red background | Head, neck, upper trunk, axillae, groin | Obstruction of sweat ducts Warmth and humidity |
| Toxic erythema (erythema neonatorum) | Red macules or papules Occasionally pustules – occurs in first few days | Maximal on trunk Spares palms and soles | Unknown Pustules contain eosinophils |
| **Vesiculobullous eruptions** | | | |
| Blistering occurs more readily in the neonate. Some of these disorders are potentially fatal, so early diagnosis is essential. Specialized techniques such as electron microscopy and immunofluorescence may be required and should be discussed with the pathologist. | | | |
| Sucking blisters | Few blisters | Fingers, lips, forearms | — |
| Bullous impetigo | Blisters become cloudy | Can be anywhere | Gram stain and culture *Staphylococcus aureus* |
| Scalded skin syndrome | Fever and malaise Generalized tender erythema with large flaccid bullae, shedding to leave raw area | Anywhere, mucous membranes spared | Gram stain and culture *Staphylococcus aureus* Histology of blister roof Superficial epidermis only |

**Table 21.1** Continued

| Condition | Clinical features | Distribution | Pathology |
|---|---|---|---|
| Epidermolysis bullosa | Depends on clinical/genetic type. Blisters at sites of trauma heal with scars in the dystrophic types | Sites of trauma and friction. Mucous membranes may be involved | Electron microscopy Immunofluorescence |
| Toxic epidermal necrolysis | Clinically similar to scalded skin syndrome. May have drug aetiology | Anywhere, mucous membranes involved | Histology of blister roof – full-thickness epidermis |
| Neonatal herpes virus infection | Blisters solitary or clustered, but can be generalized and mimic epidermolysis bullosa | Anywhere | Electron microscopy Viral culture |
| Burns, irritants | History of exposure, trauma, use of skin-cleansing agents, sticky tape, ECG electrodes, etc. | Anywhere | History |
| Bullous insect bites | Lesions often grouped | Anywhere | Puncture marks evident Exposure feasible (fleas, scabies) |
| Incontinentia pigmenti | Usually female Linear pattern of blisters, evolve into verrucous lesions, with grey-brown pigmentation. May have eye and CNS anomalies | Especially trunk and extremities | Eosinophils in vesicles |

**Table 21.1** Continued

| Condition | Clinical features | Distribution | Pathology |
|---|---|---|---|
| Epidermolytic hyperkeratosis | Erythroderma with bullae Dominant | | Histology – vacuolization of upper epidermal cells |
| Acrodermatitis enteropathica | Blisters evolving into crusts and pustules Glossitis, stomatitis Diarrhoea | Hands, feet, face and genital area | Low serum zinc |
| Mastocytosis (1) Diffuse | Thickened yellowish skin readily blisters with trauma May have flushing, abdominal and respiratory symptoms | Anywhere | Histology – excess mast cells |
| (2) Urticaria pigmentosa | Multiple reddish lesions which blister when rubbed | Anywhere | Histology – excess mast cells |
| (3) Mastocytoma | One or a few nodules which may blister when rubbed | Anywhere | Histology – excess mast cells |

**Pustular disorders**

Infection must always be considered. Most of the pustular dermatoses can be diagnosed by Gram and Giemsa stains, and a KOH preparation. Biopsy, bacterial and viral culture of pustule contents are also needed.

**Table 21.1** Continued

| Condition | Clinical features | Distribution | Pathology |
|---|---|---|---|
| **Non-infectious disorders** | | | |
| Pustular toxic erythema | Red macules and papules becoming pustular<br>Onset 24–72 hours old, lasts up to 1 week | Mainly on trunk | Smear – eosinophils |
| Pustular miliaria | See miliaria<br>Often high temperature and humidity | Flexures and clothed sites | Histology – pustules in relation to sweat ducts |
| Acropustulosis of infancy | Itchy pustules<br>Crops may continue for 2–3 years | Hands and feet | Giemsa – neutrophils in pustules |
| Neonatal pustular melanosis | Transient<br>Mainly black<br>Present at birth<br>Pustules last a few days, followed by melanotic macules which may last for months | Chin, neck, palms, soles | Giemsa – neutrophils in pustules |
| **Mild infections** | | | |
| Candidiasis<br>Congenital | Present at birth<br>Macules, papules, pustules | Widespread | KOH preparation – pseudohyphae.<br>*Candida* on culture |

**Table 21.1** Continued

| Condition | Clinical features | Distribution | Pathology |
|---|---|---|---|
| Neonatal | After first week<br>Pustules at periphery of moist red area | Oral<br>Napkin area | KOH preparation – pseudohyphae.<br>*Candida* on culture |
| Staphylococcal impetigo | Vesicles, bullae and pustules on erythematous base | Anywhere | *Staphylococcus aureus* on culture<br><br>Gram-positive cocci on smear |
| Scabies | Erythematous papules, vesicles and pustules<br>Scabies in mother or other close contact | Widespread | Mites seen on microscopy of scraping |
| **Severe infections** | | | |
| Bacterial infections<br>  *Staphylococcus aureus*<br>  Group B streptococci<br>  *Pseudomonas*<br>  *Haemophilus influenzae*, etc. | Pustules with fever, signs of septicaemia, meningitis, etc. | Widespread | Gram stain<br>Positive culture from pustule ± blood |

**Table 21.1** Continued

| Condition | Clinical features | Distribution | Pathology |
|---|---|---|---|
| Congenital syphilis | Vesiculopustular eruption ± hepatosplenomegaly, chorioretinitis, periostitis, etc. Nasal discharge | Involves palms, soles, face and genitalia | Smear – dark ground micro or direct immunofluorescence to show spirochaetes Serum, antitreponemal IgM Fluorescent treponemal antibody |
| **Viral infections** | | | |
| *Herpes simplex* | Vesicles, often grouped, precede pustules Associated lethargy, irritability, etc. | Widespread | Smear – electron microscopy, direct immunofluorescence or Giemsa |
| *Varicella zoster* | Chicken pox lesions Severe if acquired less than 5 days before or up to 3 days after delivery | Widespread | As *Herpes simplex* |
| Cytomegalovirus | Variable rash, usually includes purpura and pustules ± hepatosplenomegaly | Widespread | Urine sediment – intranuclear inclusions Virus isolation from blood, urine, CSF, chorioretinitis, etc. |
| Candidiasis, disseminated | Like congenital candidiasis plus low birthweight, respiratory distress, etc. | | *Candida* cultures from blood, urine, CSF |

**Table 21.1** Continued

| Condition | Clinical features | Distribution | Pathology |
|---|---|---|---|
| **Erythrodermas** | | | |
| Harlequin fetus | Markedly thickened skin<br>Ectropion<br>Everted lips<br>Hair and nails dysplastic or absent | Generalized | Clinical appearance |
| Collodion baby | Encased in shiny membrane<br>Ectropion<br>Everted lips<br>Normal hair and nails<br>Membrane shed in 2–12 weeks, revealing underlying ichthyoses | Generalized | Clinical appearance |
| Ichthyoses | Various patterns of scaling with underlying erythema<br>Associated skeletal and neurological disorders in some types | Generalized | Clinical appearance<br>Histology<br>Histochemistry |
| Seborrhoeic dermatitis | Red scaly patches<br>No itch or impairment of general health | Maximal on scalp, face, intertriginous areas | Clinical appearance |

**Table 21.1** Continued

| Condition | Clinical features | Distribution | Pathology |
|---|---|---|---|
| Leiner's disease | Starts off like seborrhoeic dermatitis but becomes generalized, with diarrhoea, failure to thrive and Gram-negative bacterial and Candida infections | Generalized | Complement deficiences |
| Psoriasis | Circumscribed scaly plaques and patches<br>May become pustular | Scalp, trunk, napkin area<br>May become generalized | Histology |
| Pityriasis rubra pilaris | Follicular papules | Islands of spared skin<br>Marked palmo-plantar hyperkeratosis | Clinical appearance |
| Scalded skin syndrome | Rapidly spreading tender erythema<br>May blister | Anywhere<br>Crusting around mouth, eyes, umbilicus and perineum | Staphylococcus aureus in swab from skin site and nose |
| Drug eruption | Maculopapular erythema | Generalized | Drug exposure |
| Citrullinaemia | Red scaly skin with moist eroded patches and plaques | Particularly perioral and napkin area | Amino acid analysis in blood and urine |
| Biotin deficiency | Similar to zinc deficiency (see below)<br>Infections, ataxia, hypotonia | Generalized<br>Perioral dermatitis | Biochemistry<br>Multiple carboxylase deficiency<br>Organic aciduria |

**Table 21.1** Continued

| Condition | Clinical features | Distribution | Pathology |
|---|---|---|---|
| **Eruptions in the napkin area** | | | |
| Primary irritant napkin dermatitis | Erythema, erosions in severe cases, maximal on the convexities | | Clinical appearance |
| Perianal dermatitis | Erythema limited to perianal skin | | Clinical appearance |
| Intertrigo | Erythema only, in flexures | | Clinical appearance |
| Seborrhoeic dermatitis | Mainly flexures<br>Also scalp, face, axillae<br>Erythema with greasy yellowish scaling | | Clinical appearance |
| Psoriasis | Well-defined red scaly plaques<br>Often elsewhere, e.g. scalp, trunk | | Clinical appearance<br>May be family history |
| Candidiasis | Glazed erythema, raised scaly edge, outlying pustules<br>Mouth may be involved | | Candida on culture |
| Miliaria rubra | Papules and vesciles | | Cultures sterile |
| Bullous impetigo | Thin-walled blisters, fluid often cloudy | | Staphylococcus aureus on culture |
| Herpes simplex | Clustered umbilicated vesicles, later ulcers | | Viral smear and culture |

**Table 21.1** Continued

| Condition | Clinical features | Distribution | Pathology |
|---|---|---|---|
| Chronic bullous dermatosis of childhood | Bullae often in annular groups Spread beyond napkin area May occur on scalp, around mouth | | Linear IgA on biopsy |
| Zinc deficiency | Glazed erythema with marginal peeling Perioral dermatitis Failure to thrive, diarrhoea, later alopecia | | Low serum zinc |
| Congenital syphilis | Brownish-red macules, papules, occasionally bullae (see palms, soles and sometimes elsewhere) ± Hepatosplenomegaly, lymphadenopathy | | Syphilis serology |
| Histiocytosis X | Papules, often purpuric Other sites include scalp, behind ears ± Hepatosplenomegaly | | Histology |

**Dermatitis**

Neonatal skin tends to produce an eczematous response to irritants, and such reactions are often short-lived. The most common patterns of dermatitis are a seborrhoeic dermatitis, atopic dermatitis which usually begins outside the neonatal period, and primary irritant napkin dermatitis. If a bleeding diathesis and evidence of susceptibility to certain infections, especially pneumococci, is present, then the Wiskott-Aldrich syndrome should be considered. Some other disorders described elsewhere in this chapter in which dermatitis can be a feature include zinc deficiency, Leiner's disease and histiocytosis X.

## TREATMENT OF NEONATAL SKIN DISORDERS

When in doubt about diagnosis or treatment, the advice of a dermatologist should be sought.

The management of the following is discussed in Chapter 17 (perinatal infections):

- bullous impetigo
- staphylococcal scalded skin syndrome;
- herpes virus infections;
- candidiasis;
- septicaemias;
- congenital syphilis.

### Scabies

It is essential that not only the patient but all close bodily contacts are treated, whether they have symptoms or not.

None of the currently available treatments for scabies are licensed for use in neonates, but experience has shown that 0.5% Malathion and 5% Permethrin in aqueous or cream bases are both effective and well tolerated. The treatment should be applied all over the skin and under the edges of nails, and the skin not washed for 24 hours after treatment.

### Seborrhoeic dermatitis

As in adults, this condition is thought to be at least in part, due to lipophilic yeast colonization of the skin. Treatment with an imidazole/hydrocortisone combination twice daily is usually effective, and maintenance can be achieved with less frequent applications.

## BIBLIOGRAPHY

Harper, J. (1990) *Handbook of paediatric dermatology*, 2nd edn. Oxford: Butterworth-Heinemann.

Weston, W.L., Lane, A.T. and Morelli, J.G. (1996) *Colour textbook of paediatric dermatology*. St Louis, MO: Mosby, St Louis.

# Growth charts and gestational assessment

Growth charts
Gestational assessment

## GROWTH CHARTS

All preterm, low-birthweight, high-risk (see Chapter 5) or sick infants should have weight, length and head circumference measured and plotted on a growth chart at birth, at least weekly until discharge from hospital, and at all follow-up appointments (see Figs 22.1 and 22.2).

**Figs 22.1 and 22.2** Growth charts for girls (Fig. 22.1) and boys (Fig. 22.2). Centiles for head circumference and weight from 23 week's gestation to estimated date of delivery. Reproduced with kind permission from the Child Growth Foundation. Copies of the charts may be obtained from Harlow Printing, Maxwell Street, South Shields, NE33 4PU, UK.

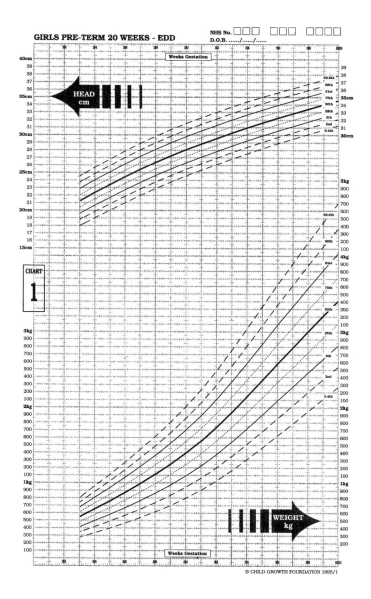

GIRLS PRE-TERM 20 WEEKS - EDD

NHS No.
D.O.B. ....../....../......

© CHILD GROWTH FOUNDATION 1995/1

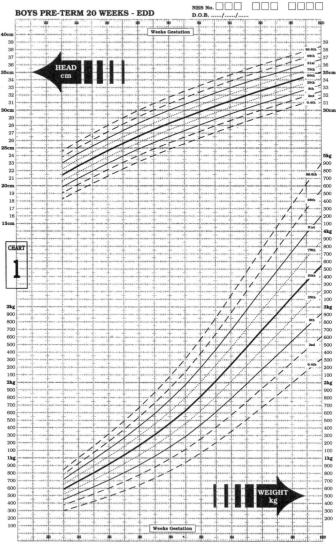

# GESTATIONAL ASSESSMENT

## Antenatal gestational assessment

The most reliable assessment of gestational age is obtained from:

1 first day of mother's last menstrual period if known (add 9 calendar months and 7 days to obtain estimated date of delivery);
2 repeated obstetric assessment of gestation before 16 weeks;
3 ultrasound assessment of fetal head size (biparietal diameter) before 20 weeks (error ± 7 days between 16 and 18 weeks).

If (1), (2) and (3) are in agreement, then the dates are almost certainly correct.

Obstetric assessment of gestational age beyond 28 weeks (including ultrasound scanning) carries a potential error of *at least* ± 2 weeks (see Chapter 1).

**Table 22.1** Assessment of gestational age: relationship between total score and gestational age (Narayanan *et al.*, 1981) (see Fig. 22.3)

| Score | Gestational age (weeks) |
|-------|-------------------------|
| 0 | ⩽ 27 |
| 1 | 28 |
| 2, 3 | 29 |
| 4 | 30 |
| 5 | 31 |
| 6 | 32 |
| 7 | 33 |
| 8 | 34 |
| 9 | 35 |
| 10 | 36 |
| 11 | 37 |
| 12 | 38 |
| 13 | 39 |
| 14 | ⩾ 40 |

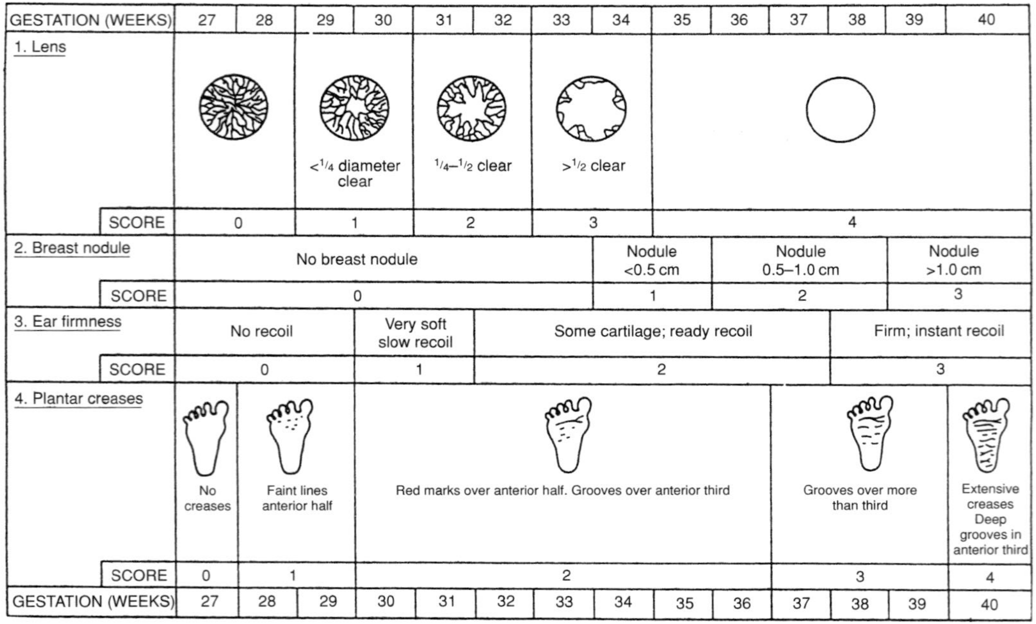

| GESTATION (WEEKS) | 27 | 28 | 29 | 30 | 31 | 32 | 33 | 34 | 35 | 36 | 37 | 38 | 39 | 40 |
|---|---|---|---|---|---|---|---|---|---|---|---|---|---|---|
| **1. Lens** | | | <¼ diameter clear | | ¼–½ clear | | >½ clear | | | | | | | |
| SCORE | 0 | | 1 | | 2 | | 3 | | | | 4 | | | |
| **2. Breast nodule** | No breast nodule | | | | | | | | Nodule <0.5 cm | | Nodule 0.5–1.0 cm | | Nodule >1.0 cm | |
| SCORE | 0 | | | | | | | | 1 | | 2 | | 3 | |
| **3. Ear firmness** | No recoil | | | Very soft slow recoil | | Some cartilage; ready recoil | | | | | Firm; instant recoil | | | |
| SCORE | 0 | | | 1 | | 2 | | | | | 3 | | | |
| **4. Plantar creases** | No creases | | Faint lines anterior half | | Red marks over anterior half. Grooves over anterior third | | | | | | Grooves over more than third | | Extensive creases Deep grooves in anterior third | |
| SCORE | 0 | | 1 | | 2 | | | | | | 3 | | 4 | |
| GESTATION (WEEKS) | 27 | 28 | 29 | 30 | 31 | 32 | 33 | 34 | 35 | 36 | 37 | 38 | 39 | 40 |

**Fig. 22.3** The assessment of gestational age (from Narayanan et al., (1981) *Indian J. Pediatr.* **18**, 715–20, reproduced with kind permission of the publisher).

## Postnatal gestational assessment

The accuracy of postnatal assessment of gestation is at best ± 10 days. Unless postnatal assessment suggests a 3- to 4-week discrepancy with the mother's dates, the latter should be accepted. Determination of gestational age may have serious medicolegal consequences, and the reasons for challenging the maternal dates should be clearly stated in the clinical notes. It is pointless to distress the mother by attempting to contradict her dates without firm reason.

External (superficial) criteria

| EXTERNAL SIGN | SCORE | | | | |
|---|---|---|---|---|---|
| | 0 | 1 | 2 | 3 | 4 |
| OEDEMA | Obvious oedema hands and feet. pitting over tibia | No obvious oedema hands and feet. pitting over tibia | No oedema | | |
| SKIN TEXTURE | Very thin gelatinous | Thin and smooth | Smooth, medium thickness. Rash or superficial peeling | Slight thickening. Superficial cracking and peeling esp hands and feet | Thick parchment-like: superficial or deep cracking |
| SKIN COLOUR (infant not crying) | Dark red | Uniformly pink | Pale pink: variable over body | Pale. Only pink over ears, lips, palms or soles | |
| SKIN OPACITY (trunk) | Numerous veins and venules clearly seen especially over abdomen | Veins and tributaries seen | A few large vessels clearly seen over abdomen | A few large vessels seen indistinctly over abdomen | No blood vessels seen |
| LANUGO (over back) | No lanugo | Abundant: long and thick over whole back | Hair thinning especially over lower back | Small amount of lanugo and bald areas | At least half of back devoid of lanugo |
| PLANTAR CREASES | No skin creases | Faint red marks over anterior half of sole | Definite red marks over more than anterior half: indentations over less than anterior third | Indentations over more than anterior third | Definite deep indentations over more than anterior third |
| NIPPLE FORMATION | Nipple barely visible: no areola | Nipple well defined, areola smooth and flat diameter <0.75 cm | Areola stippled, edge not raised: diameter <0.75 cm | Areola stippled, edge raised: diameter >0.75 cm | |
| BREAST SIZE | No breast tissue palpable | Breast tissue on one or both sides 0.5 cm diameter | Breast tissue both sides: one or both 0.5–1.0 cm | Breast tissue both sides: one or both 1.0 cm | |
| EAR FORM | Pinna flat and shapeless, little or no incurving or edge | Incurving of part of edge of pinna | Partial incurving whole of upper pinna | Well-defined incurving whole of upper pinna | |
| EAR FIRMNESS | Pinna soft, easily folded, no recoil | Pinna soft, easily folded, slow recoil | Cartilage to edge of pinna, but soft in places ready recoil | Pinna firm, cartilage to edge, instant recoil | |
| GENITALIA MALE | Neither testis in scrotum | At least one testis high in scrotum | At least one testis right down | | |
| FEMALE (with hips half abducted) | Labia majora widely separated. Labia minora protruding | Labia majora almost cover Labia minora | Labia majora completely cover labia minora | | |

| TOTAL SCORE | GESTATION AGE (WEEKS) |
|---|---|
| 5 | 26 |
| 9 | 27 |
| 13 | 28 |
| 16 | 29 |
| 20 | 30 |
| 24 | 31 |
| 27 | 32 |
| 31 | 33 |
| 34 | 34 |
| 38 | 35 |
| 42 | 36 |
| 45 | 37 |
| 49 | 38 |
| 53 | 39 |
| 56 | 40 |
| 60 | 41 |
| 63 | 42 |
| 67 | 43 |

(Abapted from Farr et al. *Develop. Med. Child Neurol.* 1966,8,507)

**Fig. 22.4** Dubowitz method of assessment of postnatal gestational age.

Neurological criteria

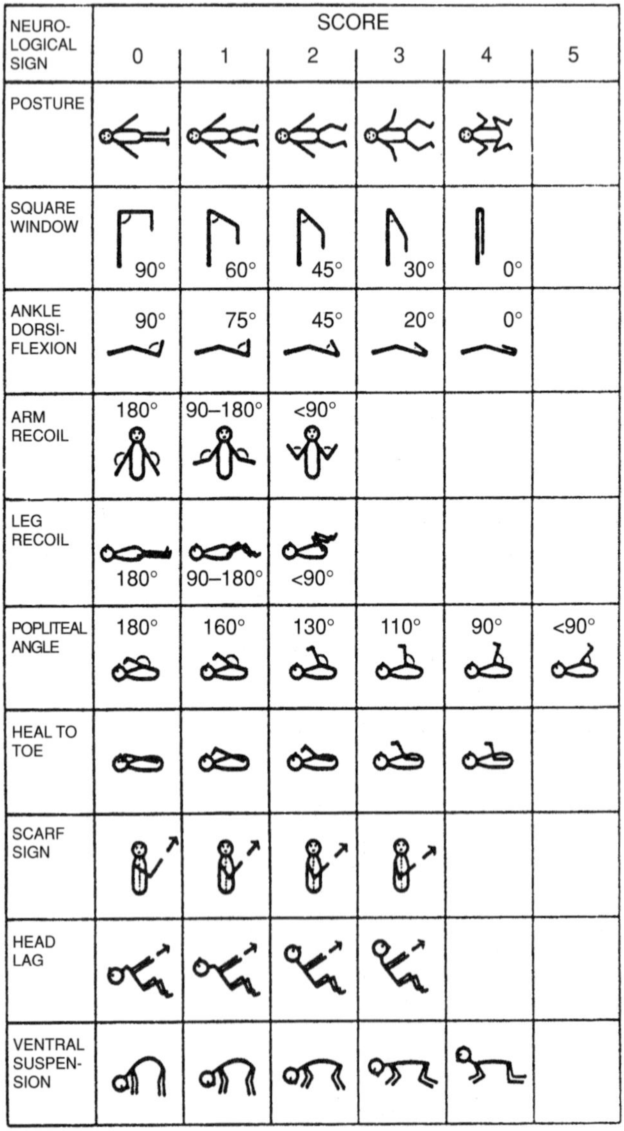

| NEURO-LOGICAL SIGN | SCORE | | | | | |
|---|---|---|---|---|---|---|
| | 0 | 1 | 2 | 3 | 4 | 5 |
| POSTURE | | | | | | |
| SQUARE WINDOW | 90° | 60° | 45° | 30° | 0° | |
| ANKLE DORSI-FLEXION | 90° | 75° | 45° | 20° | 0° | |
| ARM RECOIL | 180° | 90–180° | <90° | | | |
| LEG RECOIL | 180° | 90–180° | <90° | | | |
| POPLITEAL ANGLE | 180° | 160° | 130° | 110° | 90° | <90° |
| HEAL TO TOE | | | | | | |
| SCARF SIGN | | | | | | |
| HEAD LAG | | | | | | |
| VENTRAL SUSPEN-SION | | | | | | |

**Fig. 22.5** Clinical assessment of gestational age by the method of Dubowitz *et al.* (1970) *J. Pediatr.* **77**, 1. See notes for methods to be used.

## Some notes on techniques of assessment of neurological criteria

POSTURE: Observed with infant quiet and in supine position. Score 0: Arms and legs extended; 1: beginning of flexion of hips and knees, arms extended; 2: stronger flexion of legs, arms extended; 3: arms slightly flexed, legs flexed and abducted; 4: full flexion of arms and legs.

SQUARE WINDOW: The hand is flexed on the forearm between the thumb and index finger of the examiner. Enough pressure is applied to get as full a flexion as possible, and the angle between the hypothenar eminence and the ventral aspect of the forearm is measured and graded according to diagram. (Care is taken not to rotate the infant's wrist while doing this manoeuvre.)

ANKLE DORSIFLEXION: The foot is dorsiflexed onto the anterior aspect of the leg, with the examiner's thumb on the sole of the foot and other fingers behind the leg. Enough pressure is applied to get as full flexion as possible, and the angle between the dorsum of the foot and the anterior aspect of the leg is measured.

ARM RECOIL: With the infant in the supine position the forearms are first flexed for 5 seconds, then fully extended by pulling on the hands, and then released. The sign is fully positive if the arms return briskly to full flexion (Score 2). If the arms return to incomplete flexion or the response is sluggish it is graded as Score 1. If they remain extended or are only followed by random movements the score is 0.

LEG RECOIL: With the infant supine, the hips and knees are fully flexed for 5 seconds, then extended by traction on the feet, and released. A maximal response is one of full flexion of the hips and knees (Score 2). A partial flexion scores 1, and miminal or no movement scores 0.

POPLITEAL ANGLE: With the infant supine and his pelvis flat on the examining couch, the thigh is held in the knee-chest position by the examiner's left index finger and thumb supporting the knee. The leg is then extended by gentle pressure from the examiner's right index finger behind the ankle and the popliteal angle is measured.

HEEL TO EAR MANOEUVRE: With the baby supine, draw the baby's foot as near to the head as it will go without forcing it. Observe the distance between the foot and the head as well as the degree of extension at the knee. Grade according to diagram. Note that the knee is left free and may draw down alongside the abdomen.

SCARF SIGN: With the baby supin, take the infant's hand and try to put it around the neck and as far posteriorly as possible around the opposite shoulder. Assist this manoeuvre by lifting the elbow across the body. See how far the elbow will go across and grade according to illustrations. Score 0: Elbow reaches opposite axillary line; 1: Elbow between midline and opposite axillary line; 2: Elbow reaches midline; 3: Elbow will not reach midline.

HEAD LAG: With the baby lying supine, grasp the hands (or the arms if a very small infant) and pull him slowly towards the sitting position. Observe the position of the head in relation to the trunk and grade accordingly. In a small infant the head may initially be supported by one hand. Score 0: Complete lag; 1: Partial head control; 2: Able to maintain head in line with body; 3: Brings head anterior to body.

VENTRAL SUSPENSION: The infant is suspended in the prone position, with examiner's hand under the infant's chest (one hand in a small infant, two in a large infant). Observe the degree of extension of the back and the amount of flexion of the arms and legs. Also note the relation of the head to the trunk. Grade according to the diagrams.

If the score for an individual criterion differs on the two sides of the baby, take the mean. *For further details see Dubowitz et al., J. Pediat. 1970, 77, 1.*

Many methods have been described. Most of them rely upon physical characteristics (e.g. Narayanan *et al.*, 1981; Fig. 22.3, Table 22.1) or a combination of physical and neurological criteria (e.g. Dubowitz and Dubowitz, 1970; Figs 22.4 and 22.5).

Neurological assessment is least likely to be accurate in sick or asphyxiated babies who tolerate handling poorly. Assessment of gestations below 27 weeks is difficult. If the eyelids are fused, the gestation is probably < 26 weeks.

# Care of the family

## PHILOSOPHY OF CARE: CURRENT CHALLENGES

Parents are encouraged to be involved as much as possible in the practical and emotional care of their newborn children. The inevitable anxieties and need for support in this role are well recognized, even if the baby's medical needs are comparatively minor. However, expectations from parents are changing. Often they are now better informed, and have in pregnancy experienced greater responsibility for the well-being of their expected child through choices concerning screening tests, hand-held notes, etc. Preparation before birth for their child to be admitted to a neonatal unit because of a known congenital malformation or unavoidable premature delivery may be beneficial.

Staff working in neonatal units spend increasing amounts of time explaining treatment and procedures, and develop a relationship with the parents and families. Explanations may require frequent repetition, and this can place significant stress on staff.

Social changes have influenced the role of fathers. Practice has been long established that, except in exceptional circumstances, both parents should be counselled together regarding the illness or disability of their child. The tacit assumption of the role of the mother as prime carer may need revision. Fathers participate more openly in the nurturing and practical care of their babies in hospital, and resources for both parents to 'room in' prior to discharge are popular. Parents in disharmony pose other dilemmas, particularly if issues relating to the care of the child become enmeshed in their dispute. Unmarried fathers can apply to the courts to recognize their parental responsibility towards the baby, but in practice a narrow legalistic view at times of high tension is a last resort.

The informed consent of both parents to treatment is always desirable. If this is withheld by the parents (e.g. Jehovah's witnesses refusing blood products for their child), this 'Specific Issue' can be brought before the Family Court by Social Services Departments. Case law is still being established regarding the extent of parental rights to refuse treatment for their child.

## TEAMWORK FOR MUTUAL SUPPORT

Sensitive and supportive care of parents and other family members is enhanced when collaborative working is an established norm. The professional group is potentially large; obstetricians, fetal medicine specialists, paediatricians, paediatric surgeons and cardiologists all have a role in the medical care. Nurse practitioners and nursing staff, particularly key nurses, have the most exposure to parental concerns, and other professional staff may be involved, e.g. physiotherapists, social workers. This care needs a structure of formal and informal meetings. Prenatal meetings to discuss likely admissions to the neonatal unit should provide information about predicted family needs, both psychological (e.g. previous death of a child) and social (e.g. accommodation, fares to visit, other pressures). During the baby's admission this collaboration remains important. If ward rounds are not confidential to an individual baby and his or her parents, an arrangement must be made to discuss such issues in a place and/or time when confidentiality can be protected.

The sharing of feelings is a strength. Debriefing of all staff in any traumatic events, particularly the death of a baby, should be routine. This may require impromptu organization outside any regular staff support group meeting. Facilitating the parental role means repeated questions, struggling to avoid unhelpful inconsistency of explanation, and at times experiencing even more pressure than the technology and high occupancy rates of neonatal units already generate.

## CHILD PROTECTION ISSUES AND THE NEWBORN

Where there is evidence of poor care, previous risk factors and a lack of commitment to put the child's needs first, then clear child protection issues are present which bind all professionals, including the paediatrician, to adhere to their local procedures. A Child Protection Conference may be convened in these circumstances (or if other matters of serious concern come to light in hospital) in which social services will take a lead role. This may involve paediatricians confronted with angry, anxious parents who demand their baby's discharge. Usually, if there is serious cause for concern, the baby can be made subject to an Emergency Protection Order preventing discharge. In practice this is unusual.

The increased incidence of illegal drug dependence in pregnancy has resulted in a rise in the number of babies needing surveillance after delivery for the effects of drug withdrawal. The risk to the baby when a parent, or parents, are drug dependent needs multidisciplinary assessment, and increasingly this is seen as an antenatal priority. After birth, babies are, if possible, cared for with their mothers to enable assessment of parenting skills and commitment. Parents may be extremely reluctant to see a social worker, underestimating their duty to provide supportive services to parents under stress, and fearing removal of the child as routine.

## THE BABY WITH A CONGENITAL ABNORMALITY

Antenatal screening and ultrasound scanning result in many prospective parents facing the diagnosis of a fetal abnormality. Some will have refused a termination. All will have a vision, based to a certain extent on the ultrasound image of how their baby will look. Such preparation and anticipatory grieving for a normal baby does not necessarily lessen the impact of facing their child outside the womb with the expected illness or disability. This is a real grief, and parents need support and to share their feelings and feel that their baby is valued.

Parents who are unprepared are likely to express a different anger in their distress, which may be directed back at the messenger and the failure of antenatal screening to detect the problem, however illogical that feeling may be. Risk counselling can be mis-remembered or ill-understood. The parents need support for such difficult feelings and the accompanying guilt and blame.

Counselling by an appropriate professional should be offered. A social worker can also identify community support and resources in the longer term, as well as self-help organizations and potential financial support.

A child from 12 weeks of age, cared for by his or her parent at home, may qualify for Disabled Living Allowance with an Invalid Carer's Allowance for the carer. The criterion used is that the child's care needs are excessive compared to those of a child of similar age.

Parents whose baby has been transferred or born in a tertiary care unit may be far from home and very torn between the care of the sick baby and their other children. They may need 'permission' to spend time with the older children. Family finances are likely to be stretched to cover visiting costs. Except for those on Income Support, there are no DSS funds to cover these expenses. The unit's social worker can attempt to procure support from charities to provide assistance in such cases.

## DISCHARGE PLANNING

Parental anxiety levels prior to discharge can be very high, particularly if the baby has been critically ill and in the neonatal unit for some weeks. Many parents will only decorate their baby's bedroom in the week before discharge – a measure of their fears. A formal meeting, attended by hospital staff, members of the primary health care team and parents can be very helpful. General practitioners and health visitors who attend such meetings more quickly gain the confidence of the parents in the care of the baby, and the paediatrician is made aware of how parents remember counselling and events that occur during their baby's time on the unit. They should be encouraged to bring prepared questions and concerns thus ensuring that their needs are the central concern. Parents may appreciate a written summary, presented in language that they can understand, of their baby's past and present problems, and special needs and any continuing treatment.

## CARE OF THE FAMILY OF A DYING BABY

Recent changes in the practice and care of parents and siblings are well known. The *Guidelines for Professionals* (2nd edn) published by the Stillbirth and Neonatal Death Society are a sensitive and comprehensive basis for care. Local information about resources and choices is best incorporated in a written pamphlet for parents.

Providing appropriate and high-quality care is demanding; it needs undivided attention and time. Parents may wish to discuss taking their baby home to die, or in a quiet place away from the high technology. They may wish to take the baby home after death. Achieving the balance of reaching out to distraught parents and siblings in a way that is supportive but not prescriptive, while at the same time coping with the professional and personal issues such deaths evoke is difficult and emotionally draining. It may be even more difficult if, occasionally, parents choose to have little time and involvement with their baby, reject mementoes and the care offered, or display anger or conflict in their own relationships, rather than sharing their feelings. Staff debriefing, both formal and informal, is essential.

Many families value the offer of early and continued contact at home. This may be available from a medical social worker, chaplain, health visitor or counsellor attached to a GP surgery. Many families find a home visit from the hospital paediatrician (perhaps with their GP or midwife) very valuable as an alternative to a follow-up visit to the hospital. Such visits can be particularly valuable in raising important issues for the parents to follow through with the primary care team, and in ensuring continuity of care.

A follow-up appointment should be arranged before the parents leave the hospital. This should be either at their home or in a suitable private place (e.g. the consultant's office or a designated room for parent interviews). It should *not* be in an out-patient clinic or a busy ward office. This follow-up should be with the most senior doctor who has been involved in the care of the infant (almost always the consultant), together with a member of the nursing or junior medical staff. This meeting should take place 2 to 4 weeks after the death, and many families value a second visit a few weeks after this.

Parents who are experiencing the effects of bereavement of their baby have the same needs for choice as before. Their sense of blame, guilt and failure can be overwhelming, and each may grieve individually. Sharing feelings may be helpful, with the couple, family, a friend or a self-help group or counsellor. They will receive a lot of advice, and it is likely to be conflicting. They may seek advice about the involvement of their older children – breaking the news, attendance at the funeral, age-related explanations and meeting the needs of their care. Knowing, for example, that there are story-books suitable for small children can be useful. Often above all else in the later counselling sessions, when post-mortem reports are shared and future pregnancies discussed, parents explore their role as carers and the choices and decisions that they may have made.

## APPENDIX 23.1 NEONATAL DEATH CHECK-LIST

1 Death certificate completed, checking correct name of child. Parents given instructions on where, when and how to register the death.
2 Consent for autopsy obtained (and form signed if necessary).
3 Parents given leaflet explaining the possible types of funeral arrangements.
4 Appointment arranged for parents to see bereavement officer (to discuss the funeral arrangements).
5 Parents given information on the Stillbirth and Neonatal Death Society (see Appendix 2)
6 Inform obstetric team.
7 GP contacted by telephone and message also left for health visitor.
8 Neonatal discharge form completed. Record both parents' full names and the names of other children.
9 Medical social worker informed.
10 Summary letter written to GP.
11 Follow-up appointment arranged for parents.
12 Community paediatric department notified.
13 ? Whole body X-ray (if not already X-rayed).
14 ? Check chromosomes.
15 Photographs and other mementoes of baby, clothed in cot, to be offered to parents at follow-up visit if not available earlier or initially refused.
16 Notes sent to pathology department with request for autopsy.

## APPENDIX 23.2 USEFUL ADDRESSES OF SELF-HELP ORGANIZATIONS

**Contact:**  Contact a Family (CAF)
170 Tottenham Court Road
London W1P 0HA
Tel: 0171 383 3555
Fax: 0171 383 0259

Publishes a directory of specific conditions and support groups. Helpline holds up-to-date information.

**Contact:**  Stillbirth and Neonatal Death Society (SANDS)
28 Portland Place
London W1N 4DE
Tel: 0171 436 5881

Leaflets on bereavement, local befriender's group.

## BIBLIOGRAPHY

Stewart A. and Dent A. (1994) *At a loss*. London: Ballierè Tindall.

Stillbirth and Neonatal Death Society (1995) *Miscarriage, stillbirth and neonatal death guidelines for professionals*, 2nd edn. London: Stillbirth and Neonatal Death Society.

Ward, B. *et al.* (1996) *Good grief: exploring feelings, loss and death with under elevens (Vol. 1). With over elevens and adults (Vol. 2)*. London: Jessica Kingsley Publishers.

# 24

# Assessment of outcome and care after discharge

## MORTALITY

Conventionally three mortality rates are ascribed to the perinatal period:

- *the stillbirth rate (SBR)* – the number of babies stillborn after 24 completed weeks of gestation per 1000 infants delivered;

- *the neonatal mortality rate (NMR)* – the number of infants dying up to and including the 28th day after delivery per 1000 livebirths;
- *the perinatal mortality rate (PNMR)* – the number of stillbirths and first-week deaths per 1000 births.

The International Federation of Gynaecology and Obstetrics has recommended the reporting of figures for populations based on these figures, but that, to facilitate international comparisons, they should be reported additionally for populations excluding lethal malformations and babies under 1000 g (Table 24.1). Terms used to describe perinatal populations require strict definition (see Table 24.2). The UK definition of 'stillbirth' changed in 1993 with the reduction in the legal limit of viability from 28 to 24 weeks. In view of the increasing medium and long-term survival of very preterm babies, for the UK population the British Association of Perinatal Medicine has additionally recommended that deaths are reported in gestational age and birthweight bands based around the first 28 days, discharge from hospital and the end of the first postnatal year. However, these recommendations do not allow for case mix differences between high-risk referral units, which accept antenatal and

**Table 24.1** FIGO recommendations for the reporting of perinatal statistics

**Data collection**

- Collect numbers of births ≥ 500 g birthweight, early and late neonatal deaths and identify stillbirths and neonatal deaths with lethal malformations and birthweight < 1000 g

**Perinatal statistics**

- Lethal malformation rate per 1000 births
- Stillbirth rate per 1000 births
- Neonatal mortality rate per 1000 livebirths
- Perinatal mortality rate per 1000 births

**Excluding lethal malformations (include babies of < 1000 g birthweight)**

- SBR, NMR, PNMR

**Excluding births of < 1000 g birthweight (includes lethal malformations)**

- SBR, NMR, PNMR

**Excluding lethal malformations and births of < 1000 g birthweight**

- SBR, NMR, PNMR

postnatal referrals, and district units. Illness severity scores (e.g. the Clinical Risk Index for Babies (CRIB) score) have been developed to correct for these differences in order to facilitate comparison, but remain at present primarily research tools. Since 1993, all deaths after 20 weeks' gestation have been reported to the Confidential Enquiry into Stillbirths and Deaths in Infancy (CESDI). This has provided regular audit of the causes of perinatal death.

The perinatal mortality in the UK in 1993 was 7.8 per 1000 births, 42% of which were neonatal deaths. The main causes of neonatal death were prematurity (49%), congenital malformation (24%), asphyxia/hypoxia or trauma (11%) and infection (7%).

**Table 24.2** Perinatal definitions

| | |
|---|---|
| **Livebirth:** | Baby with signs of life observed after complete expulsion from the mother, irrespective of the duration of pregnancy (signs of life include breathing, heart beat, cord pulsation or voluntary movement) |
| **Stillbirth:** (or late fetal death) | Fetal death prior to complete delivery of a baby born after the 24th week of pregnancy (168 days after the first day of the last menstrual period (LMP)) |
| **Abortion:** | A conceptus born without signs of life before the end of the 24th week of pregnancy (< 168 days from LMP) |
| **Birthweight:** | The first weight of the fetus or newborn infant obtained after birth (preferably within the first hour) |
| **Gestational age:** | The duration of gestation measured from the first day of the LMP and expressed in complete weeks or days |
| **Preterm:** | < 37 completed weeks (< 259 days) |
| **Term:** | From 37 to < 42 completed weeks of gestation (259–293 days) |
| **Post-term:** | 42 completed weeks or more (> 293 days) |
| **The neonatal period:** | First 28 days after delivery |
| **Lethal congenital malformation:** | Death primarily due to congenital malformation (WHO *International Classification of Diseases*, Chapter XIV) |

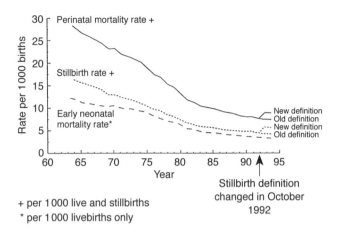

**Fig. 24.1** Perinatal Death Rate in England, Wales and Northern Ireland, 1960–1994. From *Confidential Enquiry into Stillbirths and Deaths in Infancy*, 3rd Report, 1995. Crown copyright is reproduced with the permission of the Controller of HMSO.

Trends in perinatal mortality rates and in the causes of perinatal death in the UK over the last 30 years are shown in Figs 24.1 and 24.2. Post-neonatal mortality rates have fallen since 1993 following the 'Back to Sleep' campaign of risk reduction for sudden infant death syndrome. Gestation-based survival figures over the past 5 years for the Bristol Neonatal Service are shown in Fig. 24.3. At or over 30 weeks' gestation, survival approximates 100% in the absence of malformation.

## MORBIDITY

### Disability and perinatal care

Impairment and disability are not uncommon among survivors of neonatal intensive care. However, two points should be stressed:

- *the vast majority of children who receive neonatal intensive care have a normal outcome;*

- *many of the subsequent disabilities in such children may not be directly related to events that occur in the perinatal and neonatal periods.*

None the less, and because of the high-risk nature of this population, most neonatal services have a follow-up programme designed to identify impairment early, in order to institute appropriate intervention, where possible, and to counsel and support parents.

Morbidity may be described in terms of impairments or conditions found as the child develops, or in terms of the degree of disability produced (Table 24.3). As there have been no standard definitions of disability in the past, guidelines have been developed which define severe disabilities at 2 years in preterm children to facilitate comparisons (*Disability and Perinatal Care: Measurement of Health Status at Two Years. Report of Two Working Groups.* National Perinatal Epidemiology Unit/Oxford Health Authority, 1994). The aim of these recommendations is to identify the group of children who are unlikely to function independently in the future, and thus represent the poor outcomes in premature populations.

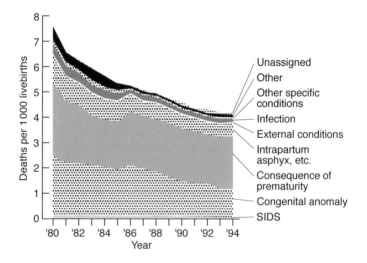

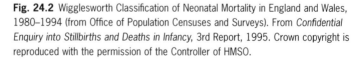

**Fig. 24.2** Wigglesworth Classification of Neonatal Mortality in England and Wales, 1980–1994 (from Office of Population Censuses and Surveys). From *Confidential Enquiry into Stillbirths and Deaths in Infancy*, 3rd Report, 1995. Crown copyright is reproduced with the permission of the Controller of HMSO.

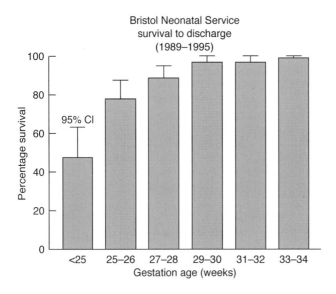

**Fig. 24.3** Gestation-based survival 1989–1995 for Bristol Neonatal Service.

**Table 24.3** WHO International Classification of Impairments, Disabilities and Handicap (1980–207)

| | |
|---|---|
| **Impairment:** | Any loss or abnormality of psychological or anatomical structure or function |
| **Disability:** | Any restriction or lack (resulting from an impairment) of ability to perform an activity in the manner or within the range considered normal for a human being |
| **Handicap:** | A disadvantage for a given individual, resulting from an impairment or disability that limits or prevents the fulfilment of a role that is normal (depending on age, sex, social and cultural factors) for that individual |

## Morbidity among preterm children

The frequency with which disabling conditions are found in this group rises with increasing prematurity (Fig. 24.4). The commonest

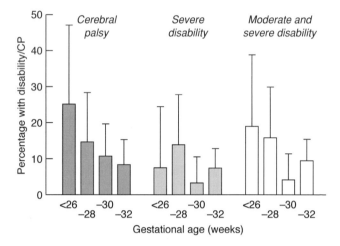

**Fig. 24.4** Frequency of disabilities at differing gestational ages among survivors studied in the Avon Premature Infant Project births 1990–1993.

impairments are cerebral palsy, developmental delay, visual impairment secondary to retinopathy of prematurity (ROP), and sensorineural hearing loss. However, many of the children with these conditions, are not severely disabled and attend normal school; only 4–6% of babies of less than 33 weeks' gestation have severe disability. In the Northern Region there is evidence that this proportion has not changed over the past 25 years. In populations of very preterm children followed up to teenage years most children are performing normally, but there is a group of children who have significant learning difficulties, motor problems and behavioural problems. The relationship of these longer-term impairments to perinatal events is unclear.

**Cerebral palsy** Occurs in about 8% of surviving children under 32 weeks' gestation, the frequency rising with decreasing gestation (Fig. 24.4). Although spastic diplegia is commonly associated with preterm birth, with increasing survival of extremely preterm infants hemiplegia and quadriplegia are now equally common. Periventricular brain injuries, detected by serial cerebral ultrasound scanning, are the best predictors of this, although in our very preterm population only 50% of the children with cerebral palsy are identified in this way.

**Developmental delay** Isolated severe developmental problems are rarely encountered in preterm children, such problems usually being found in association with other disabilities. Although, when compared to term babies, developmental scores may be slightly lower in non-disabled preterm children, some of this disadvantage relates to socio-economic factors, which are themselves associated with prematurity.

**Hearing loss** Approximately 4% of Avon children aged < 32 weeks have sensorineural hearing loss, although the reasons for this are obscure. Hearing screening is thus recommended for this population (see below).

**Visual impairment** ROP develops in the smallest and least mature children, but severe impairment is rare (1% of Avon children aged < 30 weeks). Recent advances in the treatment of this condition mean that severe visual impairment is potentially preventable by early screening and treatment (see Chapter 20).

**Other impairments** Post-haemorrhagic hydrocephalus may follow intraventricular haemorrhage and require treatment or drainage (see Chapter 12). Chronic lung disease requires special consideration – about 1–2% of ventilated very preterm babies will be discharged home on oxygen for up to several months (see below).

## Small-for-gestational-age infants

The outcome for this group is currently unclear. The presence of an abnormality or congenital infection usually confers a poor outcome. Many studies based on children without such problems, but born with weight below the 10th or 3rd percentiles for gestational age, have yielded conflicting results. Generally the risk of severe disability relates to the degree of prematurity, rather than the fetal growth retardation. No cognitive disability has been consistently associated with SGA babies. Increasing expertise in fetal assessment has led to an increase in survival for very growth-retarded fetuses (> 3SD below mean birthweight for gestation). It is too early to determine whether the same outcomes apply to this group, or whether particular children are at developmental risk, e.g. those with demonstrable hypoxia.

## Neonatal encephalopathy

Hypoxic-ischaemic encephalopathy may be graded as mild, moderate or severe (see Chapter 12). Outcome is best defined by the worst grade of encephalopathy encountered. Children with mild encephalopathy have a normal outcome in most studies. For those with severe encephalopathy, most die in the neonatal period or have severe disability at follow-up. For the intermediate moderate group, most children have no major deficit, and about 15–20% die or develop severe disability. Factors which are useful in predicting poor outcome are difficulty in controlling seizures, delay in establishing sucking feeds and CT abnormalities detected in the second postnatal week. The commonest adverse outcome is a spastic quadriplegia with athetoid features and cognitive impairment. Central visual impairment and hearing loss are also frequently found.

## Other at-risk groups

Small numbers of children develop impairments following other perinatal problems, such as severe hypoglycaemia, surgically corrected abnormalities or meningitis. Close attention to follow-up and early detection of impairment are equally important for these groups.

## FOLLOW-UP AFTER NEONATAL CARE

Follow-up of babies who have had perinatal problems and are at high risk of neurodevelopmental impairments is important for the following reasons:

- to give appropriate advice and counselling;
- to provide continuity of care and advice to parents;
- to detect and institute treatment for medical and neurodevelopmental problems;
- to provide ongoing care for specific problems (dislocated hips, anomalies, etc.).

This service must complement and not duplicate the community care provided by the primary care team. Ideally, follow-up clinics should be organized at the community level, but constraints of service provision rarely make it possible to hold clinics in local health centres. Many neonatal services have developed specialist outreach nursing support to provide home-based support for parents over the first few weeks after discharge.

## Infants requiring special follow-up

- Gestation < 32 weeks.
- Birthweight < 1500 g for gestation.
- Babies with moderate or severe encephalopathy (see Chapter 12).
- Babies who have needed intensive care (see Chapter 5).
- Babies with recognized congenital anomalies.
- Babies with specific neonatal problems (e.g. congenital infection, heart murmur, dislocatable hips, urinary tract infection).

Within these groups special attention must be paid to the follow-up of children with recognized perinatal complications which have prognostic implications (e.g. cerebral ultrasound abnormality (see Chapter 12), chronic lung disease (see below), retinopathy, etc.). Where appropriate, early referral to the relevant district paediatric specialty for assessment and care of specific disorders is essential. This referral can often be made before discharge, obviating the need to duplicate out-patient appointments.

## The follow-up appointment (see Table 24.4)

### Parents

The consultation is an opportunity for parents to discuss their specific concerns and time should be allocated for this. Taking home a child who has received intensive care is a daunting prospect for many parents, who may find difficulty in expressing their anxieties. It is important to be positive with respect to their child's progress and not deliberately overcautious.

### Frequency of appointments

The frequency of follow-up visits is determined by the support needed by each family. Standard ages allow for familiarity with developmental patterns at each age. Visits should start within 2–4 weeks of discharge from hospital and subsequently, if all is well, children are seen at 4, 8, 12 and 24 months *post-term*, although earlier discharge is usual for those at low risk of long-term sequelae. There should be a clear route of referral to community disability teams when a disability is identified. Formal disability assessment at

**Table 24.4** Follow-up checklist

---

- What are the parental concerns?
- Recent illness/problems
- Plot growth on charts
- Are diet and vitamin supplements still required?
- Medication
- Immunizations
- Development
- Physical examination, especially:
  - Murmurs
  - Vision
  - Hearing
  - Neurology
  - Hips
- Record information given to parents
- Next visit – is it really necessary? When? Who to see?

---

2 years using published guidelines is recommended for audit purposes (National Perinatal Epidemiology Unit/Oxford Health Authority, 1994).

### Correcting for prematurity
Calculation of age from expected date of delivery is essential for the assessment of growth and development in infancy and early childhood.

### Growth
Growth must be assessed at each visit, and weight, length and OFC plotted on percentile charts.

### Developmental assessment
At each visit developmental progress should be assessed. Formal estimation of DQ is time-consuming and unnecessary unless research data are being collected. A simple screening test such as the Denver Developmental Screening Test or the Schedule of Growing Skills may be of value. This should be combined with sensory assessment (see below).

### Visual testing
All babies of < 32 weeks' gestation or < 1500 g birthweight should have an ophthalmic assessment before discharge from the NICU as a screen for retinopathy (see Chapter 20). Visual assessment is part of

routine follow-up and an important component of the assessment of fine motor development.

Any child with a recognizable eye abnormality or a squint at follow-up should be referred for further assessment. Visual acuity may be assessed from 6–7 months using visual following or reaching for a 1-mm cake decoration ('hundreds and thousands') at 60 cm.

### Hearing

All children at high risk for hearing impairment should be identified to the district audiology services. Many hospitals have established screening tests while the child is an in-patient using oto-acoustic emissions or evoked responses. Indications for referral (high-risk) are:

- < 32 weeks' gestation;
- moderate/severe encephalopathy;
- exchange transfusion for hyperbilirubinaemia;
- meningitis;
- cranio-facial malformations or family history of deafness.

Hearing is assessed at each clinic visit. Stilling to sound is observed at 6 weeks. Distraction tests become most reliable after 6 months. In a quiet room the infant is seated upon his or her mother's lap whilst the examiner attracts the child's attention visually. An assistant then rolls a Manchester rattle gently on each side of the infant. At 6 months children turn to sounds presented level with each ear at a distance of 45 cm, and at 9 months they turn to sounds presented at 1 m.

### Physical examination

This involves a general physical examination, including examination for signs of persisting patent arterial duct, sequelae of intensive care and neurological abnormality. We have found a standardized neurological assessment to be useful. Children who have equivocal or abnormal neurological signs should be referred early for specialist assessment and intervention as appropriate.

### Attendance at clinic

Parents often find it difficult to attend the clinic for many reasons, such as change of address, lack of transport or illness. Consideration should be given to providing special assistance if possible for those with particular problems. The clinic may be less appealing if there is a poorly organized appointments system, a long wait, no play area for siblings, or no literature is available.

For non-attenders always arrange a further appointment (usually in 2–4 weeks). Further non-attendance should be followed up with a request for the GP or health visitor to visit the family. If families are persistent non-attenders with problems that merit follow-up, ensure that the GP is fully informed of the situation.

## Immunization

The current Department of Health recommendations are that all children should receive full immunization unless there are specific contraindications. For preterm babies this should start at 2 months of age *uncorrected for prematurity.* For some babies this will mean starting immunization before discharge from hospital. Premature babies form a special risk group who should be immunized as a matter of priority. Immunization with live oral polio vaccine is delayed until the day of discharge from hospital.

A child with neurological abnormality during the neonatal period is considered to have a problem history. It is our policy to offer pertussis immunization to all babies who have received intensive care, including those with intraventricular haemorrhage, periventricular leucomalacia and hydrocephalus. It is essential for babies who have bronchopulmonary dysplasia.

## The infant with chronic lung disease

Infants with chronic lung disease (CLD) or bronchopulmonary dysplasia (BPD) (see Chapter 10) may encounter a number of potential problems following their discharge from the neonatal unit. In addition, CLD is more common in extremely preterm infants, and thus follow-up must include consideration of the neurodevelopmental outcomes discussed above.

Problems specific to children with CLD include:

- long-term respiratory morbidity and mortality;
- recurrent respiratory infections;
- cardiovascular sequelae of hypoxaemia;
- growth and nutrition problems.

Infants who are on supplemental oxygen treatment at home should have their oxygen status assessed at every clinic visit and following any change in their oxygen prescription. This should include an assessment of $SaO_2$ during wakefulness, sleep and feeding.

It is our practice to perform 24-hour studies in the infant's home prior to a clinic visit.

Parents should be given clear instructions on what to do in the event of a clinical exacerbation of the infant's respiratory disease:

- whom to contact;
- when to increase oxygen flow;
- what to do with medication (e.g. increase inhaled budesonide, diuretic therapy);
- when to start antibiotics;
- when they should expect immediate readmission to hospital.

*Infants with BPD must be fully immunized according to the standard protocol, unless there is a specific contraindication. It is not our practice to give influenza vaccine to these infants.*

*At each clinic visit:*

- *assess growth and nutrition* – dietetic assessment of intake, and supplements; gastro-oesophageal reflux is common – review investigations and treatment;
- *respiratory assessment* – including saturation trace; consider referral to ENT if upper airway problems are present;
- *cardiovascular examination* – look for signs of pulmonary hypertension; consider ECG, review by cardiologist;
- *neurodevelopmental assessment* (see above);
- *review drugs and oxygen treatment* – arrange repeat $SaO_2$ monitoring if oxygen prescription is changed.

### When to discontinue oxygen therapy

Low-flow oxygen is gradually reduced, depending on assessment and progress. Once the infant requires 50–100 mL/min $O_2$ and $SaO_2$ has been demonstrated to be satisfactory (92–94%), consideration can be given to discontinuing oxygen for periods of the day. Our practice is to increase gradually the number of hours each day off $O_2$, and initially to continue $O_2$ during sleep. Oxygen may need to be recommenced, especially during intercurrent viral respiratory infections. Thus, when the infant no longer requires oxygen, the $O_2$ delivery system should be left with the parents for a further 3–6 months.

Many children with BPD have persistent abnormalities of pulmonary function. These include increased residual volumes and evidence of airway reactivity, often requiring bronchodilator therapy.

Consideration should be given to long-term follow-up by a paediatric pulmonologist.

## AUDIT

The collection of standardized perinatal mortality or morbidity data facilitates local and international comparisons, and is a good example of prospective clinical audit. Audit provides a mechanism whereby the efficacy of clinical care can be assessed against standards, which may be set externally, by professional organizations or management, or internally, after a review of published data. It facilitates assessment of and quality assurance in patient care, enhances medical education by promoting discussion of practice and the development of evidence-based protocols or guidelines. Although sometimes referred to as medical audit, neonatal care involves many professionals other than doctors. Clinical audit should involve all professional groups in a multidisciplinary process.

Three aspects of clinical care may be addressed:

- *structure* – the quantity and type of resources available;
- *process* – what is done to the patient or by the staff;
- *outcome* – the result of clinical intervention.

The audit process has several important components:

- observation of practice;
- setting of standards of practice;
- comparison of practice against standard;
- implementation of changes based upon this comparison;
- re-observation of practice following changes;
- feedback of information to staff.

Sometimes referred to as the audit cycle, this process has the capacity for continually updating and maintaining standards of practice. To facilitate audit, several professional publications have set standards or suggested methodology which may be used in the audit process (see Table 24.5).

Each hospital should develop its own series of guidelines for the process of neonatal care, and update them regularly following discussion and audit, as appropriate.

**Table 24.5** Examples of professional guidelines and audit tools (full references can be found in bibliography)

**Structure**

- Standards for Hospitals providing Neonatal Intensive Care (British Association of Perinatal Medicine, 1996)
- Neonatal Resuscitation (British Paediatric Association, 1993)

**Process**

- Categories of babies receiving neonatal care (British Paediatric Association/ NNA, 1992)
- Audit of clinical notekeeping (British Paediatric Association, 1989)
- Surfactant (British Association of Perinatal Medicine, 1994)
- Respiratory distress syndrome (Soll et al., 1993)
- Use of antenatal steriods (Crowley et al., 1990)
- Resuscitation of babies at birth (RCPCH/RCOG, 1997)

**Outcome**

- Clinical Risk Index for Babies (CRIB) (Scottish Consultants' Collaborative Group, 1995)
- Minimal dataset for neonatal intesive care (British Association of Perinatal Medicine, 1997)
- Disability and perinatal care: measurement of health status at 2 years (NPEU, 1994)

# BIBLIOGRAPHY

Amiel Tison, C. and Stewart, A. *Video: Neurological examination in childhood*. London, UCL.

British Association of Perinatal Medicine and Neonatal Nurses Association (1992) *Categories of babies receiving neonatal care. Report of the Working Group of the British Association of Perinatal Medicine and Neonatal Nurses Association. Arch. Dis. Child.* **67**, 868–9.

British Association of Perinatal Medicine (1994) *The use of exogenous surfactant in newborn infants. Report of a British Association of Perinatal Medicine Working Party*. London: British Association of Perinatal Medicine.

British Association of Perinatal Medicine (1996) *Standards for hospitals providing neonatal intensive care*. London: British Association of Perinatal Medicine.

British Association of Perinatal Medicine (1997) *Report of a Working Party. Minimal dataset for neonatal intensive care.* London: British Association of Perinatal Medicine.

British Paediatric Association (1989) *Clinical audit in paediatrics.* London: British Paediatric Association.

British Paediatric Association (1993) *Neonatal resuscitation. Report of a BPA Working Party.* London: British Paediatric Association.

Crowley, P., Chalmers, I. and Keirse, M.J.N.C. (1990) The effects of corticosteroid administration before preterm delivery: an overview of the evidence from controlled trials. *Br. J. Obstet. Gynaecol.* **97**, 11–25.

Department of Health and Social Services (1992) *Immunisation against infectious disease. Report of the Joint Committee on Vaccination and Immunisation.* London: HMSO.

Dunn, P.M. and McThwaine, G. (eds) (1996) *Perinatal audit.* Carnforth: Parthenon Publishing Group and European Association of Perinatal Medicine.

Egan, D.F., Illingworth, R.S. and MacKeith, R.C. (1969) *Developmental screening 0–5 years.* London: William Heinemann Medical Books Ltd.

Frankenberg, W.K. (1991) *Denver Developmental Screening Test-II.* Denver, CO: Denver Developmental Materials Inc.

National Perinatal Epidemiology Unit/Oxford Health Authority (1994) *Disability and perinatal care: measurement of health status at two years. Report of Two Working Groups.* Oxford National Perinatal Epidemiology Unit.

Royal College of Paediatrics and Child Health (1997) *Resuscitation of newborn babies at birth. Report of a Multidisciplinary working party.* London: B.M.J. Publishing Group.

*Schedule of Growing Skills.* Windsor: NFER Nelson Publishing Co.

Scottish Neonatal Consultants Collaborative Group and International Neonatal Network (1995) CRIB, mortality and impairment after neonatal intensive care. *Lancet* **345**, 1020–22.

Soll, R.F. and McQueen, M.C. (1992) Respiratory distress syndrome. In Sinclair, J.C. and Bracken, M.B. (eds), *Effective care of the newborn infant.* Oxford: Oxford University Press, 325–55.

# 25

# Medical ethics and the severely malformed or handicapped infant

General principles
Guidelines on decisions to withhold or withdraw support

## GENERAL PRINCIPLES

A doctor has two main duties: to act in the interest of the patient and to preserve life and health. When these two duties are in conflict, they give rise to ethical dilemmas of great complexity and difficulty, especially in relation to infants with severe malformation, those with irreversible brain damage, and those of extreme prematurity. Modern medicine provides the means to prevent death in circumstances in which prolonged life may not be considered to be in the interests of the patient. While adults in sound mind may exercise their right to refuse life-saving treatment, such a right does not exist in law for children and newborn infants. In practice in the UK (and in many other countries) doctors and parents have always used their discretion, and the law has been content to permit this provided that no direct action is taken to end life. In recent years, however, concerned pressure groups have sought to deny this discretion and hence deprive infants of the 'right to die' from natural causes. Despite this, attempts to invoke the strictest interpretation of the law to prosecute doctors for murder in such circumstances have been unsuccessful, and society has indicated its wish to leave these difficult decisions in the hands of the parents and their medical advisers as long as they act responsibly and within the consensus view of what is currently considered acceptable. The view of society in this respect is not immutable, but evolves in response to changing attitudes and conditions, such as advances in medical care.

It has been suggested that the law should be modified to protect doctors involved in the withholding or withdrawing of medical care from the severely malformed or handicapped infant. The problem is that there are so many variables between and within each individual case that such a law would be most difficult to frame and interpret. Probably it is preferable for the doctor to continue to strive to serve the interests of the patients in these ethical dilemmas, knowing at the same time that he or she may be called upon to defend and justify these actions before the law.

Another suggestion that has been made is that decisions in individual cases should be decided by ethical committees. However, experience has shown that such committees tend to be ponderous and insensitive, and that they also tend to err on the side of continued life-support. The wider discussion and even publicity that may result is also capable of causing great distress to the already grief-stricken family. While parents and doctors may wish to seek advice from a variety of sources, their final and usually agonizing decision is best reached after private discussions.

## GUIDELINES ON DECISIONS TO WITHHOLD OR WITHDRAW SUPPORT

The following guidelines are suggested.

- Advice and decisions on the withholding (or withdrawal) of medical/surgical measures required to preserve life should be made by the most senior doctor available, usually the consultant.
- In an emergency, as at resuscitation in the delivery room, a junior doctor must exercise clinical judgement. If in any doubt, resuscitation care should be given until further investigations can be made and the opinion of a senior doctor sought.

- Advice and decisions on the withholding of medical care should be based on careful clinical examination, supplemented by appropriate special investigations. The findings should always be carefully documented. Photographs are an important part of the record.
- Whenever possible, a second opinion should be sought from another senior doctor. This is particularly desirable when the patient's medical problem would normally necessitate assistance from another discipline (e.g. spina bifida and neurosurgery).
- The doctor responsible for the patient would also be wise always to discuss his or her thoughts on the management options with other members of the medical and nursing team, and in turn to listen to their views. They, too, are involved in the outcome of any ethical decision, even though it is the leader of the team who takes final responsibility for the decision.
- The parents should be as fully informed as possible of their baby's condition and prognosis, and also of the management options. They should be encouraged to seek advice, if they so wish, from others such as their general practitioner, and should always have the opportunity to talk together alone before reaching a decision. In many instances the doctor will not be seeking a decision, but rather will be trying as sensitively as possible to gain insight into the parents' wishes should some life-threatening event arise. A skilful and sensitive doctor who is prepared to spend time with the parents can acquire this knowledge while sparing them much avoidable distress and feelings of guilt (see Chapter 23).
- In reaching a decision to withhold medical care, both doctor and parents should have only one aim in mind – *to act in the interests of the baby*. While the interests of the family cannot be completely discounted, those of society should be. In obtaining the considered views of the parents, the doctor should convince himself or herself that their decision is a loving one in their child's interest, as well as being medically justifiable.
- Doctors giving advice in this area of clinical dilemmas must be careful not to impose their own cultural and religious prejudices on those whose beliefs and practices may be different from their own, bearing in mind the legal requirements.
- The withholding of medical or surgical care, which may be partial or complete according to the circumstances, does not of course imply withdrawal of love or of the routine non-medical care to which all human beings are entitled. Parents should be

encouraged to maintain close contact with their child. They will of course need continuing support.

- The pain and distress of a severely malformed or handicapped infant may be such that parents may ask their doctor to take active steps to end the child's life. Such appeals should be sympathetically but firmly resisted. Neither medical ethics nor the law permit doctors to undertake actions which have the intention of shortening the life of or killing the patient, however much this may appear to be in his or her interest. On the other hand, no patient should be allowed to suffer unnecessarily, and in the circumstances under discussion it would be wrong to withhold drugs capable of relieving pain or distress (even though they may also on occasion shorten life).

- The reasons for the decision to withhold care and the outcome of discussions with the parents should be carefully documented. The clinical progress should be regularly annotated, as should the reasons for giving drugs such as analgesics or sedatives.

- In the event of the baby's death, permission should be sought from the parents for a post-mortem examination. The results of the latter are required not only to confirm that the decision to withhold treatment was correct, but also to enable optimal advice to be given to the parents concerning the likely outcome of future pregnancies.

Most maternity hospitals with Neonatal Units hold regular peri-natal mortality conferences, attended by all members of the health-care team, at which the individual circumstances of all infants dying in the perinatal period are presented and discussed in confidence. It is particularly important that cases involving ethical dilemmas and decisions should be fully and frankly discussed at such meetings.

The personal qualities required by doctors who help parents to reach acceptable decisions with regard to these ethical dilemmas are compassion, humility and courage. Doctors must be prepared to accept that they will occasionally make mistakes, and they must be prepared to live with their doubts. As the great physician William Osler wrote: 'Errors of judgement must occur in an art which consists largely of balancing probabilities'. Thus it is inevitable that the doctor will wonder and question from time to time the correctness of some of the decisions he or she has made. These doubts should be shared with his or her colleagues.

The parents of a malformed infant are likely to suffer shock, denial, guilt and anger as well as sadness – feelings that may be made stronger in the knowledge that a decision has been made to withhold or withdraw medical care. In these circumstances, the doctor has therefore, an even greater responsibility than usual to comfort and support the parents and to counsel them during the following weeks and months.

Each Neonatal Unit should have a written policy covering these issues and, in establishing this policy, it may be helpful to involve a Consultant in Medical Ethics.

## BIBLIOGRAPHY

Berseth, C.L. (1983) A neonatologist looks at the baby Doe rule: ethical decisions by edict. *Pediatrics* **72**, 428.

British Medical Association (1983) *Handbook of medical ethics.* London: BMJ Publishing. Modified as *B.M.J.* **2** 1593 (Medical ethics: severely malformed infants).

Campbell, A.G.M. (1982) Which infants should not receive intensive care? *Arch. Dis. Child.* **75**, 569.

Campbell, A.G.M. (1983) The right to be allowed to die. *J. Med. Ethics*, **9**, 136–40.

Campbell, A.V., Charlesworth, M., Gillett, G. and Jones, D.G. (1997) *Medical ethics.* Oxford: Oxford University Press.

Duff, R.S. and Campbell, A.G.M. (1973) Moral and ethical dilemmas in the special care nursery. *N. Engl. J. Med.* **289**, 890.

Dunn, P.M. (1993) Appropriate care of the newborn: ethical dilemmas. *J. Med. Ethics* **19**, 82–4.

Illingworth, R.S. (1974) Some ethical problems in paediatrics. In Apley, J. (ed.), *Modern trends in paediatrics.* London: Butterworths, 329–57.

Lorber, J. and Salfield, S.A.W. (1981) Results of selective treatment of spina bifida cystica. *Arch. Dis. Child.* **56**, 822.

Rennie, J.M. (1996) Perinatal management at the lower margin of viability. *Arch. Dis. Child.* **74**, F214–F218.

Versluys, Z. and de Leauw, R. (1995) A Dutch report on the ethics of neonatal care. *J. Med. Ethics* **21**, 14–16.

Weir, R. (1994) *Selective non-treatment of handicapped newborns.* Oxford: Oxford University Press.

Working Party (1975) Report of a Working Party. Ethics of selective treatment of spina bifida. *Lancet* **i**, 85.

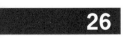

# 26

# Perinatal pathology

## THE PURPOSE OF PERINATAL POST-MORTEM EXAMINATION

The perinatal post-mortem seeks to explain why a baby died, and to predict risks for future pregnancies. It is both a retrospective and a prospective examination and it differs fundamentally from adult necropsy. The objectives of the examination are as follows.

### (1) To determine the cause of death
In perinatal medicine there is often no single cause of death, but a sequence of causes starting in pregnancy and compounded by events in parturition and the neonatal period. One-quarter to one-third of neonatal deaths are due to withdrawal of intensive care. Although necropsy may sometimes reveal a clear 'cause of death' unsuspected in life, expectation of this in every case leads to a falsely low impression of the value of the examination.

### (2) To provide information about growth, maturity, and mode and time of death
With stillbirths the pathologist will be able to tell whether pregnancy had been proceeding normally until the point of death, or whether intrauterine growth was impaired. It may be possible to determine the mode of death (e.g. sudden and asphyxial, or prolonged and

associated with uteroplacental vascular insufficiency) and the approximate time of death (e.g. before the mother entered the hospital, before the onset of labour, or during labour). Among neonatal deaths the pathologist's estimate of maturity may give valuable retrospective support to a difficult clinical decision not to offer intensive care to a very immature neonate.

### (3) To detect diseases with implications for future pregnancies
This may involve further delineation of conditions recognized in life (e.g. histological demonstration that cystic kidneys were of the autosomal recessive infantile type) or discovery of unsuspected disease which did not cause the baby's death (e.g. an incidental finding of microscopic evidence of cystic fibrosis).

The post-mortem examination is an opportunity to collect samples for DNA analysis from abnormal babies in case an antenatal diagnostic test becomes available in the future. DNA can be extracted from many tissues or, more expensively, from fibroblast cultures.

### (4) To monitor iatrogenic disease
All medical treatment may have unwanted effects. In the perinatal period these may result from obstetric procedures, obtaining vascular access, maintaining oxygenation and intravenous alimentation.

### (5) Teaching, research and epidemiology

### (6) Psychosocial objectives
For some parents the post-mortem helps them to accept the fact of their children's death. It is an opportunity to provide mementoes (photographs, locks of hair, handprints, identity bracelets, etc.). Investigation by an uninvolved third party may resolve parental and professional doubts about what might or might not have been done, and restore a doctor–parent relationship that has been strained by the baby's death.

### (7) Medicolegal objectives
A properly performed perinatal post-mortem, including examination of the placenta, is the best protection against ill-informed litigation.

### (8) To provide a basis for counselling parents
*This is the single most important purpose of the examination*, and may draw on any of the above. Parents gain much reassurance from the documentation of *normality*, which may acquire fresh significance in the light of subsequent abnormal pregnancies.

**Table 26.1** Agreement between clinical diagnoses and diagnoses after post-mortem examination in a series of 300 perinatal necropsies

| Clinical vs. pathological diagnosis | Stillbirths (%) (n = 150) | Neonatal deaths (%) (n = 150) |
|---|---|---|
| Agree | 40 | 19 |
| Agree, but additional information* from post-mortem | 34 | 66 |
| Clinical diagnosis incorrect | 26 | 15 |

From Porter and Keeling (1987) *J. Clin. Pathol.* **40**, 180–4.
* Additional information = information important for counselling parents or care of babies in the future.

*There is no such thing as a perinatal post-mortem which does not show anything. It is unacceptable not to offer a post-mortem because you think you know the cause of death* (Table 26.1).

## CONSENT FOR POST-MORTEM EXAMINATION

Every parent of a child who has died must be offered a post-mortem examination, and it is equally their *right* to refuse, unless the case has been referred to the Coroner.

Consent for necropsy is required for all liveborn infants regardless of gestation age, except in cases referred to the Coroner, when he or she will usually order a post-mortem to be carried out. The rules for referral are the same as for adults (see Table 26.2). Consent for a hospital post-mortem is usually recorded on a form provided by the hospital. Although written consent is not required by law it is a wise precaution, and should include explicit consent to retention of whole organs such as the brain or heart if this is intended. Verbal consent (e.g. by telephone) should be given to two witnesses who must record it in the clinical notes.

Consent is most likely to be obtained if the purpose and benefits of post-mortem examination are sympathetically explained to the parents by the most senior doctor they know well, and who knew their child. They can be reassured that the post-mortem will not delay the funeral and that, although the examination involves incisions, the baby will not be disfigured, and can be seen and held

**Table 26.2** Some circumstances in which deaths must be reported to H.M. Coroner (the list is not exhaustive, and if in doubt you should discuss a case with the Coroner or his Officer)

---

(1) Dead on arrival in hospital or within 24 hours of admission
(2) Unattended stillbirths*
(3) Deaths within 24 hours of an operation, anaesthetic or invasive procedure
(4) Deaths as a result of accident
(5) Unnatural, criminal or suspicious deaths, e.g. neglect, child abuse or poisoning
(6) Deaths as a result of drugs, whether prescribed or not
(7) Deaths as a result of medical or surgical mishap (the doctor should also inform his or her defence organization)
(8) Deaths in which the doctor is so uncertain of the disease leading to death as to be unable to sign a death certificate

---

* The Coroner is not responsible for stillbirths, but in unattended births he or she must establish that the child was in fact stillborn.

by them afterwards (exceptions are some second-trimester fetuses and very macerated stillborn babies).

Some parents may decline a full examination. Key clinical questions can often be answered by a limited post-mortem, e.g. excluding examination of the brain, or limited to the body cavity or organ in question. Even needle biopsies may be helpful. Restriction must be prominently stated on the consent form.

The views of religious groups should be respected. Sikhs usually have no religious objection to post-mortem examinations, but the latter are not encouraged by strict Hindus or Muslims.

A baby should not be referred to the Coroner as a second line when consent is refused by the parents.

## REQUIREMENTS FOR OPTIMAL POST-MORTEM EXAMINATIONS

The pathologist will require the following.

### (1) A clear history
This is most easily provided in a standard request form supplemented by the mother's and baby's notes. The junior doctor should remember that he or she is requesting a consultant opinion.

## (2) The placenta

Almost all neonatal deaths follow an abnormal pregnancy or delivery, and every maternity hospital should have a system for collecting all of these placentas for the pathologist in case the baby dies.

## (3) The baby

Ideally the baby should be sent straight to the mortuary with all tubes still in place. Except in Coroner's cases where this rule is absolute, there is room for compromise between the pathologist's needs and those of the parents, e.g. by tying and cutting off tubes close to the skin.

If there is likely to be a delay before the post-mortem is carried out (or there is no enthusiastic perinatal pathologist!), then the paediatrician should consider doing the following him- or herself if indicated:

- blood cultures (from the sagittal sinus);
- CSF culture (from the cisterna magna);
- samples for virology (e.g. needle biopsy of liver);
- chromosomes (skin biopsy, tissue from the fetal aspect of the placenta if the baby is at all macerated);
- photographs (any external anomalies);
- X-rays (essential in skeletal dystrophies. Gas emboli disappear from vessels within 12 hours of death).

In any case the paediatric team should be informed of the time of the examination and attend to give clinical details, to ensure that essential questions are answered, and to educate and encourage the pathologist.

## SPECIAL POST-MORTEMS

Immediate post-mortem sampling is required when an inborn error of metabolism is suspected. This should be anticipated by obtaining consent before the child's death, warning the pathologist and discussing the samples required with an experienced paediatric chemical pathologist. The tests used are changing rapidly, but if expert advice is not available then the following samples should suffice.

### (1) Unexplained metabolic acidosis or hyperammonaemia, etc.

- Blood (plasma or serum)
- CSF
- Urine
- Liver
- Kidney          } Samples snap frozen at − 80°C.
- Skeletal muscle
- Myocardium
- Spleen
- Culture and save skin fibroblasts.

NB Arrange to save all samples taken in life, including blood films.

### (2) Suspected storage disorder: in addition to the above

- Liver
- Kidney
- Skeletal muscle  } In glutaraldehyde
- Myocardium          for electron microscopy.
- Spleen

If the storage disorder (or a demyelinating disorder) affects the central nervous system, then a frontal pole of the brain should be frozen and pieces of rectum saved frozen and in glutaraldehyde.

These lists are no substitute for expert advice, which will considerably reduce the number of samples required.

A full post-mortem examination with microbiology and histology must be carried out at leisure, as in many of these cases the metabolic abnormalities are secondary to some other disorder, such as infection or congenital heart disease.

**Table 26.3** A clinicopathological classification of perinatal deaths (Wigglesworth, 1980): the five categories may be further broken down by birthweight or gestational age

(1) Normally formed macerated stillbirth
(2) Congenital malformation
(3) Conditions associated with immaturity
(4) Asphyxial conditions developing during labour
(5) Specific conditions other than the above

## AFTER THE POST-MORTEM EXAMINATION

A provisional report should be available within a few days and a final report within 6 weeks. The report may be shown to the parents, but the pathologist's consent should be obtained before they are given a copy. The Coroner's reports are confidential to him or her and should not be disclosed to a third party without the Coroner's consent. However, the parents are entitled to a copy from the Coroner, and in practice he or she usually allows the pathologist discretion to give a copy to the paediatrician concerned.

The post-mortem report must be available for the monthly perinatal mortality meeting held in all good units, and is essential for accurate clinicopathological classification of the death. The classification of Wigglesworth (1980) is widely used because it draws attention to particular aspects of patient care (see Table 26.3).

## BIBLIOGRAPHY

Becker, M.J. and Beck A.E. (1989) *Pathology of late fetal stillbirth.* Edinburgh: Churchill Livingstone.

Grunewald, O. and Minh, H.N. (1960) Evaluation of body and organ weights in perinatal pathology. 1. Normal standards derived from autopsies. *Am. J. Clin. Pathol.* **34**, 247–53.

Keeling, J.W. (1993)*Fetal and neonatal pathology*, 2nd edn. London: Springer-Verlag.

Keeling, J.W., MacGillivray I., Golding, J. *et al.* (1989) Classification of perinatal death. *Arch. Dis. Child.* **64**, 1345–51.

MacPherson, T.A., Valdes-Depena, M. and Kanbour, A. (1986) Perinatal mortality and morbidity: the role of the anatomical pathologist. *Semin. Perinatol.* **10**, 179–86.

Porter, H.J. and Keeling, J.W. (1987) Value of perinatal necropsy examination. *J. Clin. Pathol.* **40**, 180–4.

Streeter, G.L. (1921) Weight, sitting height, head size, foot length and menstrual age of the human embryo. *Contrib. Embryol.* **55**, 143–70.

Wigglesworth, J.S. (1980) Monitoring perinatal mortality: a pathophysiological approach. *Lancet.* **ii**, 684–6.

Wigglesworth, J.S. (1996) *Major problems in pathology. No. 15. Perinatal pathology*, 2nd edn. Philadelphia P.A.: W.B. Saunders.

Winter, R.W., Knowles, S.A.S., Bieber, F.R. and Baraitser, M. (1988) *The malformed fetus and stillbirth. A diagnostic approach.* Chichester: John Wiley & Sons.

# 27

# Practical procedures

Blood sampling
Insertion of intravenous lines
Intraosseous infusions
Insertion of arterial lines
Exchange transfusion
Intubation
Thoracentesis
Pericardial aspiration
Intracardiac injection
Cardiac massage
Lumbar puncture
Ventricular tap
Subdural tap
Intramuscular injections
Suprapubic bladder tap
Abdominal paracentesis
Bone marrow aspiration
Peritoneal dialysis
Haemofiltration

**Before performing any practical procedure**

1 Ensure all equipment is prepared.
2 Ensure any assistants are familiar with the procedure.
3 Maintain thermal care – use a supplementary overhead heater if the incubator is to be open for any length of time.

Do not persist after three failed attempts – seek a colleague's help or take a break and try again later.

**Remember:** The procedure is in the *infant's* interest – do not cause avoidable disturbance or trauma.

## BLOOD SAMPLING

Routine precautions for protection against hepatitis B and HIV must be observed. Protective gloves should be worn and particular caution taken with the disposal of needles and sharps.

### Capillary samples

See Fig. 27.1 for site of sampling.

• Warm or rub the area for 1–2 min to increase perfusion.

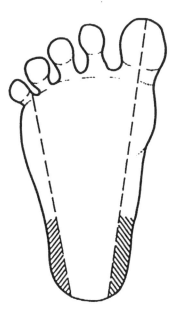

**Fig. 27.1** Sites for heel-prick capillary blood sampling. Puncture heel (shaded area) on plantar surface, beyond the lateral and medial limits of the calcaneus, to avoid damage to the bone (Blumenfeld et al., 1979).

- Clean the skin surface.
- Puncture the skin with a stilette (to a depth of 2–3 mm only), preferably using an Autolet or similar device. This has been shown to reduce the stress caused to the baby by heel-prick sampling.
- *Gently* massage the heel to encourage blood flow.
- Avoid adhesive dressings to the area – they keep it moist and increase the risk of infection.

## Venous samples

The safest sites are the *antecubital fossa* or the *back of the hand*. Small veins on the *dorsum of the foot* are also suitable.

For blood cultures, clean the skin with an iodine-containing solution and preferably use a butterfly needle (23 or 25 G) with syringe attached. Use a new sterile needle to inject the blood into each blood-culture bottle. (NB Beware the anaerobic bottle! It may take *all* of the blood sample before you can prevent it!)

### Other sites for venepuncture

*External jugular vein* This should not be used in infants with respiratory distress. Great care is needed to minimize trauma. The infant is wrapped and held with the head slightly lower than the trunk, and the neck flexed away from the side of the venepuncture. The vein is clearly seen, and the sample should be taken through a 21 or 23 G needle with a syringe attached (to minimize the risk of air embolism). After removing the needle, apply firm pressure and sit the infant up.

*Femoral vein* This site should be *avoided if at all possible*, as the needle may enter the hip joint and cause septic arthritis. The femoral artery is palpable at the mid-inguinal point, and the vein is medial to this. Clean the skin very carefully and insert the needle vertically, applying gentle suction. Stop advancing the needle as soon as blood is obtained.

## Arterial samples

Suitable sites for arterial sampling are the radial, posterior tibial and dorsalis pedis. Brachial and temporal arteries are best avoided for routine sampling (see below). Femoral arterial puncture carries a risk of septic arthritis of the hip, and is not recommended.

### Radial artery

- Check that there is an ulnar artery (it is absent in 1–2% of the population) either by transillumination or by squeezing the hand whilst occluding the sites of the radial and ulnar arteries. If the hand rapidly goes pink when the ulnar artery site is released, the ulnar artery is patent.
- Hold the wrist in neutral position, or at most slightly extended, with the palm of the hand upwards.
- Locate the radial artery by palpation or transillumination – situated at the mid-point of the lateral third of the wrist.
- Enter the artery just proximal to the wrist crease, at an angle of 25–30°. Use either a heparinized 23 or 25 G scalp-vein needle or a 23 G needle on a heparinized 2-mL syringe.

### Posterior tibial artery

- Hold the foot in neutral position or slightly dorsiflexed.
- Locate the artery by palpation or transillumination (behind the medial malleolus).
- Sampling technique is as for radial artery.

### Dorsalis pedis artery

- Partially plantar flex the foot.
- Locate artery by palpation or transillumination (between first and second metatarsals).
- Sampling technique is as for radial artery.

### Brachial artery
(NB The brachial is an end artery and should not be used as a routine site.)

- Hold the arm with elbow extended.
- Palpate the artery just proximal and medial to the antecubital fossa.
- Sampling technique is as for radial artery.

### Temporal artery
(NB Do not insert a cannula into the temporal artery because of the risk of reflex spasm or embolization of other branches of the external carotid, especially the middle meningeal artery.)

Branches of the temporal artery can be palpated and samples taken through a 25 G butterfly needle.

## INSERTION OF INTRAVENOUS LINES

### Peripheral veins

#### Site

Veins on the dorsum of the hands and feet, antecubital fossa, long saphenous vein and scalp veins are most often used.

#### Technique

Identify the site. It is often helpful to warm peripheral sites, such as hands and feet, for 1–2 min prior to starting. Try to aim for veins which have a clear, relatively linear course and which are reasonably fixed, e.g. by the joining of two or more tributaries. It is sometimes helpful to occlude the vein proximally, e.g. with the forefinger of your non-dominant hand.

- Clean the skin with antiseptic solution.
- It is sometimes necessary to puncture the skin overlying the vein. Be careful not to enter the vein and cause a haematoma. Most modern cannulae will slide through the skin without 'catching'.
- Advance a 24 G or 22 G intravenous cannula through the skin at an angle of about 30° to the skin until a 'flashback' of blood is seen. Advance the cannula over the needle to enter the vein.
- If the needle has transfixed the vein, it may be impossible to advance the cannula. This can occasionally be rectified by (1) withdrawing the needle, (2) gently pulling back on the cannula until blood flashes back into its distal portion and (3) then advancing the cannula into the vein lumen.
- Infuse a small quantity of normal saline through the cannula to ensure that the cannula is in the vein.
- Tape the cannula securely in place, ensuring that the site of the cannula tip remains visible. Immobilize the i.v. site with a suitable splint.

### Scalp veins

These should be avoided if possible, as the sight of an intravenous line in the head is often distressing to parents. Hair which is shaved off may take months to regrow.

If a scalp vein must be cannulated, first ensure that it is not an artery by direct palpation.

## Umbilical vein

This vein may be used for emergency vascular access during re-suscitation, e.g. for administration of plasma and drugs, and occasionally for exchange transfusions.

### Technique

- Use full aseptic technique (gown and gloves), carefully clean the cord and surrounding skin, and drape the abdomen with a sterile towel.
- A tie may be placed around the base of the cord to control bleeding.
- Cut the cord to 1.0–1.5 cm.
- Identify the vein (large, thin-walled, solitary structure) and clamp the cord sheath adjacent to the vein.
- Attach a three-way tap to a 5FG end-hole catheter and flush with heparinized saline (0.5–1.0 unit/mL). Pass the tip of the catheter into the vein, gently exerting counter-traction on the clamped cord sheath.
- Advance the catheter so that its tip lies between the diaphragm and the right atrium. This distance is estimated from the shoulder-to-umbilicus length.
- The final position of the catheter should be checked by X-ray. Unless required for emergency resuscitation (adrenaline, plasma and blood can be administered), the catheter can then be fixed in place by a suture through the cord sheath and tied around the catheter.
- *Ensure that the infant is not left lying in a puddle of alcohol/iodine solution used to clean the skin, as this can cause severe burns to the skin.*

## Percutaneous long-line insertion

### Silastic 'through-the-needle' cannula
These fine, silastic cannulae are ideal for medium-term parenteral nutrition and administration of other fluids and drugs. They are not generally suitable for blood product administration.

**Site** Antecubital fossa or long saphenous vein anterior to the medial malleolus.

### Technique

- Use full aseptic technique (gown and gloves).

- Perform a venepuncture with a 19 G butterfly needle (supplied with cannula). It is important to try and enter the vein cleanly and not to transfix the vessel.
- Using a pair of fine, non-toothed forceps, feed the silastic cannula through the butterfly needle and into the vein. Problems may be encountered due to brisk backflow of blood 'flushing' the cannula out of the needle; release any obstruction proximal to the needle entry site.

### Position of the cannula

There are two possible positions for the tip of the cannula.

1 Insert the cannula 2–3 cm. In this position, blood flow is fast enough to allow safe, long-term infusion of hypotonic fluids, but does not carry the risk associated with central venous lines.
2 Insert the cannula so that the tip lies in the subclavian vein or superior vena cava for antecubital lines, or the inferior vena cava for saphenous lines. The insertion distance can be judged by measuring on the surface prior to the procedure. This line will last for several weeks if meticulous anti-infective measures are taken. If this 'central' position is used, the position of the catheter tip must be checked with an X-ray.

Once the cannula is inserted to the correct length, withdraw the needle from the vein and over the cannula. Insert the reinforced free end of the cannula into the connector hub and tighten the connector to clamp the rubber 'O-ring' on to the cannula. If a leak appears at this site, check that the 'O-ring' is present and re-tighten the connection.

Secure the cannula in place using sterile transparent surgical dressing (e.g. Opsite or Tegaderm). Spare lengths of silastic cannula can be 'coiled' under the dressing.

### Seldinger technique

A percutaneous long line may be inserted using this technique for the indications stated above, and during emergency resuscitation for rapid vascular access to a major vein. However, even in skilled hands this will take considerably longer than establishing an intraosseous or umbilical venous infusion; these are the recommended initial routes of access.

**Site** In larger babies, antecubital and long saphenous veins may be used. Other sites include the femoral vein and external/internal jugular; these should be avoided by the non-expert.

### Technique

- A 22 G intravenous cannula (6 or 10 cm in length) is recommended.
- Use full aseptic technique (gown and gloves). Thoroughly clean the skin around the insertion site and drape with sterile towels.
- Cannulate the vein with a sterile 22 G intravenous cannula or with a 21 G sterile butterfly needle.
- Take the J-wire from the cannula pack and retract into the introducer to straighten the wire. Put the introducer into the hub of the needle/cannula and advance the wire for a few centimetres so that it is well beyond the needle tip. *The wire should always be checked before the procedure to ensure that it fits through the needle or cannula used.*
- Holding the wire securely in the vein, withdraw the needle/cannula completely. Thread the 22 G cannula over the wire and up to the skin. *Ensure that the wire protrudes from the proximal end of the catheter.* If not, gradually withdraw the wire from the vein until it does protrude.
- It may be necessary to make a small 'nick' in the skin; this can be done with the point of a sterile 21 G needle. Continue to thread the cannula over the wire and into the vein with a slight twisting motion.
- When the cannula is in position (*v.s.*) remove the wire and attach a three-way tap and 10-mL syringe filled with heparinized saline (1 unit/mL). Pull back on the syringe to ensure free aspiration of blood, and flush with a small amount of heparinized saline.
- Apply a transparent surgical dressing to secure the cannula.

### Care of the long line

- Change the i.v. fluid containers, giving set and tubing (excluding the T-piece) daily (use full aseptic technique). An i.v. 'set-saver' filter will extend the life of the set so that it only needs changing every 3 days.
- Spray the T-piece with iodine-containing antiseptic before connecting the new tubing.
- When the long line is removed, culture the tip.
- Any infant with a percutaneous long line *in situ* should have blood cultures taken if there is any suspicion of sepsis, e.g. raised WCC, acute phase reactants, fever. Consideration should be given to removal of the line.

## INTRAOSSEOUS INFUSIONS

For emergency vascular access in infants in whom the cord has separated and no peripheral access is possible, the intraosseous route may be used. This is a temporary route for resuscitation and is replaced with a definitive intravenous line when the patient is stabilized.

### Technique

The landmarks for intraosseous infusions are (1) the anterior surface of the tibia, 2–3 cm below the tibial tuberosity, or (2) the antero-lateral surface of the femur, 3 cm above the lateral condyle.

- Clean the skin over the chosen site.
- Insert the intraosseous needle at 90° to the skin and advance until a 'give' is felt as the cortex is penetrated.
- Attach a syringe and aspirate to confirm correct positioning.
- Volume boluses can be infused using a 50-mL syringe (note that fluids will not run under gravity alone, and must be actively infused). Most resuscitation drugs can be given by this route, but bicarbonate infusion should be avoided as it may precipitate in the tissues.

## INSERTION OF ARTERIAL LINES

## Peripheral arteries

### Site

Radial artery or posterior tibial artery. The temporal, brachial and femoral arteries should usually be avoided, as they are end arteries.

### Technique

- Check the patency of the ulnar collateral circulation before inserting a radial arterial line.
- Localize the artery by palpation or by fibre-optic transillumination. The latter technique is more successful in smaller infants.
- *Radial artery.* Position the wrist as for arterial sampling. The wrist should not be flexed or overextended, as this will compress the radial artery. It is sometimes useful to gently extend the wrist over a dental roll or similar object. The radial artery is

found at the mid-point of the lateral third of the wrist at the proximal skin crease.

- *Posterior tibial artery.* The ankle is slightly plantar flexed and everted. The artery is palpable immediately posterior to the medial malleolus.
- Clean the skin over the artery with antiseptic solution.
- Enter the skin over the artery at approximately 30° and continue to advance until a flashback of blood is seen. Either advance the cannula over the needle *or* continue to advance the needle until the artery is transfixed. Then withdraw the needle and gently withdraw the cannula until blood flows freely up the cannula. Advance the cannula into the artery. Connect a syringe of heparinized saline (1 unit/mL) or a prepared 10-cm line with a three-way tap. Aspirate to ensure that the line is correctly positioned, and then gently flush the cannula.
- Cover the cannula with a clear surgical dressing (e.g. Opsite or Tegaderm) or tape to the wrist or ankle, ensuring that the fingers or toes are clearly visible so that any evidence of ischaemia may be observed.
- Immobilize the wrist or ankle with an appropriate splint.

*NB Infusions of heparinized saline (0.45% or 0.9% NaCl with heparin 0.5–1 unit/mL) should be taken into account when calculating the daily fluid and sodium requirements.*

## Umbilical artery catheter

### Technique

- Use full aseptic technique (gown and gloves). Carefully clean the cord and surrounding skin, and drape the abdomen with a sterile towel.
- Tie a loose ligature around the base of the cord to control bleeding. Alternatively, place a purse-string suture through the cord sheath near the skin and leave the ends loosely tied. Be careful not to transfix a vessel when suturing the cord.
- Cut the cord transversely about 1.0–1.5 cm above the skin and identify the arteries as two thick-walled structures which usually stand proud of the cut surface of the cord.
- Clamp the edge of the cord with a pair of forceps adjacent to the site of the artery. Place two clamps tangentially to the cord sheath on either side of the cord to give maximum control, and stabilize the cord with the second and third fingers of the non-

preferred hand. Gently dilate the lumen of the artery with a blunt dilator or a pair of fine forceps to a depth of 5 mm. Proceed slowly and carefully at this stage; it is easy to strip the arterial intima and create a false passage.

- *Insert a 3.5FG or 5.0FG catheter. Connect the catheter to a three-way tap and 5-mL syringe. Pre-fill/charge catheter with heparinized saline (1 unit/mL) into the arterial lumen* and advance it slowly into the aorta. Success is indicated by blood flowing or being easily aspirated up the catheter.
- The catheter tip may be located either between L3 and L4, i.e. just rostral to the aortic bifurcation and below the origin of the inferior mesenteric artery, or between T8 and T10, i.e. above the level of the coeliac axis and renal artery origins. The distance to insert can be calculated from the formula:

$$3 \times \text{weight (kg)} + 9 \text{ cm (from abdomen wall,}$$
$$\text{therefore add length of remaining cord stump).}$$

- The catheter is held in place by a purse-string suture and tape. The position of the catheter must be checked by an abdominal X-ray.

### Problems

**1** The catheter will not pass through into the aorta. Sometimes this is due to resistance where the umbilical artery joins the iliac artery; gentle sustained pressure for 30–60 sec will overcome this problem. Otherwise, a false passage has been created and the cannula has passed out of the arterial lumen. In this case, the other artery should be cannulated.

**2** The catheter passes into the aorta but a 'white or blue leg' or 'blue toes' develop. This is due to vasospasm and the catheter must be removed. Try the other artery and consider using a smaller catheter – 3.5FG if a 5FG was used previously.

### Catheter removal

- The infusion through the catheter is stopped approximately 1 hour prior to removal, and a ligature is tied around the umbilical stump.
- The catheter is removed slowly over a period of approximately 5 min, to allow time for vasospasm of the umbilical artery and

thus minimize bleeding. Tighten the ligature when the catheter has been removed completely.

• Send the catheter tip for culture.

## EXCHANGE TRANSFUSION

The most common indication for an exchange transfusion is severe hyperbilirubinaemia. Other indications include polycythaemia (see Chapter 19) and septicaemia (see Chapter 17). For hyperbilirubinaemia a 'two-volume exchange' is performed, i.e. the volume of blood exchanged is equal to twice the infant's blood volume, that is $2 \times 80$ mL/kg = 160 mL/kg. This will replace approximately 80% of the infant's blood. 'Priming' the infant with albumin (1 g/kg given i.v. over 30–60 min as a 10% solution 2 hours before the exchange) may increase the removal of bilirubin.

### Technique

Fresh blood (CMV-negative) should be used that is less than 4 days old and cross-matched against the mother's blood. It should be partially packed to a PCV of 60%. There are two ways of performing the procedure.

1 *In-out method.* This used to be the commonest way of performing an exchange, but is now used less often. Aliquots, 5 or 10 mL, of infant blood are withdrawn via an umbilical venous catheter and replaced by an equal volume of donor blood in a serial manner via a three-way tap – 10 mL out, 10 mL in, 10 mL out, etc. – until the calculated volume has been exchanged. This method has a higher incidence of complications.

2 *Continuous flow method.* This is the preferred technique. Insert peripheral arterial and venous lines; if this is not possible, umbilical artery and vein or a combination of peripheral and umbilical vessels can be used. Donor blood is infused at a constant rate through the vein via a blood warmer using a volumetric pump. Baby's blood is withdrawn at the same rate from the arterial line using a 50-mL syringe. It is essential to balance the rate of withdrawal with the infusion rate.

No matter which method is used, a two-volume exchange (160 mL/kg) should take 1.5 hours to complete, i.e. a slower rate in a smaller baby. A deficit of 10 mL in the baby should be left at the end of the exchange.

## Monitoring

One operator should record the volumes of the blood exchanged, and check vital signs, e.g. heart rate, respiratory rate and temperature, at regular intervals.

In sick or low-birthweight infants, blood gas and blood sugar measurements should be checked once or twice during the exchange. If a UVC is used in sick or unstable babies central control venous pressure can be measured intermittently and BP should be checked.

If there is evidence of hypocalcaemia (irritability, tachycardia, prolonged Q-T interval) the infant should be given 0.5 mL of 10% calcium gluconate solution i.v. over 5–10 min. In the absence of such signs, the hazards of calcium administration (bradycardia or cardiac arrest) outweigh its usefulness.

## Blood samples

The *first 10 mL* of blood removed should be sent for estimation of bilirubin, haematocrit and any other investigations needed (e.g. enzyme assays for glucose-6-phosphate dehydrogenase or galactosaemia, liver-function tests, viral studies, etc.).

The *last 10 mL* of blood removed should be sent for estimation of blood sugar, electrolytes, bilirubin, calcium, blood gases and haematocrit.

Check capillary blood sugar 1, 2 and 4 hours after the exchange, as reactive hypoglycaemia may occur.

## Feeding

Do not feed infants for 2–4 hours before exchange transfusion (to reduce the risk of aspiration) and for 2–4 hours afterwards (to reduce the risk of necrotizing enterocolitis). Give maintenance fluids i.v. during this period.

## Complications

- Vascular – embolization (air or clots) and thrombosis.
- Cardiac – arrhythmia; volume overload or depletion; arrest.
- Electrolyte – hyperkalaemia, hypernatraemia, hypocalcaemia, acidosis or alkalosis.
- Infective – bacteraemia, hepatitis B, CMV.

- Miscellaneous – hypothermia, hypoglycaemia, necrotizing enterocolitis (metronidazole is sometimes given as a prophylaxis against necrotizing enterocolitis).

## INTUBATION

Endotracheal intubation should be performed as a controlled procedure in an infant who has been well pre-oxygenated with bag-and-mask ventilation using 100% oxygen.

Do not let the infant become hypoxaemic during the procedure. If you are unable to intubate within 30 sec, stop immediately and ventilate with a bag and mask. (Hold your breath at insertion of the laryngoscope and stop the attempt when you need to take a breath yourself.)

### Equipment required

- Suction devices.
- Straight-blade laryngoscopes (it is preferable to have two available).
- Endotracheal tubes of appropriate diameter (see Table 27.1).
- Introducers and connectors for ET tube.
- Bag and mask connected to 100% oxygen supply.
- Magill's forceps.

### Technique

- The airway is opened by positioning the head in the 'neutral' position, in line with the body. Remember that the larynx is anterior in an infant, and extending the neck will make intubation difficult or impossible.

**Table 27.1** ET tube sizes

| Baby's weight | Gestational (weeks) | ETT size (mm) | Distance from upper lip (cm) |
|---|---|---|---|
| < 1000 | < 30 | 2.5 | 7 |
| 1000–2000 | 30–34 | 3.0 | 8 |
| 2000–3000 | ≥ 35 | 3.0 or 3.5 | 9 |
| > 3000 | | 3.5 | 10 |

- Pre-oxygenate the infant by ventilating with a bag and mask. An oral Guedel airway of appropriate size may be used in addition.
- Insert the laryngoscope blade into the mouth, pushing the tongue to the left and advancing the blade into the posterior pharynx. There are two alternative approaches to visualizing the larynx.
    **1** Continue to advance the laryngoscope blade past the epiglottis into the proximal oesophagus. Gently lift the blade upwards (*towards the ceiling*) and retract slowly; this will 'lift' the epiglottis out of the field of vision and the vocal cords will appear (Fig. 27.2).
    **2** Advance the laryngoscope blade until the epiglottis is seen. The tip of the blade then lies in the vallecula. Lift the epiglottis upwards by exerting traction parallel to the laryngoscope handle (*not* by tilting the blade upward).
- Visualization of the cords may be improved by exerting gentle cricoid pressure. This may be achieved using the little finger of the left hand, or by employing an assistant.
- Insert an oral endotracheal tube along the line of the laryngoscope blade and through the vocal cords for a distance of approximately 2 cm. For nasotracheal intubation, insert the tube, bevel downward into the anterior nares and direct posteriorly

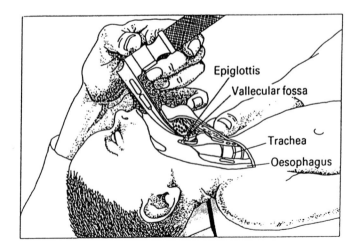

**Fig. 27.2** The technique for endotracheal intubation.

(directly towards the occiput). The tube will curve around and appear in the posterior pharynx. Grasp the tip of the tube with Magill's forceps and advance through the vocal cords for approximately 2 cm.

- Ensure correct ET tube placement by:
  - watching the chest rise during positive pressure inflations (symmetrical movement?);
  - observing the infant's colour (remains pink?);
  - auscultation over both lung fields (breath sounds symmetrical?) and over the stomach;
  - confirming the ET tube position on chest X-ray. The tip of the tube should lie approximately 1–2 cm above the carina with the head in the mid-line.
- If the infant does not respond to IPPV within 30 sec, check that the ET tube is not blocked or dislodged.

## Tube fixation

The endotracheal tube should be fixed securely in position. This can be achieved either by using a proprietary device included in the ET tube pack (remember to allow for the length of some devices when cutting the tube), or by using the following technique.

**1** Cut two pieces of 1-inch tape to a length equivalent to approximately half the distance between the mastoid process of the infant.

**2** Make a longitudinal cut in each tape for about half its length.

**3** Stick the uncut part of the tape to the infant's cheek and stick one half of the cut section to the philtrum above the upper lip.

**4** Wind the other cut half around the ET tube twice, and then stick it firmly to the tape affixed to the cheek.

**5** Repeat the procedure from the opposite side.

## Common errors

- The condition of the infant is ignored during the procedure.
- The vocal cords are not properly visualized before intubation is attempted.
- The infant's upper gum may be lacerated by excessive pressure of the laryngoscope blade. This is more likely if the blade is not *lifted* but *tilted*, using the alveolar margin as a fulcrum.
- The endotracheal tube is advanced too far down and into the right main bronchus.

### Technique for endotracheal suctioning

*Aim* To remove excess secretions from the respiratory tract by the insertion of a catheter and application of a negative pressure, resulting in improved respiratory function.

*Indication* Routine suction should *not* be performed.
Decision should be made following individual assessment, which may include:

- airway resistance (decreasing tidal volume);
- auscultation of lungs;
- nature of secretions;
- tolerance to procedure;
- visible signs of secretions.

### Technique

1 Check that vacuum pressure is correctly set (for birth weight < 1500 g use 40 mm $H_2O$, for > 1500g use 60 mm $H_2O$).

2 Use an appropriate-sized catheter for the diameter of the endotracheal tube (size 6 for 2.5–3.5 FG, size 8 for 4.0–5.0).

3 Connect the catheter to the suction tubing from the vacuum pump.

4 Observe oxygen saturation – preoxygenate 10–20% above normal requirements if necessary.

5 Wash hands and apply a non-sterile glove, (or gloves) that will be used to introduce the catheter into the ETT.

6 Ensure correct depth of suction by measuring the catheter against a pre-measured tape, so that the catheter will pass to the end of the ETT (and not more than 1cm beyond this point).

7 Disconnect the ETT from the ventilator and insert the catheter to predetermined length using gloved hand.

8 The total procedure whilst disconnected from ventilator should take no longer than 15 sec, with negative pressure applied for no longer than 5 sec.

9 Gently remove the catheter and reconnect the ventilator.

10 Check for breath sounds on both sides of the chest.

11 Monitor post-procedure saturation and heart rate, and adjust oxygen accordingly.

12 Dispose of rubbish, clear suction tubing using sterile water, and wash hands.

**13** Record the effectiveness of the procedure in the infant's records.

NB The use of advanced humidification systems in ventilation reduces the accumulation of tenacious and dry secretions, and means that the routine use of saline as an irrigant is no longer necessary. Should individual circumstances require, normal saline at 0.1–0.2 mL/kg should be instilled prior to applying negative pressure.

## THORACENTESIS

### Chest transillumination

In a low-birthweight infant, a pneumothorax may be demonstrated by increased transillumination of the hemithorax. Use a fibre-optic light source in a darkened room, or put a dark cover over the incubator. Apply the light source to the posterior chest and compare transillumination of the right and left hemithorax.

### Needling the chest

Used for the emergency relief of a tension pneumothorax or suspected pneumothorax with critical deterioration in the clinical condition of the infant. Less commonly used for draining pleural effusions.

#### Technique

- Attach a 21 G butterfly needle to a 10-mL syringe and three-way tap.
- Clean the skin over the third/fourth intercostal space in the mid-axillary line.
- Insert the needle at 90° to the skin and just above the rib below. If free gas is present, it will aspirate easily. The three-way tap allows for repeated aspiration without disconnecting the syringe from the needle.
- If a pneumothorax is found, the tap should be connected to an extension tube with the free end secured 2–3 cm under the surface of a bottle of sterile water (at least 20 cm below the level of the baby). The tap is then opened to allow drainage of the

pneumothorax through this temporary system until a definitive chest drain is inserted.

## Chest drain insertion

***Site*** See Fig. 27.3.

**1** *Lateral* – third to fifth intercostal space in the anterior axillary line.

**2** *Anterior* – third intercostal space in the mid-clavicular line, direct tip anteriorly. *The nipple and breast bud must be avoided.*

   • The drain works best if the tip lies in the anterior pleural space. The anterior insertion site is more successful in achieving an anterior position of the tip (Allen, R.W. *et al.*

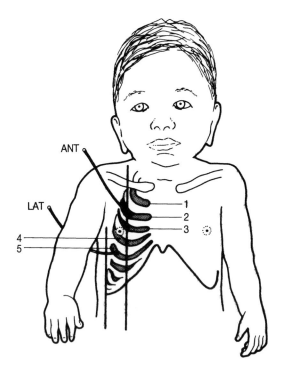

**Fig. 27.3** Sites for insertion of chest drains to relieve pneumothorax. Adapted from Allen, R.W., Jung, A.L. and Lester, P.D. (1981) *J. Pediatr.* **99**, 629–34.

(1981) *J. Pediatr.* **99**:629–34), but a more discrete scar is obtained with a lateral approach.

- Clean the skin over the insertion site and infuse a small amount of local anaesthetic (1% lignocaine) through the tissues down to the parietal pleura.
- Make a small incision through the skin parallel to the rib.
- With a pair of forceps, bluntly dissect through the intercostal muscles down to and *including* the parietal pleura. A soft hiss of gas may be heard as the pleura is breached.
- Use a size 8FG, 10FG or 12FG chest drain. Remove the trocar, discard, and grasp the tip of the drain with a pair of forceps. Push the drain and forceps through the chest wall. Release the forceps and advance the drain, aiming anteriorly. The use of a trocar during insertion risks impaling/penetrating the lung.
- Connect the drain to an underwater seal; observe for air bubbles and swinging on respiration.
- If necessary, connect the drain to $-10$ cm $H_2O$ suction pressure.
- Place a suture through the skin adjacent to the drain and tie it around the drain. Finally, tape the drain in position.
- Arrange for a chest X-ray to check the position of the chest tube and its effectiveness.

### Chest drain removal

- Once the lung has re-expanded and the drain is no longer functioning, remove it. There is no rationale for clamping intrathoracic drains.
- Withdraw the drain and close the wound with steri-strips. *Do not* use a purse-string suture, as this will result in a permanent, disfiguring scar.
- Arrange a chest X-ray after drain removal.

# PERICARDIAL ASPIRATION

This is performed if cardiac tamponade, usually due to pneumopericardium, occurs.

## Technique

- Use a 23 G needle attached to a 10-mL syringe and three-way tap.
- Clean the skin overlying the xiphisternum and subxiphoid area.
- Puncture the skin to the left of the xiphisternum and angle the needle upwards at 45°. Aim for the tip of the left scapula and advance the needle, aspirating continuously. The pericardium is entered at a depth of 1 cm.
- Observe the ECG monitor for signs of myocardial injury.
- Once the pericardium is entered, air or fluid is withdrawn. *Note that if it is possible to withdraw limitless amounts of blood, the ventricle has been entered.*

## INTRACARDIAC INJECTION

The entry point and landmarks are the same as for pericardial aspiration. The needle is inserted until blood is easily aspirated. When the myocardium is reached, pulsation can be felt through the needle and syringe.

NB In resuscitation from cardiac arrest, it is possible to give adrenaline by the endotracheal route.

> initial i.v./intracardiac bolus, 10 mcg/kg, (0.1 mL/kg 1:10 000 adrenaline);
> initial endotracheal bolus, 100 mcg/kg, (0.1 mL/kg 1:1000 adrenaline).

There is little convincing evidence that intracardiac adrenaline is more efficacious in the treatment of cardiac arrest than i.v. adrenaline. There is also no evidence that endotracheal bolus is effective.

## CARDIAC MASSAGE

Ensure that an adequate airway is established and positive pressure ventilation with 100% oxygen is being given.

The landmark for cardiac compression in infants is one finger-breadth below a line joining the two nipples.

## Technique

- Compressions can be given using the index and middle fingers of one hand, or by encircling the chest with both hands and applying pressure with the thumbs (see Fig. 27.4).
- Compress the chest wall to a depth of 1.5–2.5 cm at a rate of 120 compressions/min. Co-ordinate cardiac compressions with ventilated breaths in a ratio of 3–5:1.

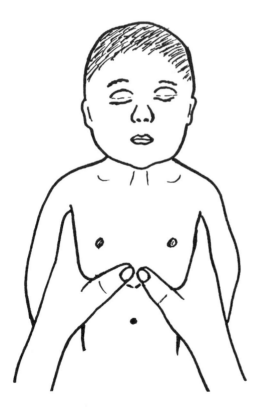

**Fig. 27.4** Hand encircling method of cardiac compression in the neonate.

## LUMBAR PUNCTURE

### Technique

- The infant is placed on his or her side and held firmly at the buttocks and shoulders, so that the lower spine is curved outwards. Care must be taken to keep the neck straight, in order not to cause airway obstruction during the procedure, and to keep the spine horizontal.
- Prepare a sterile field and drape the area with sterile towels.
- Use a 22 G LP needle with trocar. Use of a 25 G butterfly needle carries the risk of causing implantation dermoid cysts.
- Using the iliac crests as a guide, insert the needle between the L3 and L4 spinous process and advance it in the direction of the umbilicus.
- Sometimes a slight 'pop' is felt as the needle enters the subarachnoid space. The internal stilette should be withdrawn frequently and the needle gently rotated to check for CSF flow. It is easy to push the needle too far and enter the anterior vertebral venous plexus.
- Once in the subarachnoid space, CSF should be collected into two or three sterile containers, depending on individual laboratory requirements.
- After removal of the needle, swab the area with collodion and cover with a small adhesive dressing.

## VENTRICULAR TAP

*This should only be carried out by experienced staff.*

### Technique

- Have an assistant firmly hold the baby supine with the nose upwards and the neck and face parallel to the mattress.
- Mark the four corners of the anterior fontanelle with an ink marker and as accurately as possible estimate the midline of the fontanelle. Measure 6 mm to one side of the midline, in the line of the coronal suture. This is the point of entry.
- Using a full sterile technique, pass a 22 G 4- or 5-cm LP needle through the marked point and advance it horizontally – and

parallel to the midline axis – for a distance of 4 to 5 cm. Do not insert the needle beyond the level of the mid-point of the eye.
- Always insert and withdraw the needle along the same track. Before reinserting the needle after a dry tap, always withdraw the needle fully and use a new needle each time.

## SUBDURAL TAP

*This should only be carried out by experienced staff.*
The subdural space is entered with a 22 G LP needle at the lateral angle of the anterior fontanelle. Use a guard on the needle to limit insertion to 5 mm. As soon as the 'give' is felt (penetration of the dura) the stilette is withdrawn. If fluid is present it will flow out but may be viscid, so the flow may be very slow.

NB *Do not* attach a syringe and aspirate subdural fluid.

## INTRAMUSCULAR INJECTIONS

The preferred injection site is the the lateral aspect of the thigh. Avoid the buttock. Do not give repeated i.m. injections, as these may cause fibrosis of the muscles.

Gently grasp a fold of skin and muscle between thumb and forefinger. Use a 25 G needle and insert it at right angles to the skin. Before injecting, attempt to withdraw to ensure that you have not entered a blood vessel. Inject steadily and withdraw the needle.

## SUPRAPUBIC BLADDER TAP

### Technique

- This should be performed at least 1 hour after the last wet nappy.
  Ultrasound scan may be used to identify a full bladder, but scanning runs the risk of inducing micturition.
- Use a 23 G needle attached to a 5-mL syringe.
- Have an assistant hold the infant firmly, immobilizing the legs and pelvis.

- Cleanse the area with an antiseptic solution and insert the needle in the midline, just superior to the pubic symphysis.
- Advance the needle at right angles to the skin. The bladder is entered at a depth of 1–2 cm. Do not insert the needle more than 2 cm.
- After withdrawing the needle, cover the area with a small adhesive dressing.

## ABDOMINAL PARACENTESIS

This can be performed via a midline or a lateral approach.

### Midline approach
The bladder must be empty before proceeding – check with ultrasound. A 21 G needle is inserted vertically through the abdominal wall 1–2 cm below the umbilicus.

### Lateral approach
The needle is inserted into either iliac fossa, keeping well lateral to the rectus muscle, as the inferior epigastric artery runs just underneath its lateral border. Take care to avoid enlarged liver or spleen.

## BONE MARROW ASPIRATION

*This should only be carried out by experienced staff.*

### Site

There are three possible sites for this procedure:

- tibia;
- anterior iliac crest;
- posterior iliac crest.

### Technique

- Use a full aseptic technique.
- Use a 19 G butterfly needle with syringe attached.

### Tibia

1 Hold the tibia firmly with the knee flexed.

**2** Enter the bone marrow at an angle perpendicular to the skin, just below and medial to the tibial tuberosity.

### Anterior iliac crest

**1** Hold the infant firmly in the supine position.
**2** Locate the iliac crest by palpation, and enter at an angle perpendicular to the skin.

### Posterior iliac crest

**1** Hold the infant in the lumbar puncture position.
**2** Enter the posterior iliac crest at right angles to the skin.

## PERITONEAL DIALYSIS

This should only be attempted in non-specialist centres when the infant is too sick to move or there are compelling contraindications to travel. Figure 27.5 shows one type of closed dialysis system which has proved effective.

### Equipment needed

Peritoneal cannula (either Cooks neonatal or neonatal Tenchkoff catheter), 1.36% and 6.36% glucose dialysis solutions (e.g. Diaflex 61 and 62), dialysis set (neonatal Kimal) and water bath at 37°C.

## Procedure

Catheterize bladder. Choose a site that avoids enlarged organs – usually the flank, level with the umbilicus and lateral to the mid-inguinal line (to avoid the inferior epigastric artery). Full aseptic technique is required. Cleanse the skin and infiltrate the site with 1% lignocaine. Introduce a 19 G butterfly needle into the peritoneum and run in 20–30mL of warmed 1.36% dialysate to fill the abdomen. Make a small scalpel incision to facilitate the introduction of the cannula. Insert guidewire through a suitable plastic cannula, withdraw cannula and introduce the peritoneal dialysis catheter over the guidewire. Ensure that there is free flow of fluid in and out of the peritoneal cavity. Run 20–30 mL/kg fluid in and out of the abdomen until the effluent is clear of blood, then 2 cycles/hour. Use 1.36% solution initially, but if a negative balance is not achieved, or if the infant is fluid overloaded, use equal volumes of 1.36% and 6.36% mixed in the filling burette. Add heparin, 500 units/L to dialysate bags until blood staining clears, and add 2–4 mmol KCl per litre if plasma $K^+$ is < 3.0 mmol/L.

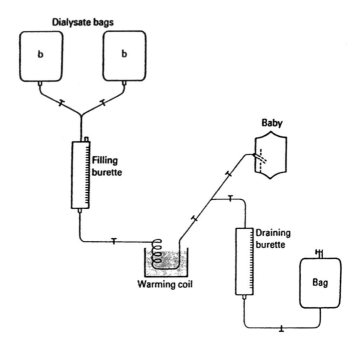

**Fig. 27.5** Diagram showing closed system for performing peritoneal dialysis in infants.

## HAEMOFILTRATION

This is a simple effective alternative to peritoneal dialysis, and may be utilized in infants in whom the abdomen cannot be used for peritoneal dialysis, e.g. post abdominal surgery, or in the presence of severe necrotizing enterocolitis. As with peritoneal dialysis, it should only be performed in a centre with the necessary local expertise.

Various sites may be used for vascular access and, although the umbilical vein and artery most reliably provide adequate transmembrane pressure gradients, femoral, brachial and jugular access may be used. Cannulae of 18–24 gauge (3.5–5 FG) will provide adequate flow. The total extracorporeal circulating volume using the Amicon minifilter is 12 mL (6 mL filter/6 mL lines). Heparinization is required, and although the standard dose of 40 units/kg followed by

10 units/kg/hour is appropriate for most patients, this can be reduced to a loading dose of 10 units/kg and maintenance dose of 5 units/kg/hour, in the presence of increased susceptibility to bleeding. The average ultrafiltration rate that is achievable is 1–2 mL/min, which would be expected to provide, in addition to ultrafiltration, adequate solute clearance for all but the most catabolic of infants. The techniques include arteriovenous haemofiltration (with or without dialysis) and pump-driven veno-venous haemofiltration. They cannot be applied to the tiniest infants, in view of the need for an extracorporeal circuit with inadequate flow rates and which is large relative to the baby's blood volume. A technique of manually operated veno-venous syringe-driven haemofiltration has been described for infants of less than 1000 g birthweight.

## BIBLIOGRAPHY

Advanced Life Support Group (1997) *Advanced Paediatric Life Support*: London: BMJ Publishing Group.

Wilkinson, A. and Calvert, S. (1992) Procedures in neonatal intensive care. In Roberton, N.R.C. (ed.) *Textbook of neonatology*, 2nd edn. Edinburgh. Churchill Livingstone, 1167–89.

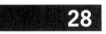

# Drugs and prescribing

Drugs in pregnancy and their effects on the fetus
Prescribing to breast-feeding mothers
Blood and blood products
Neonatal drug doses and administration

## DRUGS IN PREGNANCY AND THEIR EFFECTS ON THE FETUS

Although only a few drugs have been shown to be definitely teratogenic, no drug should be regarded as completely safe, particularly during the first trimester. After the embryonic stage of development, drugs may have toxic side-effects on the fetus, influencing growth and development. Drugs given shortly before delivery may carry over their effects into the newborn period. Remember that not all drugs are prescribed; self-medication is common and drug abuse is an increasing problem. Table 28.1 lists some of the drugs for which adverse effects are known or suspected. In some cases the benefits of maternal medication may outweigh the risk to the fetus, e.g., malarial prophylaxis or anticonvulsant therapy.

## PRESCRIBING TO BREAST-FEEDING MOTHERS

Most drugs are excreted in breast milk, but are usually present in tiny amounts that are unlikely to harm the child (see references in

**Table 28.1** The effects on the fetus and neonate of maternal drugs during pregnancy (for a more detailed list see *British National Formulary*)

| Drug | Possible effect on fetus and neonate |
| --- | --- |
| Alcohol | Fetal alcohol syndrome (see Chapter 1) |
| Aminoglycosides | Eighth nerve damage |
| Aminophylline | Neonatal irritability |
| Aminodarone | Goitre |
| Anticoagulants (oral) | Malformations; fetal and neonatal haemorrhage |
| Antimalarials | Possibly teratogenic |
|    Primaquine | Haemolysis; methaemoglobinaemia |
|    Pyrimethamine | Possibly teratogenic |
|    Quinine | Teratogenic in high doses |
| Aspirin | Fetal and neonatal haemorrhage; rash; kernicterus; metabolic acidosis. High doses could close ductus arteriosus in the fetus |
| β-adrenoceptor blockers | Hypoglycaemia; bradycardia |
| Barbiturates | Neonatal withdrawal syndrome (see Chapter 5) |
| Benzodiazepines | Respiratory depression; hypotonia; hypothermia |
| Carbimazole | Goitre; hypothyroidism |
| Chloramphenicol | Grey-baby syndrome |
| Clofibrate | Reduced fetal growth |
| Corticosteroids | High doses may cause adrenal suppression |
| Cytotoxic drugs | Teratogenic; possible immune suppression |
| Diazoxide | Impaired glucose tolerance |
| Diuretics | Reduce placental perfusion |
| Ergotamine | Oxytocic effects, vomiting, convulsions |
| Flucytosine | Possibly teratogenic |
| Indomethacin | Closure of fetal ductus arteriosus and persistent pulmonary hypertension |
| Iodides | Goitre; hypothyroidism |
| Local anaesthetics | Large doses may cause respiratory depression, hypotonia and bradycardia |
| Lithium | Malformations; goitre; hypertonia and cyanosis |
| Narcotics | Respiratory depression; withdrawal syndrome |
| Naproxen | This and other non-steroidal anti-inflammatory drugs have the same effects as indomethacin |
| Phenobarbitone | Malformations; fetal and neonatal haemorrhage (see Chapter 1 and Chapter 19); sedation |
| Phenothiazine derivatives | Occasional extrapyramidal effects |
| Phenytoin | Malformation; fetal and neonatal haemorrhage (Chapter 1 and Chapter 19) |

**Table 28.1** Continued

| | |
|---|---|
| Podophyllum | Possibly teratogenic; neonatal death |
| Propylthiouracil | Goitre; hypothyroidism |
| Radioiodine | Destruction of fetal thyroid |
| Reserpine | Bradycardia; nasal stuffiness |
| Rifampicin | Neonatal haemorrhage |
| Sex hormones | Virilization of female fetus (see Chapter 16); possibly teratogenic |
| Stilboestrol | Vaginal carcinoma |
| Sulphasalazine | Haemolysis and jaundice |
| Sulphonamides | Haemolysis and methaemoglobinaemia; risk of kernicterus |
| Sulphonylureas | Hypoglycaemia |
| Tetracyclines | Retarded skeletal growth; enamel hypoplasia and stained teeth |
| Thiazides | Thrombocytopenia |
| Tricyclic antidepressants | Tachycardia; irritability; muscle spasms |
| Trimethoprim (and co-trimoxazole) | Possibly teratogenic; same effects as sulphonamides |
| Valproate sodium | Possibly teratogenic (neural tube defects; see Chapter 1) |

footnote to Table 28.2). Studies have tended to use only a single dose, which does not reflect clinical use. The newborn metabolize and excrete drugs very inefficiently. Preterm babies are at greater risk. Where practicable, all drugs should be avoided during breast feeding, and mothers should be warned about self-medication. Recommendations for a nursing mother are probably over-cautious, and mothers who need treatment should not be prevented from breast feeding if the drug is likely to be safe. Drugs that are known to have produced adverse effects include cancer chemotherapy drugs, radiopharmaceuticals, carbimazole, lithium, ergotamine and phenindione. Others are relatively contraindicated because they reach high concentrations in milk and/or have effects which could harm the infant.

Table 28.2 gives information on drugs which nursing mothers *can* use. It includes at least one drug for each condition likely to require medication.

**Table 28.2** Drugs and breast feeding

| Category (as in BNF) | Drugs which may be used | Comments* |
|---|---|---|
| **(1) Gastrointestinal** | | |
| Antacids | Aluminium hydroxide, magnesium carbonate and trisilicate | Little absorbed by mother |
| Antispasmodics | Mebeverine; propantheline | |
| Ulcer-healing drugs | Cimetidine ⎱ Ranitidine ⎰ | Significant amounts enter milk, but safety is not known |
| | Sucralfate | Not absorbed by mother |
| | De-Nol | Absorption of bismuth too low to cause harm |
| Antidiarrhoeals | Kaolin | Not absorbed |
| | Codeine phosphate | Prolonged use of high doses could constipate and sedate infant, and cause dependence* |
| | Loperamide | Mother absorbs little |
| | Sulphasalazine | Risk of haemolysis in glucose-6-phosphate dehydrogenase-deficient infants, and of kernicterus in jaundiced infants* |
| Laxatives | Bran, methylcellulose | Not absorbed by mother |
| | Bisacodyl; senna | Large doses could cause diarrhoea in baby* |
| **(2) Cardiovascular** | | |
| Cardiac glycosides | Digoxin | Minimal amounts in milk Excretion of other glycosides unknown |
| β-Adrenoceptor | Atenolol; metaprolol; nadalol; oxprenolol; propranolol; sotalol | Look for signs of beta-blockade in infant (bradycardia, hypoglycaemia) if mother is on a large dose |
| Antihypertensives | Labetalol; methyldopa; hydralazine | |
| Diuretics | Bendrofluazide; chlorothiazide Frusemide (orally) | May decrease milk production Avoid parenteral use |
| Anticoagulants | Heparin | Not present in milk |
| | Warfarin | No apparent effect on infant's haemostasis |

**Table 28.2** Continued

| | | |
|---|---|---|
| Haemostatics | Tranexamic acid; ethamsylate | Present in milk |

### (3) Respiratory system and allergy

| | | |
|---|---|---|
| Bronchodilators | Salbutamol; isoprenaline | Use by inhalation if possible |
| | Theophylline; aminophylline | Can make infant irritable |
| Corticosteroids Anti-asthmatics | Beclomethasone Sodium cromoglycate | Preferable to oral corticosteroids |
| Antihistamines (H₁) | Chlorpheniramine; promethazine; clemastine | Infant may become drowsy |
| Nasal decongestants | Ephedrine; pseudoephedrine; xylometazoline | Irritability and disturbed sleep reported with *oral* ephedrine |
| Cough suppressants | Codeine; pholcodine | Small doses are safe (see Section 1 above). |

### (4) Central nervous system

| | | |
|---|---|---|
| Hypnotics and sedatives | Benzodiazepines | Drowsiness and poor feeding occur with regular use or high doses |
| | Chloral hydrate; dichloralphenazone | May cause drowsiness |
| Antipsychotics | Chlorpromazine; fluphenazine; flupenthixol; haloperidol | Little in milk. Drowsiness and other CNS effects* may occur with high oral doses or parenteral preparations |
| Antidepressants | Amitriptyline; imipramine; mianserin | Very little in milk |
| Anti-emetics | Metoclopramide | Very little in milk |
| | Cyclizine; promethazine | Risk of drowsiness* |
| Anticonvulsants | Carbamazepine; phenytoin; phenobarbitone; primidone | May cause drowsiness. Control maternal blood levels closely |
| | Sodium valproate | Very little in milk |
| | Ethosuximide | Significant amounts in milk |
| Analgesics Non-narcotic | Paracetamol Aspirin | Safe for occasional use. Dosage exceeding 3 g/day risks metabolic acidosis. Regular use could affect platelet function and prolong the bleeding time* |

**Table 28.2** Continued

| | | |
|---|---|---|
| Narcotic | Codeine Dihydrocodeine; pethidine; morphine | Avoid prolonged use of high doses; monitor infant for CNS depression |
| **(5) Infections** | | |
| Antibacterials | Penicillins; cephalosporins; aminoglycosides | Induction of hypersensitivity* possible. Intestinal bacteria could develop resistance* |
| | Erythromycin; trimethoprim | Significant amounts of milk |
| | Sulphonamides | Avoid in glucose-6-phosphate dehydrogenase-deficient infants |
| | Co-trimoxazole | Risk of kernicterus in jaundiced infants* |
| | Metronidazole | Makes milk taste bitter and child may stop suckling. Where single-dose therapy is suitable, a 24-hour break in breast feeding may avoid this |
| Urinary tract | Nitrofurantoin | Avoid in glucose-6-phosphate dehydrogenase-deficient infants* |
| Antituberculous | Rifampicin | Present in milk but not known to cause harm |
| | Isoniazid | Significant amounts in milk. Risk of neurotoxicity.* Mother and baby should be given pyridoxine |
| | Ethambutol | Very little in milk. Risk of ocular toxicity* |
| Antifungals | Nystatin | Not absorbed from gut. Safety of systemic antifungals (amphotericin, flucytosine, miconazole, etc.) unknown |
| Antimalarials | Chloroquine and proguanil | For prophylaxis |
| | Pyrimethamine | Avoid Maloprim and Fansidar in glucose-6-phosphate dehydrogenase-dependent infants* |
| Anthelmintics | Mebendazole | Poorly absorbed from the gut |
| **(6) Endocrine system** | | |
| Antidiabetics | Insulins Glibenclamide | Possible hypoglycaemia,* monitor infant's blood glucose |

**Table 28.2** Continued

| | | |
|---|---|---|
| Thyroid hormones | Thyroxine | Might interfere with screening of infant for hypothyroidism* |
| Antithyroid drugs | Propylthiouracil | Probably too little in milk to affect infant, but use propanolol instead if possible |
| Corticosteroids | Prednisolone | Probably safe in doses not exceeding 10 mg/day. Larger doses might cause adrenal suppression* |
| Sex hormones | | |
| Oestrogens | Ethinyloestradiol | Doses above 50 mcg/day decrease milk production and may cause feminization in male infants |
| *Oral* contraceptives | Combined oestrogen/ progestogen | Established lactation is not affected by low-dose preparations (< 50 mcg ethinyloestradiol) |
| | Progestogen only | Does not suppress lactation. Too little in milk to affect baby |

**(7) Vitamins and minerals**

| | | |
|---|---|---|
| Vitamins | Vitamin A | High doses (> 2500 units daily) risk hypervitaminosis |
| | Vitamin D | High doses (> 500 units daily) risk hypervitaminosis |
| | Vitamin B group Ascorbic acid Folic acid | |
| Iron salts | Ferrous sulphate, etc. | |

**(8) Musculoskeletal system**

| | | |
|---|---|---|
| Anti-inflammatory analgesics | Naproxen; ibuprofen Ketoprofen; mefenamic acid; fenbufen | Very little in milk |

* Indicates a theoretical risk.
BNF, *British National Formulary*. Information about specific drugs (especially if marketed recently) can often be obtained from the manufacturer or the NHS Drug Information Centres. The BNF gives further information about drugs contraindicated during breast feeding.

## BLOOD AND BLOOD PRODUCTS

It is essential that all blood and blood products are tested and shown to be negative for cytomegalovirus, hepatitis B, C and HIV before administration.

### Human albumin solution 4.5%

- 10–15 mL/kg i.v. as a volume expander for treating hypotension.
- 30 mL/kg i.v. for dilutional exchange.

### Blood

- Volume for transfusion = body weight in kg × required rise in Hb × F:
  where F = 6 for 'whole blood' (PCV = 40%);
  4 for 'partially packed cells' (PCV = 60%);
  3 for 'packed cells' (PCV = 80%).
- Six mL of donor whole blood (3 mL of packed cells) per kg body weight will raise the haemoglobin of the baby by 1 g/100 mL.
- For very preterm babies who may need several transfusions, a multi-pack system collected from a single donor is recommended.

### Platelets

- One unit of platelets will raise the peripheral platelet count by approximately 50 000 (give no more than 20 mL/kg).

### Plasma (fresh frozen)

- For dilutional exchange, 30 mL/kg (HAS 4.5% can be used as an alternative).

*Comment*: whole blood/packed cells/platelets should be given using a syringe pump or volumetric infusion pump, but *never* by peristaltic infusion pump.

# NEONATAL DRUG DOSES AND ADMINISTRATION

**Table 28.3** Suggested neonatal drug doses and administration

| Drug | Single dose/kg | Frequency | Route | Comments |
|---|---|---|---|---|
| Acetazolamide | 5 mg | 12-hourly | Oral; i.v. | As a diuretic |
| Acetylcysteine | 10 mL | 6-hourly | Gastric tube | 5% solution used in treatment of meconium ileus |
| | 20 mL | Daily | Enema | |
| Adenosine | 50 mcg | Once | i.v. fast bolus and flushed with saline | See Chapter 11 Repeat as required after 2 min with higher dose (100–250 mcg/kg) |
| Adrenaline | 0.5 mcg | Per minute | i.v. infusion | For severe hypotension (range 0.05–2 mcg/kg/min) |
| | 10 mcg | Once | i.v. | For cardiac arrest use 1:10 000. Can be repeated (see Chapter 11) |
| | 100 mcg | Once | Endotracheal | Higher doses may be required. May be repeated. Efficacy uncertain |
| Alfacalcidol (1-alpha-vitamin D) | 0.05 mcg | Daily | Oral | |
| Aminophylline | 6 mg | Loading dose | Oral; i.v. | Alter dose according to blood levels |
| | 2 mg | 12-hourly | | Therapeutic range for neonatal apnoea is 28–55 μmol/L |

| Atropine | 10 mcg | Once | i.v.; i.m. | Not used in neonatal resuscitation |
|---|---|---|---|---|
| Atracurium | 0.5 mg<br>5–10 mcg | Once<br>Per minute | i.v.<br>i.v. infusion | |
| Budesonide | 200–400 mcg per dose by metered dose inhalation | 12-hourly | Inhaled via spacer (e.g. Aerochamber) | |
| Caffeine citrate | 20 mg | Loading dose | i.v.; oral | i.v. dose over 20 min Therapeutic range is 25–100 μmol/L |
| | 5 mg | Daily maintenance | oral; i.v. | Plasma levels may persist for 7–9 days after stopping treatment |
| Calcium gluconate (10% solution) | 1–2 mL (0.2–0.4 mmol) | Once<br>8 hourly | Slow i.v. infusion<br>Oral | Use ECG monitoring |
| Captopril | 250–500 mcg<br>300 mcg | Once<br>8- to 12-hourly | Oral | Single test dose See manufacturer's literature |
| Carbamaza-pine | 5 mg | 12-hourly | Oral | Increase over 2 weeks to maximum of 15 mg/kg 12-hourly |
| Chloral hydrate | 45 mg | Once | Oral | Single hypnotic dose for EEG or CT scan |
| | 10–30 mg | 8-hourly PRN | Oral | |

**Table 28.3** Continued

| Chlorothiazide | 10 mg | 12-hourly | Oral | Usually given with spironolactone 1 mg/kg |
|---|---|---|---|---|
| Chlorproma-zine | 1 mg | 8-hourly | Oral | For drug withdrawal symptoms. Do not exceed total daily dose of 6 mg/kg |
| Cimetidine | 5 mg | 6-hourly | i.v. over 10 min | $H_2$ antagonist |
| Cisapride | 0.2–0.4 mg | 6- to 8-hourly | Oral – 30 min before feed | *Not* to be given with erythromycin or imidazole. milonazole or triazole anti-fungal agents |
| Dexametha-sone | 0.2 mg | 8-hourly | i.v.; oral | 7-day course for BPD. A further tapering 9-day course may be needed |
| | or 0.5 mg | Daily | | |
| Diazoxide | 5 mg | 12-hourly | Oral | $Na^+$ retention. Oedema. Hyperglycaemia |
| Diamorphine | 180 mcg | Once | i.v. | Loading dose |
| | 15 mcg | Hourly | i.v. infusion | Maintenance |
| Disopyramide | 2 mg | Once | i.v. | Loading |
| | 400 mcg | Hourly | i.v. infusion | Maintenance |
| | 1–2 mg | 8-hourly | Oral | |
| Digoxin | *Term baby* | | | Check blood levels. Toxicity uncommon below 3.5 ng/mL |
| | 5 mcg | 12-hourly | Oral | |
| | *Preterm baby* | | | |
| | 4 mcg | 12-hourly | Oral | |
| Dobutamine | 1–20 mcg | Per minute | Continuous i.v. infusion | Start with lowest dose (see Chapter 10) |

**Table 28.3** Continued

| Dopamine | 1–20 mcg | Per minute | Continuous i.v. infusion | Vasodilation of mesenteric, renal coronary and cerebral blood vessels at lower doses ($<$ 5 mcg/kg/min). Increased cardiac output and BP at higher doses with vasoconstriction ($>$ 5–10 mcg/kg/min). High dose may cause gangrene |
|---|---|---|---|---|
| Doxapram | 2.5 mg | Once | i.v. over 5–10 min | See *Pediatrics* (1987) **80**, 22 |
| | 0.3–1.5 mg | Per hour | i.v. infusion | |
| Edrophonium | 0.5 mg | Once | i.m./slow i.v. | Test for myasthenia. If causes bradycardia, antidote is atropine |
| Epoprostenol | 5–20 ng | Per minute | Continuous i.v. infusion | Beware of hypotension. Change infusion every 24 hours. Doses up to 40 ng/kg/min may be used |
| Ethamsylate | 12.5 mg | 6-hourly for 16 doses | i.m.; i.v. | To reduce risk of cerebral haemorrhage in preterm baby |
| Fentanyl | 15 mcg | Once | i.v. | Loading dose |
| | 5 mcg | Hourly | Continuous i.v. infusion | Tolerance and withdrawal develop if treat-ment continues for more than 3 days |

**Table 28.3** Continued

| | | | | |
|---|---|---|---|---|
| Flecainide | 1–2 mg<br>2–3 mg | 8-hourly<br>8-hourly | i.v. over 30 min⎫<br>Oral ⎭ | Unpredictable.<br>Measure levels |
| 9-α-Fludro-<br>cortisone | 0.05 mg total<br>dose | Daily | Oral | See Chapter 16 |
| Gaviscon | One dose<br>(half dual<br>sachet) | With each feed | Oral | Babies of > 5 kg.<br>Not<br>recommended<br>for preterm<br>babies, but half<br>a sachet has<br>been used |
| Glucagon | 200 mcg | Once | i.v.; i.m. | Starting dose.<br>May cause<br>rebound<br>hypoglycaemia |
| | 0.3 mcg | Per minute | i.v. infusion | |
| Glyceryl<br>trinitrate | 1–10 mcg | Per minute | i.v. infusion | |
| Heparin | 100 units<br>50 units<br>25 units | 12-hourly<br>Loading dose<br>Per hour | i.v.<br>Infusion | Modify dose<br>according to<br>clotting studies |
| Hepatitis B<br>vaccine | 10 ng<br>(0.5 mL) | Once | i.m. | Within 24 hours of<br>birth. Repeat at<br>1 and 6 months<br>(see Chapter<br>17) |
| Hydro-<br>cortisone | 2.5 mg | 6-hourly | i.v.; i.m. | Maintenance dose.<br>Physiological<br>dose 1 mg/kg/<br>hour infusion |
| | 25 mg | Once | i.v. | For shock |
| Hydralazine | 0.5 mg | 8-hourly | Oral; i.m.; i.v. | Modify dose<br>according to<br>response.<br>Beware of<br>hypotension.<br>Maximum 2–3<br>mg/kg every 8<br>hours |

**Table 28.3** Continued

| Indomethacin | 0.1 mg | 24-hourly to a maximum of 6 doses | i.v.; oral | For closure of PDA. Renal toxicity |
|---|---|---|---|---|
| Insulin | 0.1 unit | According to blood glucose levels | s.c.; i.m.; i.v. infusion | Beware hypoglycaemia. Neonatal diabetes (0.5–3.0 units/kg/daily) |
| | 0.3–0.6 units | Per hour | i.v. infusion (+ glucose infusion) | Hyperkalaemia |
| Ipratropium bromide | 40–80 mcg per dose (by metered dose inhaler) | 6- to 8-hourly | Inhalation by spacer device (e.g. Aerochamber) | |
| | 0.25–1.0 mL (250 mcg/mL solution) diluted to 4 mL | 4- to 6-hourly | Nebulized | |
| Isoprenaline | 5 mcg | Once | i.v. bolus | For bradycardia and hypotension |
| | 0.02–1.0 mcg | Per minute | Continuous i.v. infusion | |
| Lignocaine | 1–2 mg | Once | i.v. slowly | For cardiac arrythmia and convulsions |
| | 20 mcg | Per minute | Continuous i.v. infusion | |
| | 3 mg (0.3 mL of 1% solution) | Once | s.c. | Local analgesia |
| Magnesium sulphate (50% solution) | 0.2 mL | 12-hourly (maximum of 3 doses) | i.m.; oral | For hypomagnesaemia and hypocalcaemia |
| | 250 mg | Once | i.v. over 10 min | Loading dose for PPH (see Chapter 10) |
| | 20 mg | Per hour | i.v. infusion | |

**Table 28.3** Continued

| | | | | |
|---|---|---|---|---|
| Mannitol | 1 g | Once | i.v. infusion over 30 min | For management of cerebral oedema (see Chapter 12) |
| Methyldopa | 2.5 mg | 8-hourly | Oral; i.v. | Increase up to 5 mg/kg according to response |
| Midazolam | 150 mcg 50–200 mcg | Once Hourly | i.v. i.v. infusion | Loading dose Halve infusion rate after 24 hours in < 33 weeks' post-conceptional age. Probably safe for 4 days |
| Morphine | 0.1 mg 5–20 mcg | Once Per hour | i.v. i.v. continuous infusion | Loading dose For sedation of babies on ventilation |
| | 0.1 mg | 6-hourly | i.v.; i.m. | |
| | 50 mcg | Once | Orally | For opiate withdrawal. May be given repeatedly if weaning is required |
| Naloxone | 10 mcg | Once, but may be repeated at 2- to 3-min intervals | s.c.; i.v. | Narcan Neonatal contains 20 mcg/mL |
| | 100 mcg | Once | i.m. | 200 mcg (0.5 mL adult Narcan) for babies of > 1.5 kg and 100 mcg for babies of < 1500 g |
| Neostigmine | 0.04 mg 1 mg | Once 6-hourly | i.m. Oral | Myasthenia test Maintenance |

**Table 28.3** Continued

| | | | | |
|---|---|---|---|---|
| Nitroprusside (sodium) | 0.5 mcg | Per minute | Continuous i.v. infusion | Beware of severe hypotension and thiocyanate toxicity. Maximum infusion rate is 8 mcg/kg/min (Benitz et al. (1985) J. Pediatr. **106**, 102–10). |
| Noradrenaline | 0.05–1.0 mcg of noradrenaline base | Per minute | Continuous i.v. infusion | Through a central line. Noradrenaline acid tartrate 2 mg/mL has 1 mg/mL noradrenaline base |
| Octreotide/ somatostatin | 1–4 mcg | Daily | Subcutaneously | Maximum of 250 mcg. May need to increase to 8–12-hourly |
| | 3–5 mcg | Hourly | i.v. infusion | |
| Omeprazol | 0.4–0.8 mg / 2 mg / 1 mg | Daily / Once / 8- to 12-hourly | Oral / i.v. / i.v. | Maximum 40 mg / Loading dose / Maintenance dose |
| Pancuronium | 50–100 mcg | As required | i.v. | |
| Paracetamol | 24 mg | 8-hourly | Oral | |
| Paraldehyde | 0.1 mL / 0.3 mL / 1 mL of 5% solution made up in 5% glucose | Once / / Per hour | Deep i.m. / Rectal / Continuous i.v. infusion. Change syringe every 12 hours | Use glass syringe With olive oil Up to 3 mL/kg/ hour may be needed to control status epilepticus. Protect from light |
| Pethidine | 1 mg | 12-hourly | i.m. | Beware respiratory depression |

**Table 28.3** Continued

| | | | | |
|---|---|---|---|---|
| Phenobarbitone | 10 mg | 2 doses, 30 min apart | i.v. over 5–10 min | see Chapter 12 for control of convulsions |
| | 2 mg | 12-hourly | i.m.; oral | Maintenance |
| Phenytoin | 20 mg | Once | i.v. over 15 min | Monitor ECG, may cause arrhythmia. See Chapter 12 for control of convulsions |
| | 2.5 mg | 12-hourly | Oral | Maintenance |
| Prednisolone | 0.5 mg | 6-hourly | Oral; i.m.; i.v. | |
| Propranolol | 0.05 mg | Once | i.v. | For hypertension |
| | 0.1 mg | Once | i.v. | For supraventricular tachycardia. *Caution.* |
| | 0.2–0.5 mg | 8-hourly | Oral | Maintenance. May need to increase dose to 1.5 mg/kg/dose or frequency to 6-hourly |
| Prostaglandin $E_1$ | 10 ng | Per minute | Continuous i.v. infusion | $E_1$ and $E_2$ are equally effective at identical doses, but $E_2$ is cheaper (see Chapter 11) |
| Protamine | 1 mg/100 units of last dose of heparin | Once | i.v. | |
| Pyridoxine | 50 mg total dose | Once | i.v. | Pyridoxine dependency |
| Ranitidine | 0.5 mg | 8-hourly | Oral; i.v. | |

**Table 28.3** Continued

| Salbutamol | 4 mcg | Over 5 min | i.v. | For hyperkalaemia |
| | 2.5 mg nebule (total dose irrespective of weight) | 8-hourly | Nebulized | For chronic lung disease |
| Sodium benzoate | 500 mcg | Per day | i.v. or oral | Acute hyperammonaemia |
| | 250 mcg | Per day delivered in small doses | Oral | |
| Spironolactone | 1 mg | 12-hourly | Oral | |
| Theophylline | 5 mg | Once | Oral; i.v. | Loading dose |
| | 1–2 mg | 8-hourly | Oral; i.v. | Adjust dose according to blood levels |
| Thyroxine | *Preterm* 8–10 mcg *Term* 5-8 mcg | Daily | Oral | See Chapter 16 |
| Tolazoline | 1 mg | Once | i.v. over 1–2 min | Beware of hypotension, G-I bleeding |
| | 0.1 mg | Per hour | Continuous i.v. infusion | May increase infusion rate to 0.5 mg/kg/hour according to response |
| Vecuronium | 100 mcg | Once | i.v. | |
| | 50–150 mcg | Hourly | i.v. infusion | |
| Vitamins | | | | See Chapter 13 |
| **ANTIBIOTICS** | | | | |
| Amikacin | 10 mg | Once | i.v. | Loading dose |
| | 7.5 mg | 12-hourly | i.v. | |
| Amoxycillin | 50 mg | 12-hourly 8-hourly after first week | oral; i.v.; i.m. | |

**Table 28.3** Continued

| Ampicillin | 50 mg | < 7 days old, 12-hourly<br><br>> 7 days old, 8-hourly<br>> 28 days old, 6-hourly | Oral; i.m.; i.v. | 100 mg/kg/ 8-hourly for meningitis |
|---|---|---|---|---|
| Azlocillin | *Preterm*<br>50 mg | < 37 weeks, 12-hourly | i.v. | Must not be mixed in same syringe or infusion as aminoglycosides |
| | *Term*<br>100 mg | < 7 days old, 12-hourly<br>> 7 days old, 8-hourly | i.v. | |
| Flucloxacillin | 25 mg | < 7 days old. 12-hourly<br>> 7 days old, 8-hourly<br>> 28 days old, 6-hourly | Oral; i.m.; i.v. | 50–100 mg for severe infection |
| Cefotaxime | 25 mg | < 7 days old, 12-hourly<br><br>> 7 days old, 8-hourly<br>> 28 days old, 6-hourly | i.m.; i.v. | In severe infections 50 mg/kg/day may be given |
| Ceftazidime | 25 mg | 12-hourly | i.m.; i.v. | 50 mg/kg for meningitis |
| Cefuroxime | 25 mg | 12-hourly | i.m.; i.v. | 100 mg/kg/day should be given for meningitis |

**Table 28.3** Continued

| Chloramphenicol | 25 mg | All infants < 14 days old, 24-hourly

>14 days old, 12-hourly | Oral; i.v. | Always monitor blood level. Therapeutic range 15–25 mg/L. Toxic level 50 mg/L. Infants' total daily dose should not exceed 25 mg/kg for infants of < 2.0 kg, regardless of age |
|---|---|---|---|---|
| Ciprofloxacin | 5 mg | 12-hourly | Oral; i.v. | Not recommended in children, but use may sometimes be justified |
| Erythromycin | 15 mg | 6- to 8-hourly depending on severity of infection | Oral; i.v. | Excreted by liver, so use with caution in presence of jaundice or immaturity |
| Fucidic acid | 5 mg | 6-hourly | Oral; i.v. | For i.v. use, dissolve powder in buffer provided and infuse dose over 6 hours |
| Gentamicin | 2.5 mg

4 mg
5 mg | *Preterm and term* < 7 days old, 12-hourly *Daily* < 35 weeks > 35 weeks | i.m.; i.v. | Montior blood levels. Peak 4–8 mcg/mL. Trough < 2 mcg/mL |
| Isoniazid | 5 mg | 12-hourly | Oral | Pyridoxine supplement should be given |

**Table 28.3** Continued

| | | | | |
|---|---|---|---|---|
| Metronidazole | 7.5 mg | 8-hourly | Oral; i.v. | |
| Netilmicin | 3 mg | *For preterm and term infants < 7 days old,* 12-hourly | i.m.; i.v. | Monitor blood levels. Peaks 6–12 mcg/mL. Trough < 2.5 mcg/mL |
| | | *For term infants > 7 days old,* 8-hourly | | |
| | 4 mg | Daily | i.m.; i.v. | |
| Penicillin G (benzyl-penicillin) | 30 mg | < 7 days old, 12-hourly | i.m.; i.v. | If meningitis, give 60 mg/kg dose (= 100 000 U/kg) |
| | | > 7 days old, 8-hourly | | |
| Rifampicin | 5 mg | 12-hourly | Oral | Use with caution in jaundiced infants |
| Teicoplanin | 16 mg 8 mg | Loading dose Once daily | i.v. i.v. over 30 min | |
| Trimethoprim | 4 mg | 12-hourly | Oral | Not recommended in first 14 days |
| | 3 mg | 12-hourly | i.v. | |
| | 2 mg | Daily | Oral | Prophylaxis |
| Tobramycin | 2 mg | < 7 days old, 12-hourly | i.m.; i.v. | Monitor blood levels as for gentamicin |
| | | > 7 days old, 8-hourly | | |
| Vancomycin | 15 mg | 12-hourly | i.v. infusion over 1 hour | Monitor blood levels. Peak 25–40 mcg/mL. Trough 5–10 mcg/mL |
| | | < 28 weeks, 24-hourly | | |

**Table 28.3** Continued

## ANTIFUNGAL AGENTS

| | | | | |
|---|---|---|---|---|
| Amphotericin (liposomal) | 1.0 mg<br><br>May be increased to 3.0 mg/kg/day | Daily | i.v. over 1 hour | |
| Fluconazole | 6 mg | Every 3 days in 1–2 weeks<br>Every 2 days over 3 weeks | Oral; i.v. | |
| 5-Flucytosine | 50 mg | 6-hourly | Oral; i.v. | Usually given in combination with amphotericin |
| Miconazole | 10 mg | 12-hourly | i.v. infusion over 1 hour | Also available as 2% gel for oral or topical use |
| Nystatin | 100 000 units (1 mL) | 6-hourly | Oral (not absorbed from gastro-intestinal tract) | Also available as cream for topical use |
| Acyclovir | 10 mg | < 7 days old, 12-hourly<br>> 7 days old, 8-hourly | i.v.<br><br>i.v. | Over 1 hour |
| Zidovudine | 2.5 mg<br>180 mg/m$^2$ | 4-hourly<br>6-hourly | i.v.<br>Oral | |

## BIBLIOGRAPHY

American Academy of Pediatrics (1994) Transfer of drugs and other chemicals to human milk. *Pediatrics* **93**, 137–50.

British National Formulary (1997) No. 33 Prescribing in Pregnancy, p. 585. Prescribing during breast feeding, p. 595. London: British Medical Association and Royal Pharmaceutical Society of Great Britain.

Neonatal Formulary (1996) *Northern Neonatal Network*. London: BMJ Publishing Group.

## Units for drug doses

1 gram (g) = 1000 milligrams (mg)
1 milligram = 1000 micrograms (mcg)
1 microgram = 1000 nanograms (ng)

When prescribing doses in micrograms or nanograms, these should be written out in full and not abbreviated.

# Normal laboratory and physiological data

Normal values for laboratory investigations in the newborn
Drugs – therapeutic range
Normal physiological values in the newborn

## NORMAL VALUES FOR LABORATORY INVESTIGATIONS IN THE NEWBORN

### Clinical chemistry

*Test and reference range*          *Comment*

Alanine aminotransferase         Not always available as a routine
  9–44 IU/L                      test since it adds no more
                                 information than aspartate
                                 aminotransferase (*qv*).
                                 Haemolysis, lipaemia and
                                 turbidity interfere.


Albumin
  24–36 g/L at birth
  34–46 g/L at 0–3 months

Alkaline phosphatase
70–260 IU/L

Reference range depends on the method used and will vary in different hospitals. Serum is the preferred specimen. Anticonvulsants cause raised values, and transient hyperphosphatasaemia is well recognized in infancy. Activity increases on storage, and EDTA samples are not suitable (they bind magnesium/zinc). Although widely measured, it is of little value on its own.

Alpha-1-antitrypsin
0.8–1.8 g/L

Reference range based on UK Protein Reference Unit data. Older nephalometric methods give higher results. May be low in respiratory distress syndrome and low birthweight infants. The genotype should be assessed if the level is below 1.1 g/L in infants with prolonged jaundice.

Alpha-fetoprotein
13–86 mg/L at birth

Levels decline rapidly after birth; plasma half-life = 3.5 days. May remain increased in neonatal hepatitis, biliary atresia and tyrosinosis. May become elevated with certain tumours.

Amino acids
Approximate upper limit of
($\mu$mol/L)
0–21 days

Quantitation is usually performed to confirm an inborn error in which levels of individual acids may be up to 10 times higher. Minor increases are of doubtful significance and should not be a cause for concern except in infants undergoing treatment for a specific amino acid disorder. Interpretation is difficult, and may be impossible, in infants receiving hyperalimentation.

*30* Aspartic acid
Citrulline
Methionine

*100* Arginine
Glutamic acid
Histidine
Isoleucine
Phenylalanine
Taurine

*150* Cystine
Leucine
Ornithine
Serine
Threonine
Tyrosine

*200* Lysine
Valine

*300* Glycine
Proline

*400* Alanine

*500* Glutamine

Ammonia
10–40 μmol/L
(venous samples)

May rise to 150 μmol/L in capillary samples even when analysed within 30 min of collection

Arterial samples may be easier to interpret

EDTA sample is usually required. Ammonia continues to rise after sample collection, and rapid separation and analysis are essential. Thus this test must be arranged with the laboratory. Results may be up to 150 μmol/L in all sick infants, and are often raised in a number of organic acidaemias in addition to urea cycle disorders. This is an important, often under-requested, investigation in sick infants.

Anion gap
6–14 mmol/L

Calculated as the sum of sodium and potassium, less the sum of chloride and bicarbonate. A raised level is highly suggestive of the presence of an unmeasured organic acid anion, e.g. phosphate, lactate, methylmalonate, etc. Many laboratories do not measure chloride and bicarbonate.

Asparate aminotransferase
3–60 IU/L

Haemolysis causes elevated results. Turbidity and severe icterus interfere with laboratory methods. Laboratory method used will affect reference range.

Bicarbonate
18–22 mmol/L

Usually measured as total $CO_2$ liberated from plasma when included with other electrolytes; otherwise see notes on acid-base studies.

Bilirubin
1–12 hour, 15–115 μmol/L
12–24 hour, 20–170 μmol/L
24–48 hour, 10–180 μmol/L
76–96 hour, 20–170 μmol/L
1–4 weeks, 0–100 μmol/L
(see Fig. 18.1)

Increased values are caused by dextrans (technical) and lower values by phenobarbitone (pharmacological). Bilirubinometer results may correlate poorly with chemical methods in infants receiving phototherapy (see Chapter 18).

β-hydroxybutyrate
0.03–0.78 mmol/L

Usually measured with lactate (*qv*). May require special container or rapid separation of plasma and prior arrangement with the laboratory.

Calcium
*Breast fed*
  1 day, 1.77–2.29 mmol/L
  8 days, 1.72–2.64 mmol/L
*Artificial feeds*
  1 day, 1.88–2.28 mmol/L
  8 days, 2.14–2.46 mmol/L
  1–6 weeks, 2.25–2.80 mmol/L

Increased by thiazides and vitamin D and decreased by phenobarbitone, phenytoin and insulin. There is often a marked fall immediately after birth lasting for 2–3 days, especially in RDS, acidosis, hypoalbuminaemia and associated with maternal diabetes. Approximately half of the total calcium is ionized, but prediction of the true ionized fraction is not possible from the total concentration even if pH, protein and albumin concentrations are known, although a crude calculation for albumin concentration is helpful. Action is required if albumin-corrected calcium falls below 1.7 mmol/L (see Chapter 16).

Chloride
  92–109 mmol/L

Cholesterol
  1.0–5.6 mmol/L

Copper
  12–27 μmol

Cortisol
  150–700 nmol/L

There is a steady rise to the adult range of 280–700 nmol/L by the end of the first week of life. The reference range is markedly method-dependent.

| | |
|---|---|
| **Creatine kinase**<br>40–470 IU/L | Apparent activity is increased by haemolysis due to adenylate kinase. There is a rapid rise and fall in plasma activity in the first 3 days of life. Birth asphyxia causes a marked increase in all CK isoenzymes, mainly CK-MM. The reference range is dependent on the method used and the temperature of incubation. |
| **Creatinine**<br>28–60 μmol/L | Results in the newborn period are often unreliable for methodological reasons. |
| **Ferritin**<br>Birth, 65–395 μmol/L<br>2 weeks, 90–630 μmol/L<br>4 weeks, 140–400 μmol/L | Increased in haemolysis. Rapid changes occur in the neonatal period. |
| **Folic acid**<br>4–24 nmol/L | |
| **Gamma-glutamyl transferase**<br>0–260 IU/L | The reference range is dependent on the temperature at which the assay is performed. It is high at birth, with a steady predictable fall with age. This is a more interpretable enzyme than alkaline phosphatase in liver disease, except that it may be induced by some drugs such as anticonvulsants. |
| **Glucose**<br>Full-term, 2.8–4.5 mmol/L<br>Preterm, 1.7–3.6 mmol/L | Although lower concentrations may be found in premature or low-birthweight infants, their interpretation as 'normal' is debatable. A glucose concentration of less than 2 mmol/L is cause for concern at any gestation (see Chapter 16). |

17-Hydroxyprogesterone
  0–36 hours, < 50 nmol/L
  Subsequently, < 18 nmol/L

The sample must be separated promptly. It is usually best to arrange this test with laboratory staff. Premature infants may have higher results which remain high for longer than in full-term infants. Usually 200 nmol/L in CAH.

Immunoglobulins
*IgA*
  0–1 week, 0–0.10 g/L
  1–4 weeks, 0–0.20 g/L
*IgG*
  0–1 week, 5.0–17.0 g/L
  1–4 weeks, 4.0–13.0 g/L
*IgM*
  0–1 week, 0.1–0.2 gL
  1–4 weeks, 0.1–0.4 g/L

Based on data from the UK Protein Reference Unit.

Iron
  14–22 μmol/L

May be much higher at birth – up to 60 μmol/L – with a rapid fall in the first few hours, followed by a modest rise over the next few weeks. Ferritin is a more reliable index.

Lactate
  1.4–2.8 mmol/L

May be higher shortly after birth, falling into the reference range by the end of the first week. Requires prior arrangement with laboratory staff as plasma needs to be separated rapidly or may need a special container.

Magnesium
  0.7–1.0 mmol/L

May be lower at birth and in infants with RDS or macrosomia due to maternal diabetes. Haemolysis elevates values. Neuromuscular symptoms do not usually occur unless below 0.5 mmol/L.

Osmolality
  Plasma 270–285 mosmol/kg

Sodium salts are the principal contributors to osmolality. There are more than 20 formulae in the literature for calculation of osmolality from other parameters, but a figure representing twice the sodium concentration approximates to the true osmolality sufficiently well for practical purposes, provided that urea or glucose are not grossly raised, except in very premature infants where the usual relationships of sodium, water and renal tubular function may not hold.

Phosphate
  1.2–2.78 mmol/L

Affected by dietary intake and the type of milk feeds. Increased by haemolysis.

Potassium
  3.6–5.2 mmol/L

Usually higher in capillary samples – up to 6.6 mmol/L in newborn infants. Affected by haemolysis and elevated in acidosis.

Protein (total)
  54–74 g/L

Pyruvate
  Up to 120 μmol/L

May be measured with lactate (*qv*), but very unreliable and of doubtful value.

Sodium
  133–143 mmol/L

30% of very-low-birthweight infants may have a sodium level of less than 130 mmol/L. Concentration depends on intake. Term infants receiving 3 mmol/kg hours at 2–6 weeks should have a sodium concentration above 130 mmol/L (see Chapter 14).

Thyroxine ($T_4$)
0–1 week, 145–325 nmol/L
1–16 weeks, 110–220 nmol/L
Free $T_4$, 10.0–23.0 pmol/L

Thyroid-stimulating hormone (TSH)
0.3–6.0 MIU/L

This test is included with the PKU screening test (see Chapter 4). The reference range quoted refers to plasma. Not age related.

Triglycerides
1.1–2.3 mmol/L

In fasting state before next feed.

Urea
1.4–5.4 mmol/L

Upper limit of reference range may be increased to 7.5 mmol/L for infants on cows' milk formulae, and may be lower than 1.4 mmol/L in the first few days of life in low-birthweight infants.

Uric acid
60–240 μmol/L

There is a transient increase in the first few days of life.

Vitamin A
0.4–2.1 μmol/L

Arrange with laboratory. Specimen must not be exposed to daylight, and must be sent to the laboratory immediately.

Vitamins $B_1$, $B_2$, $B_{12}$ and E

Adequate information in newborn infants is not available.

Zinc
9.2–29.1 μmol/L

Clotted samples give higher values.

## DRUGS – THERAPEUTIC RANGE

*Note that the half-life of all drugs is greater in preterm infants.*

Digoxin
1–2.5 nmol/L

Therapeutic dose may be higher than that used in adults. Blood levels also tend to be higher relative to dose, but are better tolerated. Blood levels must be assessed when blood and tissue concentrations are in equilibrium

– usually 4–6 hours after i.m. dose.

Phenobarbitone
45–110 μmol/L

Although 50% is protein bound in older children, this is not the case in jaundiced neonates, where up to 70% of the drug may be free. Cerebrospinal fluid concentrations approximate to the free plasma concentration. Toxicity levels are poorly defined. Half-life is 67–95 hours.

Phenytoin
40–80 μmol/L

Only 10% or less of the drug is free in plasma. Newborn infants have diminished capacity to eliminate phenytoin, especially if premature. Half-life is up to 60 hours. Exhibits saturation kinetics with time to peak 4–8 hours.

Theophylline
25–80 μmol/L

The distribution of this drug is equal between red cells and plasma, so haemolysed samples can be assayed unless haemolysis directly interferes with the assay – ask the laboratory staff. Half-life is 24–30 hours. Peak time after dose is 2–3 hours.

Valproic acid (sodium valproate)
350–700 μmol/L

There is no recognizable relationship between blood levels and therapeutic effect, although there is for toxic effects. Half-life is very variable.

## Haematological values in the newborn

NB See Chapter 19 for investigation of bleeding/clotting disorders. Table 29.1 shows mean haematological values in term infants and Table 29.2 shows differential counts in term and preterm infants.

**Table 29.1** Mean haematological values during the first 2 weeks of life in term infants (95% ranges are shown in parentheses)

| Value | Cord blood | Day 1 | Day 3 | Day 7 | Day 14 |
|---|---|---|---|---|---|
| Haemoglobin* (g/dl) | 16.8 (13.7–20.1) | 18.4 (14–22) | 17.8 (13.8–21.8) | 17.0 (14–20) | 16.8 (13.8–19.8) |
| Venous haematocrit (%) (capillary values 2–3% higher) | 53 | 58 | 55 | 54 | 52 |
| Red cells ($10^3$/mm$^3$) | 5.25 | 5.8 | 5.6 | 5.2 | 5.1 |
| MCV (fl) | 107 (96–118) | 108 | 99 | 98 | 96 |
| MCH (pg) | 34 (33–41) | 35 | 33 | 32.5 | 31.5 |
| MCHC (%) | 31.7 (30–35) | 32.5 | 33 | 33 | 33 |
| Reticulocytes (%) | 3–7 | 3–7 | 1–3 | 0–1 | 0–1 |
| Nucleated RBC/mm$^3$ | 500 | 200 | 0–5 | 0 | 0 |
| Platelets ($10^3$/mm$^3$) | 290 (150–400) | 192 | 213 | 248 | 252 |

MCV, mean corpuscular volume.

MCH, mean corpuscular haemoglobin.

MCHC, mean corpuscular haemoglobin concentration.

Nucleated RBC counts may rise very rapidly with stress (e.g. fetal distress, birth asphyxia, infection, RDS), as well as after haemorrhage. Counts may rise to 10 000/mm$^3$ within 6 hours (Slade, 1990).

* Haemoglobin values in preterm AGA infants are lower (mean cord Hb 15 g/dl at 32 weeks' gestation), and values in SGA infants are commonly higher (see Chapter 19).

From Oski and Naiman (1982) *Haematological problems in the newborn*, 3rd edn. London: W.B. Saunders.

## Cerebrospinal fluid values in infants without meningitis

Table 29.3 shows CSF values in infants without meningitis.

**Table 29.2** Differential white cell counts in term and preterm infants ($10^3$ cells/$mm^3$)

| Age (hours) | Total WBC | Neutro-phils | Bands Metas | Lymphocytes | Monocytes | Eosinophils |
|---|---|---|---|---|---|---|
| **Term infants** | | | | | | |
| 0 | 10.0–26.0 | 5–13 | 0.4–1.8 | 3.5–8.5 | 0.7–1.5 | 0.2–2.0 |
| 12 | 13.5–31.0 | 9.0–18.0 | 0.4–2.0 | 3.0–7.0 | 1.0–2.0 | 0.2–2.0 |
| 72 | 5.0–14.5 | 2.0–7.0 | 0.2–0.4 | 2.0–5.0 | 0.5–1.0 | 0.2–1.0 |
| 144 | 6.0–14.5 | 2.0–6.0 | 0.2–0.5 | 3.0–6.0 | 0.7–1.2 | 0.1–0.8 |
| **Preterm infants** | | | | | | |
| 0 | 5.0–19.0 | 2.0–9.0 | 0.2–2.4 | 2.5–6.0 | 0.3–1.0 | 0.1–0.7 |
| 12 | 5.0–21.0 | 3.0–11.0 | 0.2–2.4 | 1.5–5.0 | 0.3–1.3 | 0.1–1.1 |
| 72 | 5.0–14.0 | 3.0–7.0 | 0.2–0.6 | 1.5–4.0 | 0.3–1.2 | 0.2–1.1 |
| 144 | 5.5–17.5 | 2.0–7.0 | 0.2–0.5 | 2.5–7.5 | 0.5–1.5 | 0.3–1.2 |

From Xanthou (1970) Leucocyte blood picture in healthy full-term and premature babies during the neonatal period. *Arch. Dis. Child* **45**, 242.

**Table 29.3** Cerebrospinal fluid values in infants without meningitis

| | Term infants | Preterm infants |
|---|---|---|
| Total white blood cell count (cells/$mm^3$) | | |
| Mean | 8.2 | 9.0 |
| Median | 5 | 6 |
| Range | 0–32 | 0–29 |
| ± 2 SD | 0–2.4 | 0–25.4 |
| Mean polymorphonuclear cells (%) | 61.3 | 57.2 |
| Protein (g/L) | | |
| Mean | 0.9 | 1.15 |
| Range | 0.2–1.7 | 0.65–1.5 |
| Glucose (mmol/L) | | |
| Mean | 2.9 | 2.8 |
| Range | 1.9–6.6 | 1.3–3.4 |
| CSF/blood glucose (%) | | |
| Mean | 81 | 74 |
| Range | 44–248 | 55–105 |

From Sarff, Platt and McCracken (1976) *J. Pediatr.* **88**, 473.

## NORMAL PHYSIOLOGICAL VALUES IN THE NEWBORN

### Blood pressure

See Figs 29.1 and 29.2 for blood pressure values.

### Blood gases

*Normal values in healthy term infants*

| Age *(hours)* | 1–4 | 12–24 | 24–48 | 48–168 |
|---|---|---|---|---|
| PaO$_2$ (mm Hg) | 50–75 | 60–80 | 65–85 | 70–85 |
| (kPa) | 6.5–9.8 | 7.8–10.4 | 8.5–11 | 9.1–11 |
| PaCO$_2$ (mm Hg) | 30–45 | 30–40 | 30–40 | 30–38 |
| (kPa) | 3.9–5.9 | 3.9–5.2 | 3.9–5.2 | 3.9–4.9 |
| *Arterial pH* | 7.30–7.34 | 7.30–7.35 | 7.35–7.40 | 7.35–7.40 |

NB Values obtained for PaCO$_2$ and pH on arterialized capillary blood are close to those given. For PO$_2$ arterialized capillary values are usually 5–10 mm Hg (0.65–1.3 kPa) lower than arterial values for PaO$_2$ < 60 mm Hg (7.8 kPa). Above this value capillary PO$_2$ does not reflect arterial PO$_2$. Capillary blood gases are unreliable in conditions of hypotension, poor peripheral perfusion, and cold stress.

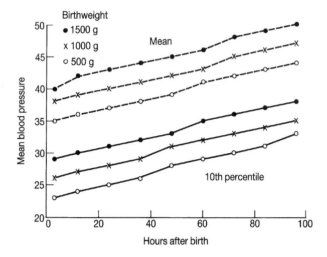

**Fig. 29.1** Mean and 10th percentile values for mean blood pressure in infants of different birthweights. From Weindling, A.M. (1989) Blood pressure monitoring in the newborn. *Arch. Dis. Child.* **64**, 444–7.

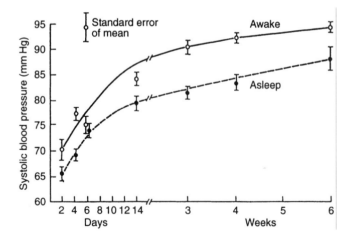

**Fig. 29.2** Increase in systolic blood pressure in healthy, term infants, awake and asleep, between the ages of 2 days and 6 weeks. From Earley *et al.* (1980) *Arch. Dis. Child.* **55**, 755–7. Reproduced with permission of the authors and publishers.

# Index

Page numbers in **bold** type refer to figures; *italic* page numbers refer to tables.

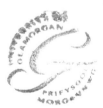